Facial Reconstruction of Unusual Facial Clefts

Nivaldo Alonso
Renato da Silva Freitas
Cristiano Tonello • Philippe Pellerin
Editors

Facial Reconstruction of Unusual Facial Clefts

A Guide to Diagnosis and Treatment

Springer

Editors
Nivaldo Alonso
Department of Plastic Surgery
Universidade de São Paulo
São Paulo, São Paulo, Brazil

Cristiano Tonello
Craniofacial Surgery Department
Universidade de São Paulo
Bauru, São Paulo, Brazil

Renato da Silva Freitas
Plastic Surgery Unit
Hospital de Clínicas, Universidade Federal do Paraná
Curitiba, Brazil

Craniofacial Surgery
Assistance Center for Cleft Lip and Palate (CAIF), Hospital do Trabalhador
Curitiba, Brazil

Philippe Pellerin
Plastic Surgery Department
University of Lille
Lambersart, France

ISBN 978-3-031-40925-7 ISBN 978-3-031-40926-4 (eBook)
https://doi.org/10.1007/978-3-031-40926-4

This Springer imprint is published by the registered company Springer Nature Switzerland AG
The registered company address is: Gewerbestrasse 11, 6330 Cham, Switzerland

Paper in this product is recyclable.

Foreword

It is a singular honor and pleasure to be asked to do this foreword on the book *Facial Reconstruction of Unusual Facial Clefts* edited and contributed by Professors Nivaldo Alonso, Renato Da Silva Freitas, Cristiano Tonello, Philippe Pellerin, and Alexandre Viera. The authors are to be commended and congratulated on tackling the task of writing a book on such rare deformities. Children born with these malformations are marginalized primarily because of the complexity of the deformities and the rarity of these disorders. These are usually quite grotesque, with each patient being different. The literature is scanty regarding managing these children, especially surgical planning and execution. Therefore, most reconstructive surgeons and even craniofacial surgeons are sometimes bewildered and at a loss when confronted with such patients. This book has compartmentalized the rare Tessier clefts detailing the deformities and management of these. The description, sequencing of surgical procedures, and results testify to the authors' vast experience and astute observations, planning, and technical surgical skill. The staging and long-term results are excellent guides to surgeons confronted with these patients.

This book will now allay fears when such patients present to craniofacial surgeons. It will long be a revered reference book that surgeons will turn to. I am so pleased and heartened that the authors have recognized this black hole in craniofacial surgery and provided an illuminating solution to treat these patients. Once again, I congratulate and thank the authors for having the courage and foresight to produce a book that is most needed and that only some would have ventured to undertake. I trust that the craniofacial fraternity will acknowledge them and duly appreciate them for their contribution.

Anil Madaree

Department of Plastic Surgery, Inkosi Albert
Luthuli Central Hospital, Nelson R Mandela
School of Medicine
University of Kwazulu Natal,
Durban, South Africa

Foreword

Craniofacial and cleft surgeons are known for their elevated attention to detail, meticulous facial analysis, deft surgical technique, and self-assurance that can make them difficult to bear. However, for most, this self-assurance wavers in the face of a Tessier facial cleft. The sheer rarity of these conditions limits their presentation to most practitioners to once every few years, limiting the ability of most surgeons to gain any meaningful clinical experience. Considering the multiple types of unusual facial clefts and the varied expression of each type, it is no wonder that these complicated patients remain a nebulous group, presenting challenges in treatment planning and predicted outcomes.

Even in this era of excessive publication, the rarity of these conditions has largely confined the literature to case series. Long-term studies are few and far between, and no dedicated surgical textbook on reconstructing unusual facial clefts exists. Thus, with a scarcity of available references and individual professional experience, cleft and craniofacial surgeons who confront patients with unusual facial clefts must leverage their collective resources to prepare for the big moment of surgery: they meticulously gather the details of the patient's presentation; reflect on lessons learned from congenital, traumatic, oncologic, and aesthetic surgery; review the sparse literature; reach out to trusted colleagues; dig deeply into their figurative toolbox; and prepare for the big day. This culmination of surgical experience into a fixed period of physical activity with profound consequences has few life comparisons. A championship match in professional sports or big wave surfing at Nazare comes to mind.

To address this gap in knowledge, the five editors (four surgeons and a craniofacial geneticist) produced *Facial Reconstruction of Unusual Facial Cleft*, the first comprehensive textbook on rare facial clefts, edited by master clinicians whom each treat more facial clefts within a couple of years than most will see in their lifetimes. The pages of this rich textbook are culled from their collective experience spanning decades, involving more than 500 patients at some of the busiest cleft centers in the world. The two Brazilian centers are Hospital de Reabilitação de Anomalias Craniofaciais (HRAC) of the University of São Paulo, commonly known as Centrinho and Centro de Atendimento Integral ao Fissurado Labiopalatal (CAIF).

The reader should note that the HRAC center "Centrinho" is the largest hospital dedicated to treating cleft and craniofacial anomalies in the Western Hemisphere and likely one of the largest in the world. The French center in Lille is represented by Dr. Phillippe Pellerin, the head of the French National Reference Center for rare craniomaxillofacial malformations between 2007 and 2012.

In comparison to past literature, including that of Paul Tessier, *Facial Reconstruction of Unusual Facial Cleft* benefits from a unity of comprehensive, advanced imaging analysis, large patient experience, interdisciplinary assessment, genetic consultation, and data on long-term outcomes. When appropriate, corrections of prior descriptions of facial clefts are made to provide clarity for future practitioners. The collective experience contained within these pages is nothing short of mind-boggling. The book offers page after page of the most challenging hard and soft tissue dilemmas affecting the face and provides a new benchmark for facial cleft reconstruction that should be on the shelf of any serious cleft or craniofacial surgeon. It is also a celebration of not only some of the best works in cleft and craniofacial surgery but also the critical contributions to our great field by a distinguished group of Brazilian craniofacial surgeons and the centers they represent.

Read. Learn. Savor. Grow.

Cleft Lip and Palate, Hansjörg Wyss
Department of Plastic Surgery, NYU Langone Health
New York, NY, USA

Roberto L. Flores

Foreword

It is with great pleasure that I write a foreword for the book *Facial Reconstruction of Unusual Facial Clefts* by professors Alonso, Da Silva Freitas, Tonello, Pellerin, and Viera. Treating a patient with rare facial clefts is one of the biggest challenges for a craniofacial surgeon. It encompasses a lack of bone, muscle, nerve, and skin tissue and specifically disturbed growth of the affected area. Surgical correction thus involves accurate reconstruction of the deficits and needs to bear in mind the growth impairment over time and the required surgery at later ages. Attempts to repair the facial cleft by inexperienced hands can have a devastating effect on the outcome. Taking care of children with such a rare condition should be left to surgeons dedicated to craniofacial surgery. This book beautifully illustrates what can be offered to these patients if performed by an expert surgeon.

Irene M. J. Mathijssen

International Society of Craniofacial Surgery
Philadelphia, PA, USA

European Reference Network Craniofacial Anomalies
and ENT Disorders (ERN CRANIO)
Rotterdam, The Netherlands

Plastic and Reconstructive Surgery and Hand Surgery,
Erasmus Medical Center
Rotterdam, The Netherlands

Preface

This book was born 37 years ago when I was a craniofacial fellow with Dr. Daniel Marchac at Necker-Enfants Malades hospital. I was impressed with all the congenital deformities treated there. I met Dr. Philippe Pellerin several times, and he was always talking about unusual Tessier clefts, and we became friends and exchanged some ideas about them. I came back to Sao Paulo and started to do craniofacial surgery at the University of Sao Paulo. One of my first patients was an unusual Tessier cleft 4; her name was Paloma. I did her surgery as was described in Tessier's book, since then I have been very passionate about these congenital deformities. I was so lucky that one of my first Ph.D. students, Prof. Renato da Silva Freitas, also turned to be a craniofacial surgeon, and we both became friends and traveled around the country and the world doing congenital craniofacial surgeries. Prof. Renato became a full professor at the Federal University of Parana and Director of one busy congenital craniofacial center in the country, Caif. Since then, we have been discussing almost all our congenital cleft cases together. After working at the University of Sao Paulo since 1987 doing craniofacial surgery, I joined one of the most famous cleft centers in the world, HRAC—Hospital de Reabilitacao de Anomalias Craniofaciais, in 2008. I have seen more unusual clefts in 1 year than in the last 20 years in Sao Paulo. Another student and fellow in craniofacial surgery, Prof. Cristiano Tonello, joined me in this big challenge and we both became craniofacial surgeons in HRAC in 2013 and turned professors at the medical school of the University of Sao Paulo Bauru campus. Four of us, Cristiano, Renato, Philippe, and I, put all our cases together with pictures and CT scans and decided to analyze all our cases critically. Prof. Alexandre, a geneticist from Pittsburg, joined us on this great journey to write this book with the most valuable collection of unusual congenital facial clefts and try to unravel their fabulous mystery and at the same time make a guide with protocols for those who have seen only a few cases during their lifetime.

São Paulo, São Paulo, Brazil — Nivaldo Alonso
Curitiba, Paraná, Brazil — Renato da Silva Freitas
Bauru, São Paulo, Brazil — Cristiano Tonello
Lambersart, France — Philippe Pellerin

Contents

Chapter 1
Introduction

Renato da Silva Freitas and Nivaldo Alonso

Craniofacial clefts are among the most disfiguring of all facial anomalies. They exist in many patterns and varying degrees of severity: patient may demonstrate an incomplete form or a microform, whereas another will display more complete skeletal and soft tissue manifestation [1].

Craniofacial clefts are rare. The exact incidence is unknown, but estimates range from 1.4 to 4.9 per 100,000 live births [2]. In a classical study, Fogh-Andersen identified the incidence of one case each of 300 regular cleft lip and palate [3]. Monasterio and Taylor related in his series 2.2 rare facial cleft each 100 common clefts [4]. Even though these are unusual facial congenital diseases, Brazil is a continental country and has very few craniofacial centers; in this book, we merge three important centers, São Paulo, HRAC from Bauru, and CAIF from Curitiba, with one of Phillippe Pellerin, who has been head of the Department of Plastic and Craniofacial Surgery in Lille between 1982 and 2013, head of the French national reference center for rare cranio-maxillofacial malformations between 2007 and 2012 and during the same period has treated such conditions during European cooperation and humanitarian mission all over the globe. Among the three centers, one common point is the protocol. The experience came from the University of São Paulo initially from Nivaldo Alonso, who has trained the other coauthors Renato da Silva Freitas and Cristiano Tonello.

Even though the phenotype may be variable, most occur along predictable embryologic lines. Tessier utilized these lines to classify these facial malformations.

R. da Silva Freitas (✉)
Plastic Surgery Unit, Hospital de Clínicas, Universidade Federal do Paraná, Curitiba, Brazil

Craniofacial Surgery, Assistance Center for Cleft Lip and Palate (CAIF), Hospital do Trabalhador, Curitiba, Brazil

N. Alonso
Plastic Surgery, Universidade de São Paulo, São Paulo, Brazil

Craniofacial Surgery, Hospital de Reabilitação Anomalias Craniofaciais Bauru USP Universidade de São Paulo, Bauru, Brazil

N. Alonso et al. (eds.), *Facial Reconstruction of Unusual Facial Clefts*,
https://doi.org/10.1007/978-3-031-40926-4_1

However, the exact cause of craniofacial clefts remains obscure. Those theories of cleft formation that apply to typical cases of cleft lip and palate may also apply to the craniofacial clefts [5]. Dursy [6] and His [7] proposed the failure of fusion theory, and Pohlann [8] and Veau [9] the failure of mesodermal penetration theory. The etiology of most of the abnormalities mentioned still needs to be discovered. It is clear, however, that these rare malformations must develop in the earliest embryonic stages [10].

Most craniofacial clefts occur sporadically [3]. Amniotic band syndrome has also been implicated in the process of facial clefting. Animal and human clinical studies have demonstrated the influence of four major categories of risk factors: radiation, infection, maternal metabolic imbalances, and drugs and chemicals [1].

Humanitarian missions frequently occur around the world, specifically in developing countries. Latin America, Africa, and Asia have several nongovernmental organizations helping people daily. Identifying patients with a rare facial cleft in these missions is possible. However, besides standard cleft lip and palate having standardized treatment, its execution continues to be a world problem. And rare facial clefts become a challenge; it is not easy to identify hospitals or surgeons that can work on treating these patients. Sieg et al. demonstrated his experience during several missions [11]. The paper discussed the difficulty of correct diagnostics, sometimes without imaging techniques (computerized tomography scan and magnetic resonance imaging) and surgical procedure planning. They are associated with the absence of facilities to perform effective procedure as craniofacial surgery and intensive care unit. And the article suggested that the best conduct should be transferring these patients to craniofacial centers. The authors have worked in humanitarian missions since very early and have faced many rare cleft patients. Specifically in Brazil, the patients are sent to continue treatment in our cleft center after the mission's first stage.

There are few articles published about rare facial clefts. The majority of them are case reports. Few numbers of clinical series are found [2, 4, 12, 13]. Associated with the significant variation in the presentation of these malformations, the proposition of treatment protocols becomes challenging. Long-term follow-up is necessary to propose any treatment sequence for any craniofacial anomalies. Evaluation of long-term results can reveal a difference in techniques, better techniques, and relapses [13]. However, these evaluations have been scarce. Patients can come to the center without any treatment at an early age and receive a staged treatment, possibly at the best time for each procedure. Or they can arrive late, with partial treatment, sometimes with nonstandardized methods, and the results will not be the best. The authors have been treating these deformities since 1987; during this period, our team could publish many papers about this topic [14–29]. Most of our knowledge about it, including pictures of the procedures, is present in this book.

Treating rare craniofacial clefts brings better results if these patients receive an interdisciplinary approach with several professionals. For example, cases of cranial involvement, such as encephalocele, will need a neurosurgeon, so as an ophthalmologist, for abnormalities of the eyes. In addition, mental retardation may be present in a few patients. In these cases, surgery should be restricted to what is necessary, and no operation should be performed if there is no real advantage to the patient [10].

The objectives of the rehabilitation of rare facial clefts must follow some principles. The initial priority is to solve possible emergencies. First, the protection of corneas, treatment of hydrocephaly, or airway management in patients with some oral mass or micrognathia (Pierre-Robin Sequence) are examples of procedures that need to be made in a short period. Second, the soft-tissue component will be addressed earlier than the bony, which usually brings a relatively normal appearance. Third, all facial features (orbital, eyelid, nose, lip, and ear malformation) must be evaluated and defined, isolated or global, depending on each case. Fourth, operating on these patients early age is optional due to the altered maxillary growth. And fifth and new, the tridimensional evaluation, including prototypes, brought new perspectives to restore normal anatomy.

References

1. Ozaki W, Kawamoto HK Jr. Craniofacial clefting. In: Lin K, editor. Craniofacial surgery: science & surgical technique. Philadelphia, PA: W.B. Saunders; 2001.
2. Kawamoto H. Rare craniofacial clefts. In: McCarthy J, editor. Plastic surgery. Philadelphia: W.B. Saunders; 1990. p. 2922–73.
3. Fogh-Andersen P. Rare clefts of the face. Acta Chir Scand. 1965;129:275.
4. Monasterio FO, Taylor JA. Major craniofacial clefts: case series and treatment philosophy. Plast Reconstr Surg. 2008;122–2:534–43.
5. Stark RE. The development of the center of the face with particular reference to surgical correction of bilateral cleft lip. Plast Reconstr Surg. 1958;21:177.
6. Dursy E. Zur Entwicklunsgeschichte des Kopfes des Menschen und der höheren Wirbelthiere. Türbigen, Verlag de H. Lauppschen—Buschhandlund; 1869. p. 99.
7. His W. Die Formentwicklung des ausseren Ohres. In: Anatomie menschlischer Embryonen; 1885. p. 211.
8. Pohlmann FE. Die embryonale Metamorphose der Physiognomie und der Mundhohle des Katzenkopfes; 1910. p. 41–617.
9. Veau V. Harelip of the human embryo 21–23 mm long. Z Anat Entscklng. 1938;108:459.
10. Schweckendiek W. Nasal abnormalities in facial clefts. J Maxillofac Surg. 1976;4(3):141–9. https://doi.org/10.1016/s0301-0503(76)80023-9.
11. Sieg P, Hakim SG, Jacobsen HC, Saka B, Hermes D. Rare facial clefts: treatment during charity missions in developing countries. Plast Reconstr Surg. 2004;114(3):640–7. https://doi.org/10.1097/01.prs.0000130934.26961.29.
12. Tessier P. Anatomical classification facial, craniofacial, and lateral-facial clefts. J Maxillofac Surg. 1976;4(2):69–92. https://doi.org/10.1016/s0301-0503(76)80013-6.
13. Versnel SL, van den Elzen ME, Wolvius EB, Biesmeijer CS, Vaandrager JM, van der Meulen JC, Mathijssen IM. Long-term results after 40 years experience with treatment of rare facial clefts: part 1–oblique and paramedian clefts. J Plast Reconstr Aesthet Surg. 2011;64(10):1334–43. https://doi.org/10.1016/j.bjps.2011.04.021. Epub 2011 Jun 1.
14. Alonso N, da Silva Freitas R. Craniofacial clefts and other related deformities. In: Guyuron B, Eriksson E, Persing JA, Chung KC, Disa J, Gosain A, Rubin P, Kinney B, editors. Plastic surgery, vol. 1. 1st ed. Oxford: Elsevier; 2009.

15. da Silva Freitas R, Alonso N, Azzolini TF, Busato L, Tolazzi ARD, Cruz GAO, Goldenberg D. The surgical repair of half-nose. J Plast Reconstr Aesthet Surg. 2008;63:15. https://doi.org/10.1016/j.bjps.2008.08.040.
16. da Silva Freitas R, Groth AK, Cruz GAO, Alonso NF, No F. 4 de Tessier: Revisão da Literatura e Relato de Casos. Arq Cat Med. 2000;29:240–2.
17. da Silva Freitas R, Contin Mansur AE, Alonso N, Busato L, Cruz GA. Hemifacial microsomia: 105 cases in 7 years. In: Proceedings of X international congress of the international society of craniofacial surgery. Monterey, CA: Medimond; 2003.
18. da Silva Freitas R, Souza RT, Calixto EC, de Biagi VM, Invitti HL, Bodnese T, Fernandes HADR, Freitas JF, Busato LS, Alonso N. Microssomia craniofacial: o espectro clínico de 163 pacientes tratados. Braz J Craniomaxillofac Surg. 2008;11(3):89–93.
19. Franco D, Franco T, da Silva Freitas R, Alonso N. Commissuroplasty for macrostomia. J Craniofac Surg. 2007;18(3):691–4.
20. da Silva Freitas R, Gaia S, Busato L, Barbosa R, Alonso N. Síndrome de Pai—characteristicas clínicas e relato de caso. Arq Catarin Med. 2003;32(1):145–8.
21. da Silva Freitas R, Bertolotte W, Shin J, Busato L, Alonso N, Grande CV, Cruz GAO. Combination micrografting and tattooing in the reconstruction of eyebrows of patients with craniofacial clefts. Ophthal Plast Reconstr Surg. 2008;24(4):340–2.
22. da Silva Freitas R, Alonso N, Shin JH, Busato L, Ono MC, Cruz E, GA. Surgical correction of Tessier number 0 cleft. J Craniofac Surg. 2008;19(5):1348–52.
23. Alonso N, da Silva Freitas R, Cruz GA, Goldenberg D, Dall'oglio Tolazzi AR. Tessier no. 4 facial clefts: evolution of surgical treatment in a large series of patients. Plast Reconstr Surg. 2008;122(5):1505–13.
24. da Silva Freitas R, Alonso N, Shin JH, Busato LS, Tolazzi ARD, Cruz GA. The Tessier number 5 facial cleft: surgical strategies and outcomes in six patients. Cleft Palate Craniofac Surg. 2009;46:179–86. https://doi.org/10.1597/07-192.
25. Buonocore S, Broer PN, Walker ME, da Silva Freitas R, Franco D, Alonso N. Macrostomia: a spectrum of deformity. Ann Plast Surg. 2014;72(3):363–8. https://doi.org/10.1097/SAP.0b013e31826aefdf.
26. da Silva Freitas R. Fissuras craniofaciais raras: Aperfeiçoamento cirúrgico no tratamento de 310 pacientes. Tese de Livre-Docência, São Paulo—SP, 118 p.
27. Tonello C, Alonso N. Rare facial clefts. In: Hamdan U, et al., editors. Interdisciplinary cleft care global perspectives. San Diego, CA: Plural Publishing; 2023.
28. da Silva Freitas R, Alonso N. Rare facial clefts. In: Chung K, et al., editors. Plastic surgery indications and practise. China: Saunders Elsevier; 2009.
29. Raposo-Amaral CE, Jarrahy R, Lim R, Alonso N. The rare facial. In: Alonso N, Raposo-Amaral C, editors. Cleft lip and palate treatment: a comprehensive guide. Cham: Springer; 2018.

Chapter 2
Genetics in Unusual Facial Clefts

Alexandre R. Vieira

2.1 Introduction

The rapid development of medicine seen in the last century allowed for a dramatic change in lifespan and a greater chance of survival from conditions that before were not manageable. From around 30 years during the dark ages to more than doubling since the Age of Enlightenment, people are living longer and more likely surviving illness [1].

The result has been a growth in the number of individuals dealing with chronic illness and other conditions. The growth was also seen in individuals surviving particularly rare conditions, which are understudied and poorly understood. It came to a consensus that these rare diseases would only be appropriately addressed with incentives for their study and development of therapies.

These conditions were defined as any disease affecting a small percentage of the population. In the United States, rare is when it affects less than 200,000 people [2]. Cumulatively, more than 7000 rare diseases affect millions of people, more than 30 million in the United States alone [3].

Several conditions that affect the craniofacial structures, including several forms of orofacial clefts, are rare. This chapter aims to describe the modes of inheritance that most likely explain rare orofacial clefts.

A. R. Vieira (✉)
School of Dental Medicine, University of Pittsburgh, Pittsburgh, PA, USA
e-mail: arv11@pitt.edu

N. Alonso et al. (eds.), *Facial Reconstruction of Unusual Facial Clefts*,
https://doi.org/10.1007/978-3-031-40926-4_2

2.2 Inheritance in Humans

Most common conditions in humans are complex, meaning they result from contributions from several genes and can be influenced by the environment. Traits like height, weight, blood sugar level, blood pressure, intelligence, behaviors, sexual orientation, or diseases such as cancer, cardiovascular risks, diabetes, asthma, arthritis, mental conditions, and many structural birth defects appearing in isolation are complex. They, therefore, have a multifactorial (or complex) mode of inheritance. Then, there are a number of exceptions due to chromosomal abnormalities or characteristics, such as the one described by Gregor Mendel, which are called monogenic conditions or single gene disorders. Finally, there are instances that an environmental agent can cause conditions, and when this agent leads to a birth defect, it is called a teratogenic agent [4, 5].

About 3500 of the 7000 total rare diseases (the average number of patients per disease is 6000) have a monogenic mode of inheritance. Of those, 1750 are diagnosable. Figure 2.1 describes the modes of inheritance of rare diseases [6].

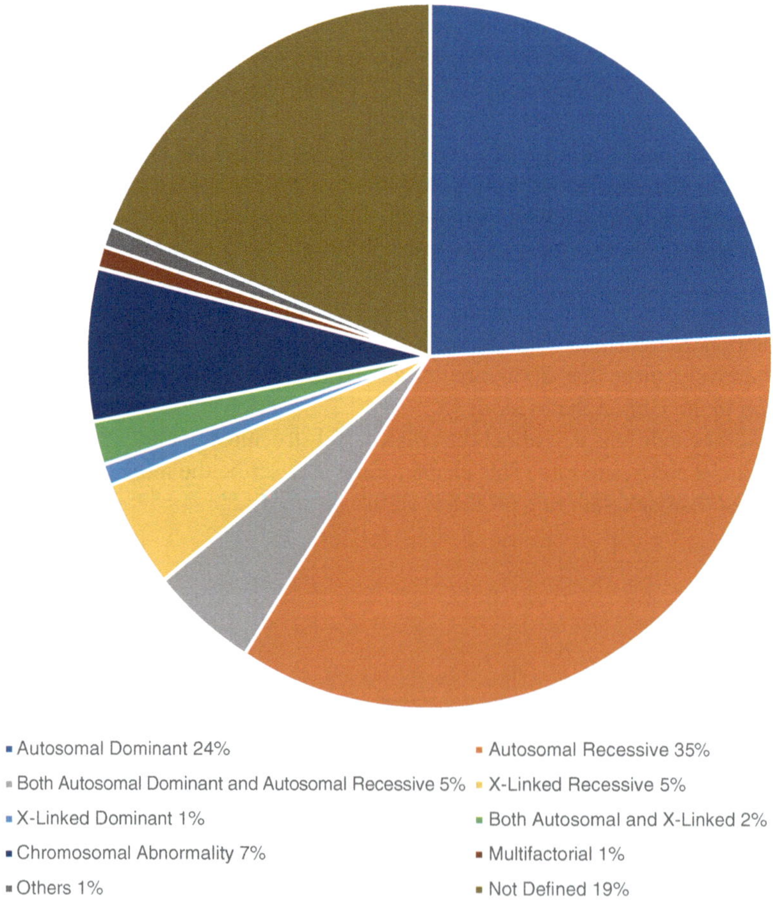

Fig. 2.1 Modes of inheritance of rare diseases (according to [6])

2.3 Orofacial Clefts

Most cases of orofacial clefts (70%) involve the lip and/or palate, constituting the only structural abnormality the child was born with. They do not present any apparent familial segregation pattern (Fig. 2.2), and many cases are sporadic. They likely have a complex or multifactorial mode of inheritance. Orofacial clefts may also be due to single gene forms of inheritance, chromosomal abnormalities, or teratogenic agents.

The remaining 30% of cases born with clefts have some additional associated condition, and more than 400 entities are described to date [7]. A subset of those entities are rare forms of clefts, and they are the objective of this book.

Most of the rare forms of clefts are sporadic cases. Counseling of those cases typically revolves around mentioning a de novo mutation and, therefore, a low recurrence risk. Technological advances have allowed the genetic counseling field the ability to attempt the detection of the hypothesized causal mutation that would explain the occurrence of the rare cleft.

Most forms of rare clefts are sporadic, and linkage approaches are inadequate since they rely on multiple affected individuals in families. On the other hand, association strategies could be better suited, too, since they rely on measuring common variants in the population and the need for many observations, which are not available since the types of clefts of interest are rare. Association study results are also of little value for counseling rare forms of clefts because these results suggest probabilities of occurrence of the condition in a particular group, and these estimates could be more helpful individually.

The hypothesis to be tested is the presence of rare genetic variants with significant effects, which can be ascertained by sequencing genomic DNA. This approach

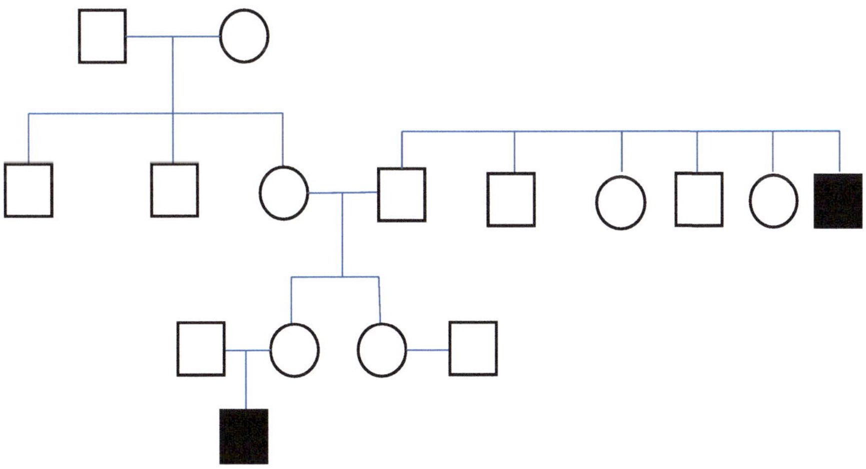

Fig. 2.2 Typical pedigree of a multifactorial condition of a family with positive history of the disease

has also been used for isolated forms of clefts from multiple distinct populations [8–14]. Sequencing can be done by targeting exons, which are the coding segments of genes, or scanning the whole genome. Typically, any given individual may be carrying dozens to hundreds of these rare variants that could be interpreted as potentially pathogenic, and evaluation of these finds require further scrutinization, taking into consideration potentially known biological roles of specific genes that may be harboring defective DNA single nucleotide changes or small deletions or duplications.

These practices are raising new ethical questions [15]. Newborn screening, which has a place when concerned with metabolic conditions, may become the screening of newborns. Sequencing has many limitations, such as the noise in the data mentioned above. Sensitive issues also exist, and limitations should be presented to and understood by parents. Keeping up with the vast amount of information is very challenging, and there needs to be a central repository of all rare and disease-associated variants. Finally, the availability of large-scale sequencing may increase testing by more cautious health professionals. Such increases would raise health care costs and lead to the physical and psychological costs of increased testing.

References

1. Roser M, Ortiz-Ospina E, Ritchie H. Life expectancy. OurWorldInData.org, 2013. https://ourworldindata.org/life-expectancy [Online Resource].
2. US Congressional Research Service. Rare diseases act of 2002. US Library of Congress; 2002.
3. National Organization for Rare Disorders (NORD). Rare diseases database. Consulted in 2023. https://rarediseases.org/rare-diseases/ [Online Resource].
4. Vieira AR. Inheritance in oral health conditions. In: Vieira AR, editor. Genetic basis of oral health conditions. 1st ed. Springer: Cham; 2019. p. 1–8.
5. Vieira AR. Basis of inheritance in humans. In: Vieira AR, editor. The overlooked individual: susceptibility to dental caries, erosive tooth wear and amelogenesis, vol. 30. Basel: Karger; 2022. p. 1–19.
6. Wakap SN, Lambert DM, Olry A, Rodwell C, Gueydan C, Lanneau V, Murphy D, Cam YL, Rath A. Estimating cumulative point prevalence of rare diseases: analysis of the Orphanet database. Eur J Hum Genet. 2020;28:165–73.
7. Murray JC. Gene/environment causes of cleft lip and/or palate. Clin Genet. 2002;61(4):248–56.
8. Vieira AR, Avila JR, Daack-Hirsch S, Dragan E, Félix TM, Rahimov F, Harrington J, Schultz RR, Watanabe Y, Johnson M, Fang J, O'Brien SE, Orioli IM, Castilla EE, Fitzpatrick DR, Jiang R, Marazita ML, Murray JC. Medical sequencing of candidate genes for nonsyndromic cleft lip and palate. PLoS Genet. 2005;1(6):e64.
9. Bureau A, Parker MM, Ruczinski I, Taub MA, Marazita ML, Murray JC, Mangold E, Noethen MM, Ludwig KU, Hetmanski JB, Bailey-Wilson JE, Cropp CD, Li Q, Szymczak S, Albacha-Hejazi H, Alqosayer K, Field LL, Wu-Chou Y-H, Doheny KF, Ling H, Scott AF, Beaty TH. Whole exome sequencing of distant relatives in multiplex families implicates rare variants in candidate genes for oral clefts. Genetics. 2014;197(3):1039–44.
10. Aylward A, Cai Y, Lee A, Blue E, Rabinowitz D, Haddad J Jr. Using whole exome sequencing to identify candidate genes with rare variants in nonsyndromic cleft lip and palate. Genet Epidemiol. 2016;40(5):432–41.

11. Basha M, Demeer B, Revencu N, Helaers R, Theys S, Saba SB, Boute O, Devauchelle D, Francois G, Bayet B, Vikkula M. Whole exome sequencing identifies mutations in 10% of patients with familial non-syndromic cleft lip and/or palate in genes mutated in well-known syndromes. J Med Genet. 2018;55:449–58.
12. Muhopadhyay N, Bishop M, Mortillo M, Chopra P, Hetmanski JB, Taub MA, Moreno LM, Valencia-Ramirez LC, Restrepo C, Wehby GL, Hecht JT, Deleyiannis F, Butali A, Weinberg SM, Beaty TH, Murray JC, Leslie EJ, Feingold E, Marazita ML. Whole genome sequencing of orofacial cleft trios from the Gabriela miller kids first pediatric research consortium identifies a new locus on chromosome 21. Hum Genet. 2020;139(2):215–26.
13. Zhong W, Zhao H, Hung W, Zhang M, Zhang Q, Zhang Y, Chen C, Nueraihemaiti Z, Tuerhong D, Huang H, Maimaitili G, Chen F, Lin J. Identification of rare *PTCH1* nonsense variant causing orofacial cleft in a Chinese family and an up-to-date genotype-phenotype analysis. Genes Dis. 2021;8(5):698–7.
14. Awotoye W, Mossey PA, Hetmanski JB, Gowans LJJ, Eshete MA, Adeyemo WL, Alade A, Zeng E, Adamson O, Naicker T, Anand D, Adeleke C, Busch T, Li M, Petrin A, Aregbesola BS, Braimah RO, Oginni FO, Oladele AO, Oladayo A, Kayali S, Olotu J, Hassan M, Pape J, Donkor P, Arthur FKN, Obiri-Yeboah S, Sabbah DK, Agbenorku P, Plange-Rhule G, Oti AA, Gogal RA, Beath TH, Taub M, Marazita ML, Schnieders MJ, Lachke SA, Adeyemo AA, Murray JC, Butali A. Whole-genome sequencing reveals de-novo mutations associated with nonsyndromic cleft lip/palate. Sci Rep. 2022;12:11743.
15. Lantos JD. Ethical and psychosocial issues in whole genome sequencing (WGS) for newborns. Pediatrics. 2019;143(Suppl 1):S1–5.

Chapter 3
Mechanisms, Etiology, and Classification of Rare Clefts

Philippe Pellerin and Renato da Silva Freitas

Pearls
Published in 1976, Tessier's classification of rare clefts imposed itself on the world of craniofacial surgeons. Forty-six years later, the tremendous progress in biology and medical imaging has permitted us to erase the question marks in his sketches and answer some of the questions that arise in his text, and propose the up-to-date issue of this classification for the twenty-first century that will be found below.

3.1 Introduction

Mechanism and etiology are other names for pathogeny.

Progresses in prenatal development knowledge led to a better understanding of numerous hereditary or environmentally produced malformations, notably craniofacial.

Seventy percent of birth defects concern the head and neck. Of these, 10% are due to chromosomal anomalies, 20% to single gene mutation, and for the most part: 70% are multifactorial [1]. Although only a few malformations directly rely upon mutations, the study of macromolecular biology phenomena involved could help apprehend this pathogeny.

P. Pellerin (✉)
Centre Hospitalier Régional Universitaire de Lille, Lille, France

R. da Silva Freitas
Plastic Surgery Unit, Hospital de Clínicas, Universidade Federal do Paraná, Curitiba, Brazil

Craniofacial Surgery, Assistance Center for Cleft Lip and Palate (CAIF), Hospital do Trabalhador, Curitiba, Brazil

N. Alonso et al. (eds.), *Facial Reconstruction of Unusual Facial Clefts*,
https://doi.org/10.1007/978-3-031-40926-4_3

3.2 Normal Biology

3.2.1 Craniofacial Phylogenesis

The science of evolution has two sections: phylogenesis, which is devoted to the evolution between the species, and whose subject is the stem history, and ontogenesis, which is interested in the development of the individual, which is embryology. One of the significant philosophical theories is that ontogenesis reproduces phylogenesis and is the cause of ontogenesis [2]. This is the Haeckelian recapitulation theory.

One could believe that there is no room for such consideration in a modern book of surgery... but we have learned from macromolecular biology that acquiring new biological characteristics is linked to the incorporation of new genes or the mutation of existing genes.

Consequently, the research in morphogenesis comes with a forward and backward movement between the comparative anatomy, comparative embryology, and the macromolecular to understand the gears of phylogenesis. The research in ontogenesis also learns from a study in phylogenesis. This global approach is the neontology [3]. Standard research on genetic disease processes is usually after recognizing a candidate gene by testing the consequences of its neutralization on an animal model. Mice and zebrafish are the most popular species for that purpose.

The understanding of mechanisms that are involved in rare clefts pathogenesis could take benefit from some pieces of knowledge in phylogenesis and ontogenesis.

From the phylogenesis, we learn the origin of the neural crest, which is involved in most craniofacial malformations. The acquisition of the neural crest has been a significant step in vertebrate evolution.

A new head: The Gans and Northcutt scenario (Fig. 3.1).

According to this theory, the apparition of the neural crest during phylogenesis concomitates the development a new head [4]. This new head is required for the acquisition of new functions. It starts after the emergence of active dispersing species, which acquired a notochord and segmented muscles. Neural crest cells (NCCs) were required to develop pharyngeal breathing (cartilage, gill capillaries, and branchiomeric muscles), to allow predation abilities (paired external sense organs and brain), to enhance the former ability by developing electroreception (external bones) and finally, the competence for biting (postotic skull, vertebra, and jaws).

This path of phylogenesis has driven the emergence of gnathostomes, the phylum to which we belong. The primitive jaws came from the differentiation of the first and second pharyngeal arches [5] (Fig. 3.2). It has taken several attempts at trying and failing and the process of natural selection, as learned from Darwin, to reach the actual form of our craniofacial skeleton.

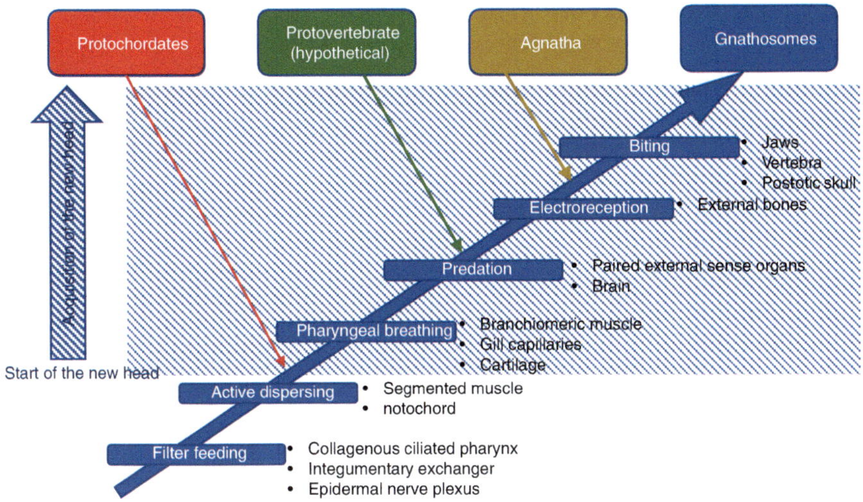

Fig. 3.1 Hypothesized transition in vertebrate evolution (after Gons); function acquisition corelated with structural changes

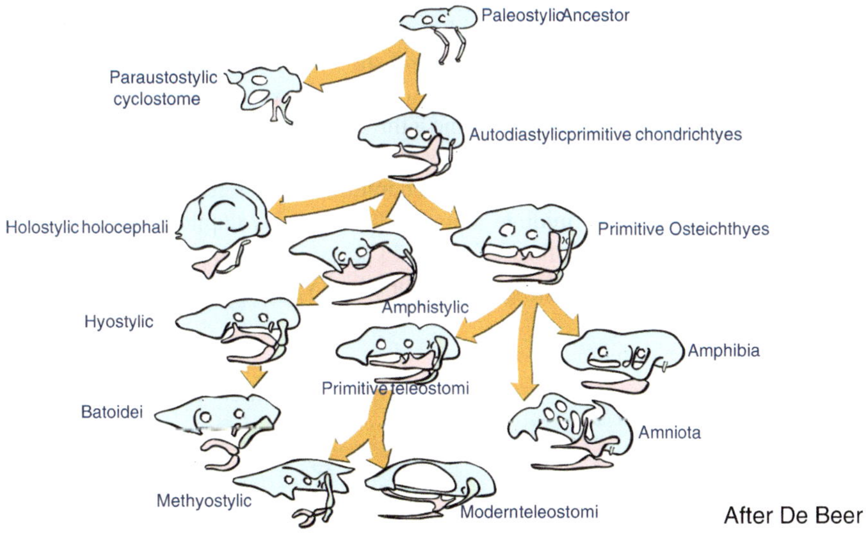

Fig. 3.2 Jaws Phylogenesis. Pink correspond to derivatives of the first pharyngeal arch. Green correspond to derivatives of the second pharyngeal arch

3.2.2 *Craniofacial Ontogenesis*

The paths and targets of pathological modifications of the embryo differ, according to the stage of development.

3.2.2.1 At the Gastrulation Stage

Two significant events occur during the organization of the midline and the ectoderm patterning.

Midline Organization: The Primitive Streak [6]

By the third week of development, the gastrulation will change the bilaminar embryo (epiblast and hypoblast) into a trilaminar embryo (ectoderm, mesoderm, and endoderm). This metamorphosis starts with the formation in the midline of the primitive streak, a groove with slightly protruding edges (Fig. 3.3). The primitive streak grows from the caudal part of the embryonic disc toward its cephalic part. Its cephalic end includes the primitive pit surrounded by the elevation of the primitive node.

Epiblast cells migrate toward the midline. They reach the primitive streak, where they detach themselves from the epiblast and slip beneath its layer in an invagination move that will locate them between the two initial layers, thus forming the third layer. Henceforth the embryo has become a three-layer one.

The initialization of the primitive streak depends on the Nodal gene. HNF-3β maintains the node and induces forebrain and midbrain structures. Misexpression of this gene results in severe midline abnormalities such as duplication or defects, which will feature a different form of cleft 14 [7].

In the chicken embryo, the injection of chickVg1 could produce an additive streak.

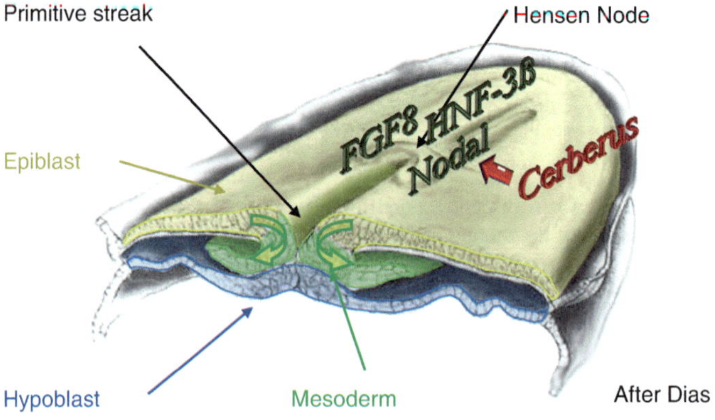

Fig. 3.3 Gastrulation: The primitive streak, the Node, the formation of the three-layer embryo

Cerberus gene code for a protein lack of which could cause the development of a supernumerary ectopic head [8].

The retinoic acid path plays an important role early during gastrulation [9]. It is essential for the morphogenetic movements that explain this molecule's teratogenic effect, which could interfere at several stages of embryogenesis.

Ectoderm Patterning

Craniofacial mesenchyme stems from the ectoderm, which migrates through the streak during gastrulation, and the neural crest cells.

First, before the NCC, the head epithelium acquires a spatial specification very early (could be during gastrulation). The cells fated to occupy the maxilla already have a specific location in the head's ectoderm before the pharyngeal arches' formation. Those cells express Fgf8 and Bmp4; those expressions require the presence of endoderm.

The patterning of the facial skeleton begins with the early migration of specific areas of the ectoderm, and the ectoderm–endoderm interactions regulate this patterning. This mechanism does not involve NCC [10].

3.2.2.2 Neurulation

During the neurulation stage, two processes could play a role in the occurrence of craniofacial clefts: the deployment of the neural crests and neural crests cells (NCCs) and the closure of the neural tube.

The Discovery and Studies of Neural Crest Cells [1, 11]

The neural crests, a transient formation, were discovered in 1868 by His [12] (Fig. 3.4). They are formed during the neurulation as two outgrowths at the epidermal and neural ectoderm boundaries. Once separated from the neuro tube and the

Fig. 3.4 His original drawing from 1868

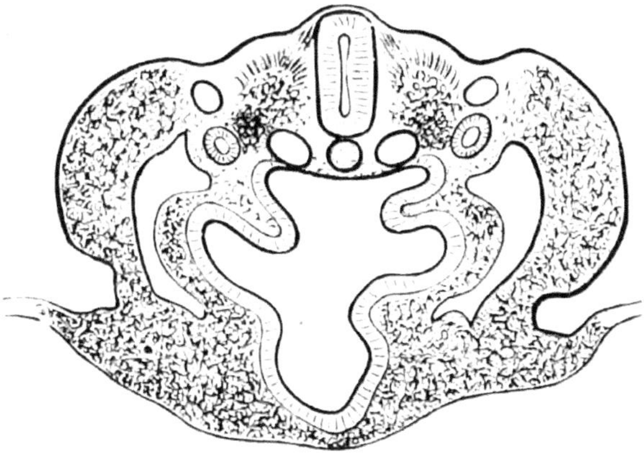

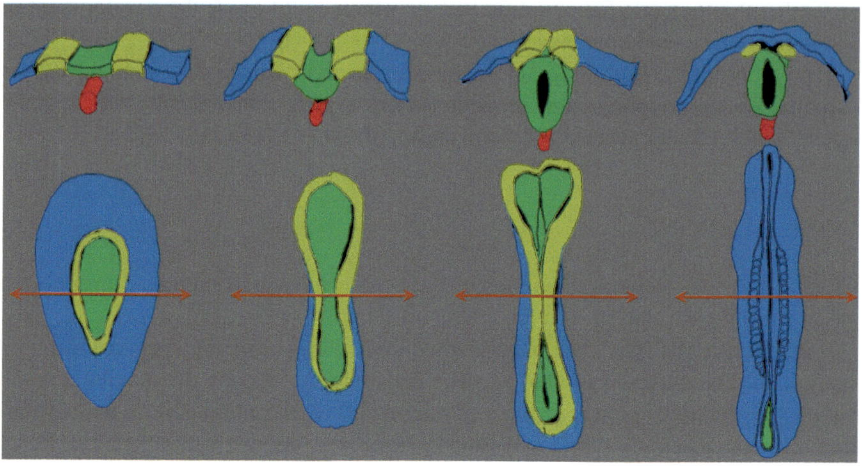

Fig. 3.5 Neural crest formation. Green-neural plaque, yellow-neural crest, green-ectoderm, red-notochord, double arrow-level of section

ectoderm, they will form two elongated stacks parallel to the neural tube (Fig. 3.5). Then they will migrate to their final destination to give rise in the head to most of the craniofacial skeleton through interaction with the mesoderm, according to different modes of patterning. The fate map of the neural crest cells (NCCs) was initially known thanks to Le Douarin's experiences with the chicken-quail chimera [11]. Moreover, new tools were developed at the beginning of the twenty-first century, which took us inside the mechanism that controls their behaviors.

As seen above in the Gans and Northcutt scenario, the neural crest would appear as a new head that would be very specific to gnathostomes.

The history of NCCs is governed by three sets of genes [13]: the first set localized at the neural plate border, so-called "cell specification genes"; the second set, "neural crest cells survivor"; and the third is "migration/differentiation neural crest genes."

Neural Crest Cells Individualization [13]

On the edges of the neural tube folds, the border of the neural plate, signals coming from the neural plate, overlying epidermis, and underlying mesoderm will induce the specification of ectodermal cells into NCCs, which will delaminate into a mesodermal–mesenchymal transition. The set of genes that orchestrates this differentiation comes from all around. The surrounding inductive tissues will issue a set of signals for the transforming cells; Notch comes from the neural plate; Wnt, FGF, and RA from the neural crest and BMP from the epidermis. Those signals activate a genetic program in the nascent NCCs involving Hairy, Msx, Dlx, AP2α, Zic, Pax3, and c-Myc.

Neural Crest Cells Survival

Once differentiated, NCCs have to maintain their specificity. Snail and Sox family of genes, as well as genes FoxD3, Id3, and Twist, are involved in this task.

Hedgehog (Hh) pathway plays an essential role in NCC's proliferation, differentiation, and survival when they have reached their destination in the craniofacial prominences [14].

Apoptosis of NCCs

Programmed cell death is one of the important mechanisms for regulating morphogenesis. For NCCs, it is a way to regulate the number of cells. For ectodermal cells along the fusion area of the processes of the primordial face, it is necessary to permit the adhesion of the mesenchyme.

NCCs Migration (Fig. 3.6)

The striking capacity to migrate that characterizes the NCCs has a series of prerequisites:

- To be free from intercell attachment [15].
- To be able to reach and cross the basal lamina.
- To be in the capacity to move through the extracellular matrix.

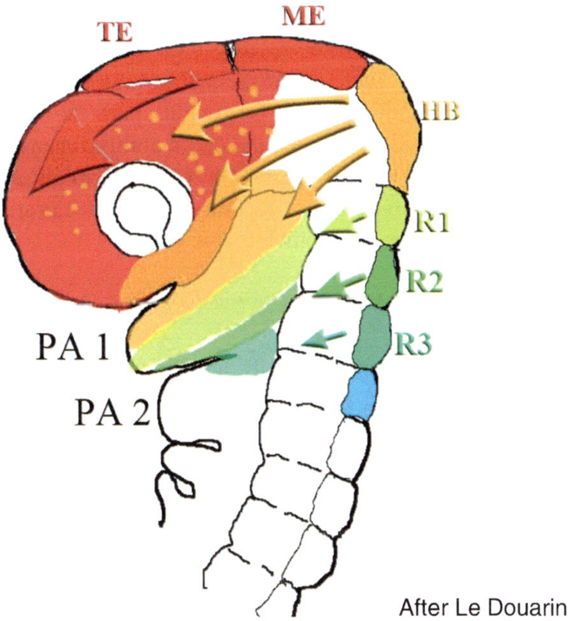

Fig. 3.6 The fate map of neural crest cells. *TE* telencephalon, *ME* mesencephalon, *HB* hindbrain, *R1* 1st rhombomere, *R2* 2nd rhombomere, *R3* 3rd rhombomere, *PA1* 1st pharyngeal arch, *PA2* 2nd pharyngeal arch

The NCCs will move to inhabit and interact with their target areas in three steps. The first step is the acquisition of oriented migration along their incoming pathways. Once the NCCs leave the neural tube, they contact the cranial mesenchyme and surface ectoderm near the hindbrain and telencephalon. This contact will allow intercell information exchanges, which permit the second step.

The second step is the streaming of cells along the dorsolateral pathways, which brings them to the frontonasal process and branchial arches.

The third step is the arrival at the frontonasal process and branchial arch and their invasion [16].

For each of these points, many protein components have been recognized to play regulating roles and their genetic control and regulation.

Genetic Coding Affecting NCC Mobility

The NCC's ability to migrate depends on several factors. First, the cells themselves must possess specific qualities. Second, the paths for their displacements must be accessible.

Cells Deformability

Cytoskeletal structures and mechanisms controlling lineage specification have been recently discovered. They yield to the organization of tissue architecture during development. We have new insights into the processes that cells use to change their cytoskeleton with specific temporal and spatial patterning in the early stage of embryogenesis [17].

The ability of cells to modify their cytoskeleton is linked to their capacity to migrate. For instance, a cytoskeletal protein synthesized under the SPECC1 gene control is mandatory in NCCs for this purpose [15]. A sufficient amount of this protein is necessary to keep the cell's ability for cytoskeletal reorganization under such signals as the WNT5 protein. SPECC1 might mediate endothelin. The endothelin pathway regulates the intracellular concentration of Ca^{++}, which affects the cytoskeletal, thus the motility of the cells.

Cells Adhesion

To start their migration, cells must release the attachments that keep them all together.

Mechanical studies [18] demonstrated that both viscosity and cell adhesion were involved in motility. Cadherin 11 plays an important role, mainly in the latter.

Epithelial–Mesenchymal Transition

The epithelial–mesenchymal transition, the first step of NCCs' appearance, changes the shape, mechanical characteristics, and polarity of cells [19], allowing their delamination and migration. Matrix metalloproteinase 4 (MMP14) plays a role in this process of early delamination.

Filopodial Motility

The NCC's motility involves filopodial extensions. There is evidence of communications between NCCs through filipodia extending between NCCs and the capacity to move forward thanks to their contractile abilities. Leading cells of the streams of the migration act as trailers [16].

Filopodial structures depend on the cytoskeleton structure. The genetic control of cytoskeletal proteinic components would affect this function.

Paths Followed by NCCs

Inside the stream of migrating NCCs, those trailing cells lead the flow. Morphologies depend on the cell's position in the path; the leading cells extend filopodia toward the ectoderm, overspreading the way, and have a bipolar shape. Advanced cells appear to have multiple filopodial extensions, some extending backward to guide bipolar cells [16].

The paths control could be driven according to several modes:

- Cell polarity.
- Local inhibition signals.
- Cell nudging (after contact, swelling of the cell opposite from the site of contact that kindly pushes forward the migrating NCC).
- Chemoattractants and chemorepulsives [20]. FGF8 in the frontal process might act as a chemoattractant for NCCs [21]. FGF8 produced in the frontonasal bud stimulates rhombencephalon NCC proliferation and migration to BA1.

The role of the extracellular matrix is enlightened by recent knowledge. A permissive extracellular matrix such as laminins and fibronectin lines routes of NCCs migration [22].

Neural Crest Cells Patterning and Differentiation

The NCCs are the source of the chondrocranium and facial bones (Fig. 3.7).

The NCC appears during phylogenesis only in vertebrate fields [4] and is primarily responsible for the development of the head.

A long-held belief was that the neural crest was the source of patterning in the face.

In the head, the NCCs are programmed before their migration [23]. The human equivalent of the mutated gene involved in disorganization in mice, which is supposed to be the GATA4 gene, is considered to play a role in this early NCC patterning.

But NCCs do not determine the formation of the skeleton all by themselves.

An epithelial–mesodermal interaction is required to develop the osteochondral tissue, forming the skull.

We could not do better than to quote the late Peter Thorogood literarily [24].

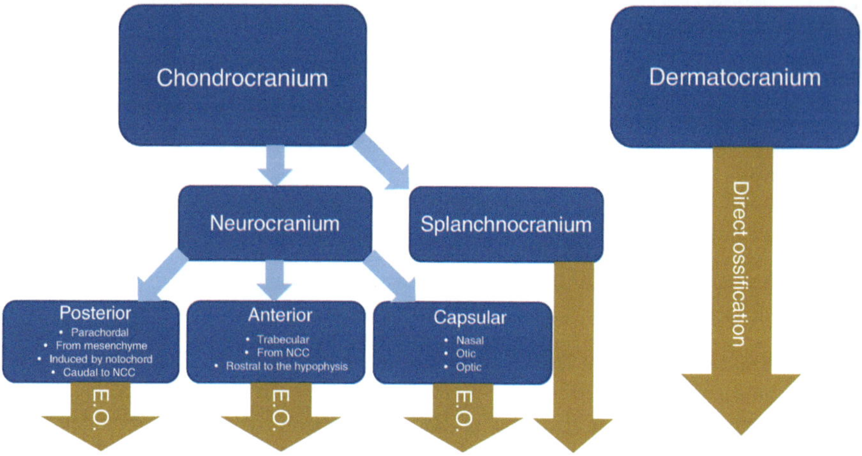

Fig. 3.7 Origin of the craniofacial skeleton

1. "The early developing head is viewed as a convoluted bag of folded epithelia enclosing an extensive extracellular compartment only sparsely populated by mesodermally-derived mesenchyme cells.
2. Into these matrix-filled spaces, NC cells migrate autonomously and opportunistically.
3. Their migratory behavior is, to some extent, controlled by extracellular matrix, particularly by epithelial-derived matrices."

Furthermore, the place and time of this interaction, which is a matrix-mediated event, control how and where this differentiation will occur.

It is as if some locations were patterned to stop the migration and kick on the differentiation.

Thorogood describes this phenomenon as the "flypaper mode". He proved that the spatial patterning of this trapping event is related to the folding of epithelium: the topography of the primordial head invaginations and evagination will create the map of the sticking area, thus the shape of the skull.

Developing hard tissues in the first branchial arch involves a combination of prepattern and epigenetic mechanisms.

The pattern of those epithelial folding could support epigenetic consequences; small shifts of parameters of both NCC motility and/or "sticking area" mapping would result in phylogenetic changes and could underlie craniofacial malformations.

The endothelin path is of most importance to what we are concerned; Sato's [25] work indicates that if the NCCs within the first pharyngeal arch (PA1) are competent to give either maxillary or mandibular structure, it is the endothelin-1 receptor type-A which switches toward one or the other morphogenetic program.

Genetic Coding Affects the Patterning Capacity of Surface Cranial Ectoderm

We will evocate two examples of the genes involved in this patterning helpful to understanding craniofacial morphogenesis.

Pax6 and the Lambda Junction [26]

Compagnucci demonstrated how Pax6 mutation affects the migration of many Hox-negative NCCs in amazing work. Those NCCs essential to forming the upper jaw and lateral nasal capsule are migrating from the anterior midbrain. Instead of reaching the devoted frontonasal area, they stack beneath the ocular area. They demonstrate that it is due to an upregulation of Hnk1-epitope (a molecule involved in cell adhesion) in the surface cephalic ectoderm of the ocular area. Hence the area became the glue of the "flypaper."

Among the ectoderm invaginations and evaginations, the lambdoid junction between the maxillary process of the first branchial arch and the lateral and medial processes of the frontonasal process is an essential area for the cross talk between NCC and surface cranial ectoderm.

Positioning the Articulation Between Mandible and Maxillary: The Hinge and Cap Model [27]

One of the main roles in patterning the NCCs is to secure the assignment of cell populations, whether to the maxilla or the mandible, thus defining a location for the forthcoming hinge, which will define the final position of the temporomandibular articulation. This arrangement supposes the existence of a hinge organization center. This area could be located at the lambdoid junction (λ), which is the place where the medial and lateral primordial facial processes converge. It is a place where complex sets of signals will organize combinations of cell multiplications and apoptosis to fulfill the program.

Fgf8 and the Frontonasal Process

Hu and Marcuccio [28] and Griffin [29] demonstrated the role of Fgf8 in the same manner for the organization of a specific area for this cross talk in the frontonasal process. They demonstrated that an early boundary between the zones of expression of Fgf8 and Shh determined a zone that they called the frontonasal ectodermal zone (FNZ).

The patterning capacity of this FNZ is such as to be able to override the prepatterning of the NSS itself. FNZ regulates both the dorsoventral patterning and the proximo-distal growth. This FNZ is established before NCC arrives at the time of neural tube closure (see primary cilia above).

Patterning Role of the Foregut Endoderm

The role of the foregut in patterning the facial skeleton has been demonstrated by Couly [30]. The endodermal cul-de-sac developed at the early stage of facial morphogenesis beneath the frontonasal bud expresses patterning signals. NCCs not expressing Hox genes will respond to those signals, while NCCs expressing Hox signals will not.

Couly concludes that bone and cartilage facial skeletons depend on their shape and position on the foregut endoderm. The relation of this endoderm to the embryonic axes would determine the relation of the skeleton.

"The Hox-negative neural crest possesses the exclusive capacity to generate the facial skeleton but does not carry the information to pattern it"—(Couly).

Closure of the Neural Tube

Closure of the neural tube is a complex process requiring strict gene expression control. Among them, two seem to be of utmost importance: GATAD2A, a transcriptional repressor, and TFAP2A, an activating enhancer.

3.2.2.3 Facial Buds: The Facial Primordia (Fig. 3.8a)

A series of buds, the facial primordia, will arise from the ventrolateral surfaces of the embryo. Notably, they are delimited by points of apposition between the ectoderm and endoderm and are filled, stereotypically, with CNCs surrounding a core of the cephalic mesoderm [1]. At the midline, between the two optical placodes, the frontonasal process will give rise to the medial and two lateral processes. The lateral process around the olfactive placode will separate into medial and lateral. Laterally at the level of the first branchial arch, two processes, the maxillary and mandibular, will grow on both sides.

Young et al. in 2014 [31] and then Hu et al. [32] demonstrated the convergence of the facial embryonic bauplan at the time of the fusion of facial buds, thus realizing a phylotypic stage in facial embryogenesis. That means the 4D development of the facial primordia: spatial geometry, and changes over time are restricted to a few combinations that only permit their fusion, especially in the lambda junction. This constraint is the reason for the convergence and the very similar aspect of the amniote fetuses of different species at this stage. Most striking is that the regulation of this 4D event is under the strict regulation of the Sonic Hedgehog (SHH) pathway.

The fusion of those processes around the oral cavity will form the face. Proper fusion of those prominences requires apoptosis or epithelial transformations at the contact surfaces. A key point is the lambda junction [10].

A key role for IRF6 was first reported in 2002 [33]. IRF6, which promotes epithelial cell death, thus removing the epithelial seam and consecutive bud fusion, acts downstream to P63 itself downstream to WNT signaling. This cascade could be hampered by expanded SHH signaling [34] (Fig. 3.8b).

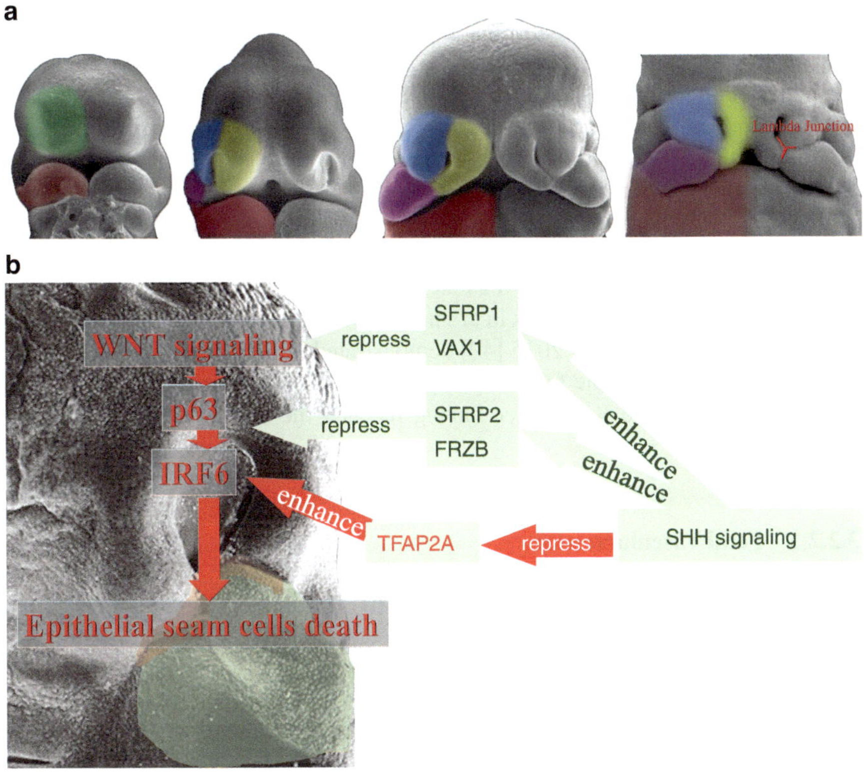

Fig. 3.8 (**a**) Coalescence of facial buds: frontal view, human embryo from 26 to 31 mm. Yellow: medial nasal process. Blue: lateral nasal process. Purple: maxillary process. Red: mandibular process. (**b**) Genetic cascade regulating the bud fusion. SHH signaling is at the heart and should have a balanced action. Shh gain of function hampers the epithelial seam removal. Shh loss of function hampers the growth of maxillary bud

3.2.2.4 The Role of Primary Cilia

The important role of primary cilia has been among the recent progress in understanding the mechanism of craniofacial malformations, including rare clefts.

Primary cilia are cytoskeleton structures that are central hubs of signal transduction for developmental pathways [35]. Some of those pathways play an essential role in craniofacial morphogenesis, notably the SHH pathway, a discovery published by Huangfu in 2003 [36]. The movement of proteins, called intraflagellar transport, into the cilia looks like an active phenomenon and could act in both directions for the SHH pathway. The WNT pathway, another one important for its role in the growth of lateral processes of facial primordia and in the releasing action of the epithelial seam at the time of fusion of facial buds, seems to be, as well concerned with the primary cilia function.

FGF signaling pathway is essential for the regulation of cilia development. Thus, indicating that craniofacial malformations related to its perturbation could be cilia related. It is stricking that FGF8, known for its role in frontonasal development, plays an essential role in determining cilia length and function [37] suggests that its action upon facial morphogenesis could be expressed through ciliary dysfunction.

Among the several signaling pathways determinant in craniofacial morphogenesis, there is an increasing interest in the planar cell polarity signaling pathway (PCP) [38]. This pathway, well known in insects, has attracted the attention of researchers toward its role in craniofacial morphogenesis. A key gene in this pathway, the gene Fuz, is known to regulate ciliogenesis [39] regulates Hh and Wnt signaling, two essential pathways in craniofacial morphogenesis.

Research by Liu et al. in 2015 [40] demonstrated, in a mice strain defective for Kif3a, which is responsible for ciliopathy, that NCCs did not rely on cilia for their migration but required Kif3a once having reached the midline to respond to the WNT signaling.

3.2.2.5 Fetal Vascularization

From Poswillo's research [41, 42] came the hypothesis that some malformations could be related to localized vascular accidents, either hemorrhage or ischemia. He quoted Braithwaite [43] and others that ischemia due to vascular anomalies would lead to more or less extensive embryo necrosis responsible for malformations.

The ontogenesis of the vascular system is as complicated as the craniofacial one [44, 45].

Mesodermal cells, through in situ differentiating processes, give rise to hemangioblast. Hemangioblasts can differentiate into hematopoietic cells or angioblasts. The transformation of angioblasts into mature endothelial cells is called vasculogenesis. Endothelial cells organize themselves in capillaries (Fig. 3.9a).

These primary vessels will be remodeled into veins and arteries under the onset of embryonic circulation. That is angiogenesis.

Angiogenesis is based on endothelial sprouting or intussusceptive microvascular growth [46].

The vascular development will involve a series of complementary processes [47]: branching, remodeling, and pruning. The new vessels are enforced by recruiting mural cells and by generating an extracellular matrix [44].

The development of subcutaneous vascular plexus in the head has been studied specifically by Finley [48]. Her research confirmed the vasculogenesis process as described above and met Hochstetter's macroscopic description [49]. She described the spatiotemporal progress of the vasculogenesis into the scalp as a wave breaking toward the top of the head to reach the midline (Fig. 3.9b).

The blood vessel growth occurs under the control of many genes [50], acting at different places at different times. Diseases related to mutations affecting those genes would lead to diffuse alterations more than to a localized defect, but consequences of local aggression could be mediated by regional angiogenesis or vasculogenesis perturbation.

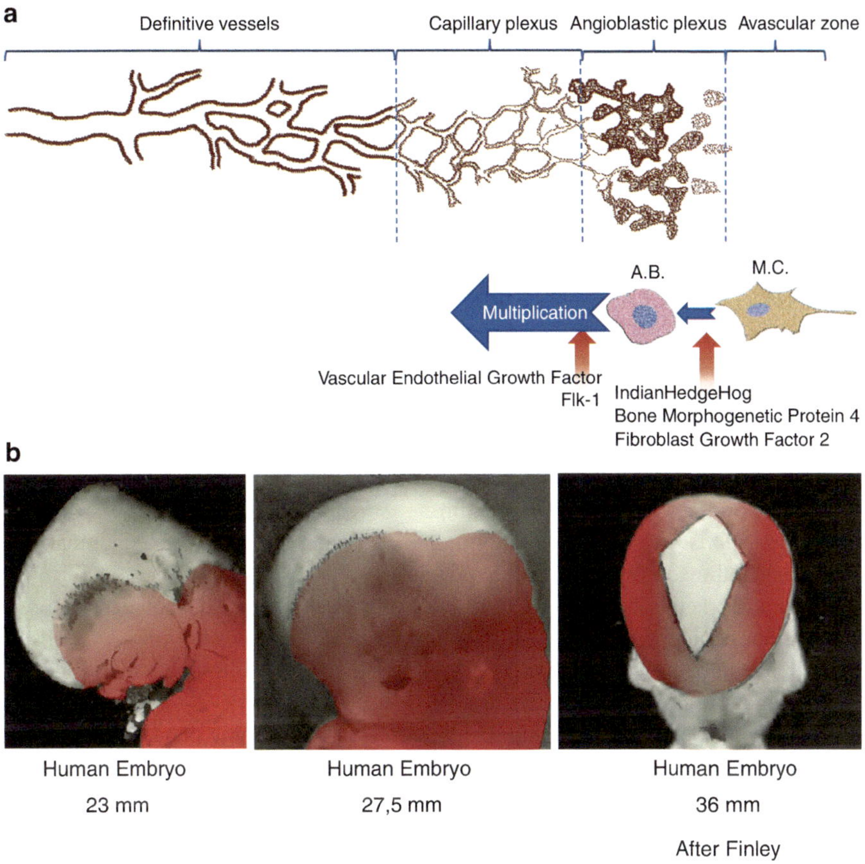

Fig. 3.9 (**a**) Vascular system ontogenesis. (**b**) Vascular system ontogenesis. Vascular invasion of the head

Segmentation

Segmentation is a highly conserved character, which the Hox gene family drives. Hox genes are expressed in the visceral arches as well as in the NCC from the hindbrain and fated to the visceral arches. The vertebrate upper jaw bones originate from Hox-negative cranial neural crest cells from rhombomeres 1 and 2, the mesencephalon, and the diencephalon [51]. Hox code is expressed in the mesoderm, transferred to rhombomeres of the hindbrain, and then migrating NCCs pass the signal to the visceral arch and finally to the pharyngeal endoderm and superficial ectoderm [52].

3.3 Pathology

We will see how the ontogenetic process could be affected to yield craniofacial malformations.

3.3.1 The Terminology for Birth Defects (Fig. 3.10)

The need for a classification of birth defects that would be pathogenetically oriented was addressed in 1982 [53]. Spranger and the international working group proposed the following:

- *Malformations*: inherited/defective developmental processes; malformations are caused by genetic and/or environmental factors acting independently or together. Most malformations occur during the third to eighth week of gestation and result in alteration, even the lack of structure.
- *Deformations*: mechanical disruptions to embryos; due to pure mechanical disturbance, they could be reversible postnatally.
- *Disruptions*: consequences of destructive processes of already formed structures. Vascular accident, as in Poswillo's hypothesis for craniofacial microsomia [41] or defects arising in amniotic band syndrome. External interference with developmental processes, when a teratogen is administered.
- *Syndromes*: design a set of anomalies occurring in the same patient relative to a common cause whose diagnosis has been made.

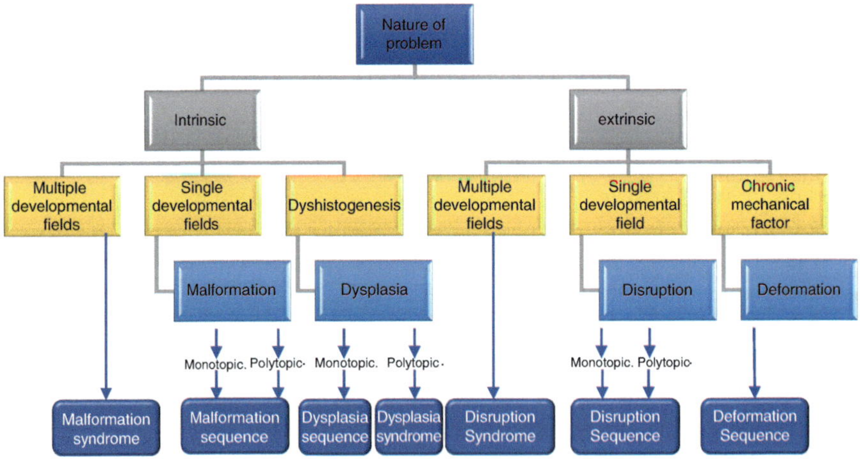

Fig. 3.10 Birth defect nomenclature

- *Associations*: design the simultaneous presence of non-stochastic anomalies because they are met more frequently than if they came randomly. CHARGE or VACTERL are examples.
- *Dysplasias*: neoplastic changes.

As an attempt at clarity, we will angle the etiology of birth defects possibly responsible for rare clefts from two directions: first, the agents of birth defects, the causal events; and second, the targets, ontological events, that those agents have to strike to get the considered birth defect.

3.3.2 The Agents of Birth Defects

3.3.2.1 Environmental Causes of Birth Defects (Fig. 3.11)

Environmental agents affecting pregnant mammals lead to birth defects in their brood. It became evident with the rise of thalidomide-related malformation.

The nature and extent of the malformation are related to the time, intensity, and duration of the exposure. It could be intricated with a genetic disposition that could explain the variability of phenotypes. A list of teratogens is displayed in Fig. 3.11. There is some evidence that the teratogenic effect would be related to the augmentation of cell deaths [54]. Panoutsopoulos [55] raises the hypothesis that dysfunction in ribosome biogenesis, which occurs in spliceosomal dysfunctions, heightens the vulnerability of NCCs to the damaging effect of alcohol.

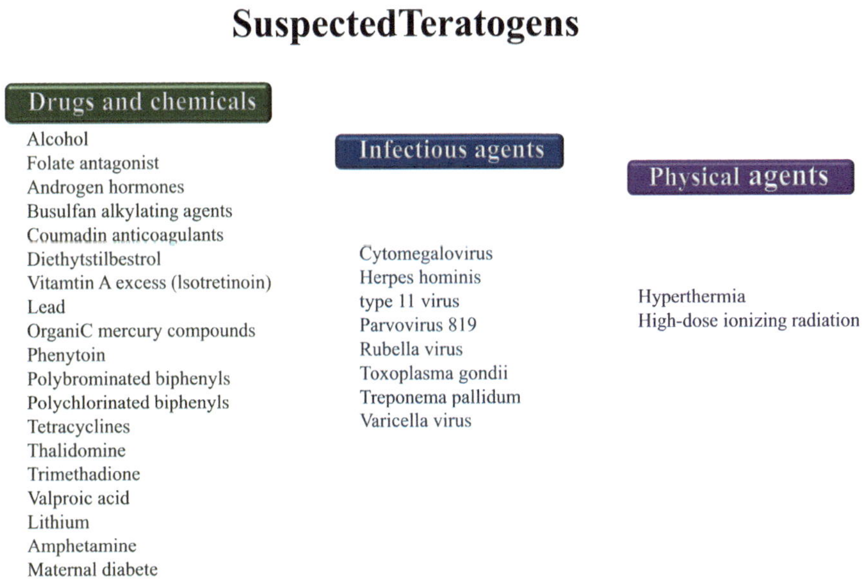

Fig. 3.11 The teratogens

Another way of action for some of the teratogens could be a specific impairment of a single gene function. This has been demonstrated, for instance, for the teratologic mechanism effect of dithiocarbamates, which affects sox9a gene expression by downregulating [56].

3.3.2.2 Genetic Causes of Birth Defects (Figs. 3.12 and 3.13)

Chromosomal anomalies or gene mutations are responsible for malformations. Gene mutations could be acquired or transmitted. An acquired mutation may be related to exposure to mutagenic agents or occur spontaneously, independently of any known cause.

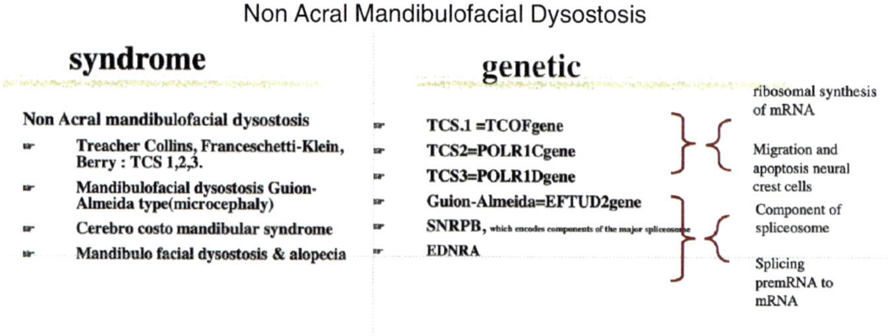

Fig. 3.12 Genes involved in non-acral dysostosis

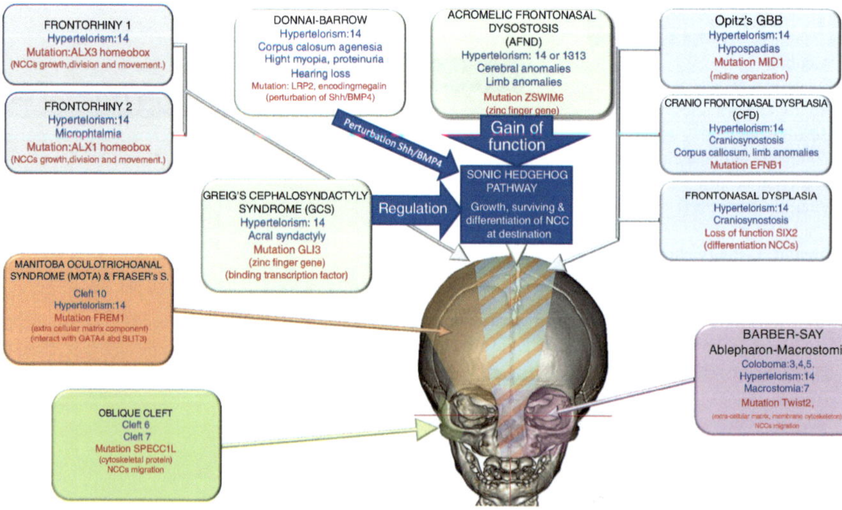

Fig. 3.13 Known gene mutations related to rare clefts

When some transmitted mutation is found in a familly it is, then,an hereditary disease and usually provoke an array of malformations belonging to a syndrome.

But in some cases, gene mutations could necessitate specific environmental conditions and/or epigenetic associations to be expressed. This multifactorial steering of birth defects is the most frequent.

3.3.3 The Targets of Birth Defects

3.3.3.1 Midline Organization

Midline Duplication

Among the cases of clefts 14, some patients present a more or less critical duplication of facial components ranging from the most severe head duplication to the lighter duplication of superior frenulum labiae associated with mesiodens. Although opposed to the defect mechanism responsible for frontonasal dysplasia, it is responsible for huge hypertelorisms [57]. A possible explanation would be a default of regulation in the control of the primitive streak, which is known to depend on Cerberus, Nodal, and HNF-3β [58].

The characteristic signs of this series of malformations are duplicated structures belonging to the frontonasal process.

Midline Dysraphia

With the term "cleft" came the image, as it occurs in the cleft lip, of a default of fusion in the midline. Anterior neuropore closure is frequently hypothesized as a cause of craniofacial midline dysraphia. Also, most of the research in teratogenesis shows that it leads to anencephaly since the neuro tube cannot bear to stay exposed during embryogenesis and disappear [59]. So, the idea of midline dysraphia through default of neuropore closure as a mechanism for malformation could be discussed.

Two genes are involved in the anterior neuropore closure: GATAD2A, a transcriptional repressor, and TFAP2A, an activating enhancer [7].

Fong et al. [60] observed in a mice strain called Tuff, a phenotype of encephalocele with midfacial cleft and hypertelorism that they found related to insufficient closure of the anterior part of the neural tube. They needed help in understanding the molecular mechanism involved.

Away from neural tube closure, some genes are known to play a specific role in midline organization as MID1—a gene whose mutation cause Opitz's GBB syndrome, which includes hypertelorism that could be seen as cleft 14 [61].

Midline Defect

Defects in the midline could occur at different times of the embryogenesis: during gastrulation. At the beginning of the third week of development, a time when the gastrulation is initiating, teratogenic insults are highly damageable. At this time, the patterning of groups of cells fated to form specific organs, such as the eyes and brain, already exists, and those populations may be damaged by teratogens. It is known, for example, that high doses of alcohol at this stage kill cells in the anterior midline of the germ disc; those cells miss the midline craniofacial structures, which results in holoprosencephaly. The question to include or not holoprosencephaly and its different manifestations is still patent: cranial manifestation is hypotelorism, which is a midline malformation, but which is the contrary to hypertelorism...

Severe facial forms, in the absence of the medial nasal process of the frontonasal process, lead to a condition mimicking the median cleft lip. Those cases are frequently published as cleft 0. They are, in fact, cases of bilateral cleft lip with the absence of medial prolabium.

3.3.3.2 Malformations Due to Neural Crest Cells Anomalies

Perturbation in NCCs Multiplication and Apoptosis

Multiplication and apoptosis are two mechanisms that determine the number of available NCCs and, thus, the quantity of craniofacial skeleton. A good example of this regulation is the Treacher-Collins syndrome (TCS). TCS has been proven to be the consequence of TCOF1 gene mutation. The pathogenetic mechanism in which it acts has been very well analyzed in Calo's publication [62]. The mutation induces ribosomopathy; TCOF is part of a cascade of events in the ribosome, which lead to rRNA synthesis; the mutation inhibits rRNA synthesis, provokes a loss of DDX21, and damages the rDNA. The combination of rDNA damage and nucleolar stress activates p53, a tumor suppressor protein that increases NCCs apoptosis. Moreover, the apoptosis-increasing activity could be sensible to in utero exposure to environmental hazards, which could explain the variability of phenotypes.

The exact path has been investigated for a strain of mice with Pak1ip1 gene loss of function [55].

All the non-acral mandibulofacial dysostosis syndromes are related to mutations involving the spliceosomal complex (Fig. 3.12).

Perturbations in NCCs Migration (Fig. 3.13)

A mutation affecting the NCCs migration will decrease the number of cells reaching their patterned destination.

- The deficiency of SPECC1L cytoskeletal protein affects the cytoskeletal of NCCs, thus affecting their migration faculty, which leads to oblique facial clefts, Tessier's cleft types 6 and 7 [15]

- SPECC1L encodes a novel coiled-coil domain-containing protein and functionally interacts with microtubules and the actin cytoskeleton, especially in mitotic spindles 21 [63].
- Frontorhiny is a frontonasal dysplasia associated with a mutation in the ALX3 homeobox gene [64]. The protein coded by this gene is a transcription factor, which attaches to DNA and controls the activity of some genes that control cell growth, division, and movement. The precise mechanism is unknown, but migration is likely affected.
- Another type of frontorhiny, the most severe and associated with microphthalmia, has been attached to a mutation in the ALX1 homeobox gene [65]. Research in a zebrafish model [66] found that ALX is necessary to ensure proper migration of NCCs toward the frontonasal region

Perturbation Affecting NCC at their Arrival Location (Fig. 3.13)

When the NCCs reach their final destination in the facial primordia processes, they still have to survive and much more to proliferate and differentiate to achieve a normal craniofacial skeleton. The hedgehog path plays an essential role in those events [14]. However, Sonic Hedgehog (SHH) is not directly expressed in the mesenchyme derived from the NCC, it is provided by the foregut endoderm. SHH loss of function increases NCC apoptosis in situ and disrupts craniofacial structures. Two hypertelorism syndromes are known to be caused by a gene mutation affecting the SHH pathway: Acromelic frontonasal dysostosis (AFND), which is related to a mutation of ZSWIM6 [67–69] and Greig's cephalopolysyndactyly related to GLI3 mutation, which acts downstream in the pathway.

Hufnagel et al. [70] reported frontonasal dysplasia due to a loss of function in SIX2, a gene critical for cell fate determination.

3.3.3.3 Complex Conditions of Unknown Origin

Amniotic Band Syndrome/ADAM/LWD

In medical literature, relations of malformations caused by amniotic membrane anomalies go way back in time. A precise description of what will be known more recently as rare clefts could be found in the nineteenth century. In 1837, Dick [71] reported a case of a stillborn 7-month-old fetus with the features of hypertelorism that looked like a bilateral cleft 13 and two facial oblique clefts, which could be cleft 6 or 7 associated with amniotic bands and multiple parietal defects involving the head with an exencephaly a thoracic defect and an abdominal defect. The fetus was missing the right superior extremity. Nowadays, this association of malformations would be classified as a limb and wall defect (LWD) syndrome.

Dick quotes St Hilaire's opinion that the band is the cause of disruption and a different opinion from Serre that the disruption is of vascular origin. Other cases of unusual craniofacial clefts occurring in the setting of amniotic band syndrome were reported in 1867 by Ross [71], in 1890 by Chavane [72], and in 1897 by Marchand [73].

Since the reports of the association between craniofacial clefts and amniotic band syndromes have been so frequent, it became a common opinion that amniotic band sequence is one of the causes of craniofacial clefting.

The nomenclature of conditions with several malformations associated with bands crossing the amniotic sac and usually attached to the placenta is confusing, mainly depending on the main author's focus. As well as confusing the supposed etiology of those conditions.

Starting with the nomenclature: congenital constricting bands; Amniotic band sequence (ABS); Amniotic deformity-adhesion-mutilation (ADAM); Streeter anomalies; limb and wall defects (LWD); Amniotic Band disruption complex. Among so many appellations, the choice is difficult; for us, it will be ABS since it looks more inclusive when LWD excludes conditions without parietal defect, ADAM excludes conditions without mutilation, and Streeter anomalies refer to a hypothesis that could be accounted for only a part of cases.

When miscarriages and terminations between 9 and 18 weeks are considered (1.78% of miscarriages and terminations have ABS), the condition is quite a frequent [74]. The malformation spectrum is extremely wide, affecting the right-left sides and cephalic-caudal extremities similarly. Since it is frequently lethal to the fetus, it is primarily a preoccupation for the fetal pathologist. When surviving and being able to benefit from surgery, most survivors have normal intellectual development.

Pathogenic Hypothesis for ABS

Many pathogenic hypotheses have been proposed to explain the lesions observed in ABS. They could be sorted into two groups: the first infers that an amniotic anomaly disrupts the embryo acting as an environmental constraint, and the second infers that the amniotic bands are side effects of the primary malformation.

ABS is Considered a Disruption Caused by Amniotic Anomalies

Congenital amputations have been well known for a long time, and many cases have been reported in the medical literature. The first explanation for the congenital amputation and the stiction bands was that a coil of the umbilical cord around a limb would dig a groove deeper and deeper until the most severe amputation. Quite rapidly, this explanation was found unsustainable because of the softness of the umbilical cord and the absence of spiral grooves [75].

Then came the hypothesis that bands supplied the pressure for those amputations and strictures. Montgomery, in 1832 (Fig. 3.14), was the first to report a case giving much attention to limb amputation and probably the first to notice a relationship between the presence of "threads" that he considered as "organized lymph" and amputation. But it is noticeable in the case drawing that craniofacial anomalies, including interorbital and lateral clefts, were present.

Fig. 3.14 Montgomery, 1832

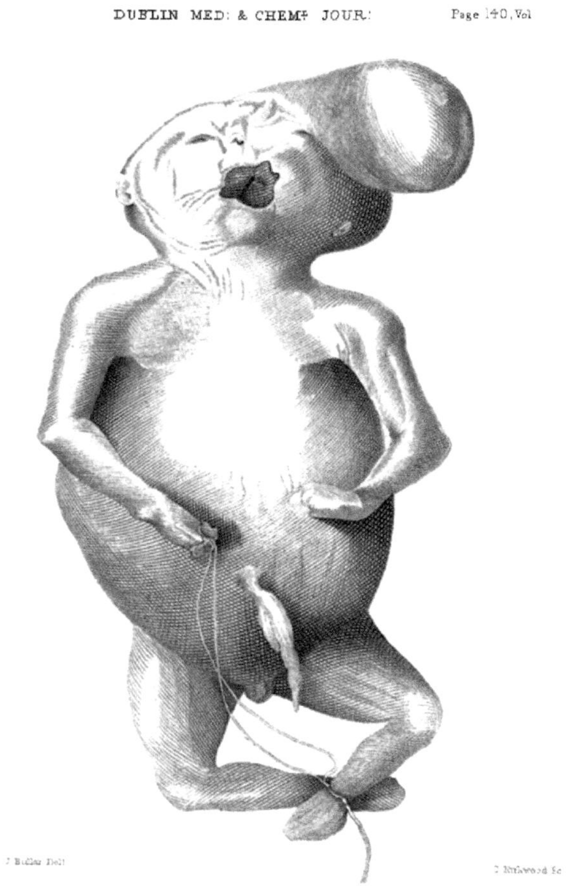

Without a precise understanding of the real cause of amniotic bands observed, it was supposed that loss, infections, or any inflammatory disease of the amniotic liquid were responsible for the formation of aberrant bands that, in their turn, would exert a mechanical strength or a tourniquet effect around limbs or segment of a limb to cause ischemia thus disruption [76].

Soon came an evolution in theory sustained by Jeanne 1886 and Raynaud 1895 that the bands were not essential but that the skin alteration came first.

Amazingly, Ballantyne's wish [75] from 1902 that the ABS pathogeny should be fully understood is not yet fulfilled.

The new theory of early amniotic rupture, or early amnion rupture sequence, brought new hypotheses and new light on the causes and consequences of band formation. It postulates that tears in the amnion are the causes for amniotic bands that may encircle part of the fetus and that this rupture produces not only the bands but crowding as well as responsible for a part of the deformation spectrum [77].

Turpin [78] gave a comprehensive description of the supposed sequence leading from the initial damage to the amniotic membrane to the constitution of bands,

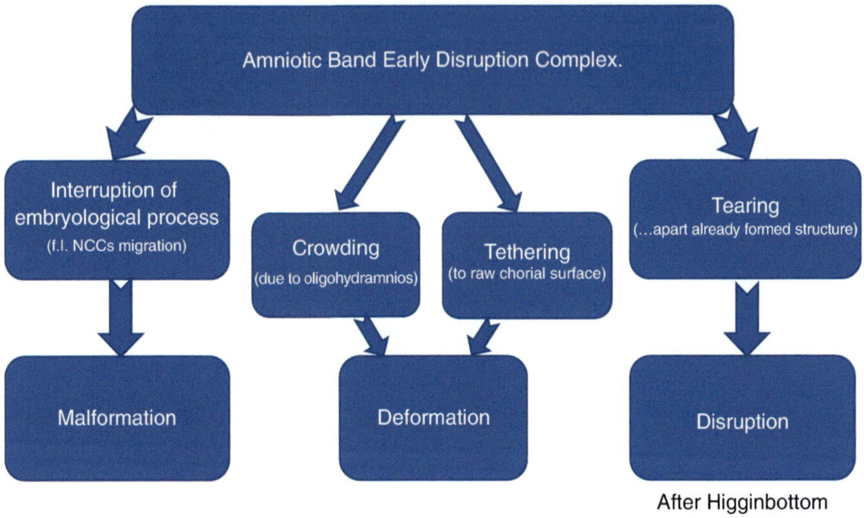

Fig. 3.15 Higginbottom organigram or ABS

transient oligoamnios and constitution of raw, abrasive surfaces of chorion to explain the observed lesions. Higginbottom [77] complemented the amniotic band disruption complex theory and produced an exciting organigram to explain the heterogeneous components of the malformation complex (Fig. 3.15).

The Streeter Hypothesis

Streeter's proposal in 1930 that ABS (which he called congenital amniotic bands) was caused by a disruption in embryogenesis at a stage as early as the embryonic disc has been widely cited in medical literature and brought up to date in Bamforth's 1992 paper [79] when they compared data of 54 ABS cases, from the literature and their one's cases to the predicted consequences of discrete local aggression to the embryo prior to 26 days post-conception. They found that observed arrays of lesions correlated with what was expected from local damages causing, at that time, disruption of established structures as well as malformations due to interrupted programs: perturbation of the anterior neuropore closure, damages to the mesonephros and local interference of NCCs migration. Bamforth established a fate map of embryonal defects resulting from known spatial and temporal aggression to the embryo and correlated the results to the different phenotypes of observed damages.

In his opinion, three strong points of the theory were as follows:

1. The spatial disposition of defects makes better sense when considering the aggression affecting the embryonic anatomical relationships than the mature one.
2. The defects are consistent in terms of a combination of malformation-disruption with understanding what was known about embryonic organization.
3. And we quote literary the third: "*The defects are those of absence. When, by chance, the disruption wave produces a group of cells large enough to sustain limited further development, this development will be ectopic and incomplete*".

3.3.3.4 Amniotic Bands as Part and Not the Cause of the Syndrome

The Vascular Hypothesis

Keith, in 1940 [80], considering Streeter's research in combination with Finley's research on the development of embryonic vascularization [48] hypothesized that a defect of vascularization led to necrosis and the formation of the bands out of exudations from the necrosed tissues and thus explain oblique facial cleft as consecutive to an avascular area between the maxillary and dental arteries. Keith explains other more complex defects and extends his theory to several border areas separating known vascular domains.

Van Allen [81], addressing more specifically the internal damages encountered in ABS, believed that early vascular disruption during the 4- to 6-week gestation and, more specifically, to the ectodermal-amnion area was responsible for the anomalies. They appear to be a spectrum of defects that result from vascular damage to the developing embryo combined with consequences of tethering to the amnion and persistence of the extraembryonic coelom.

Opitz, in 2018, made up his mind out of an extensive review of the literature [74]. His opinion sides with Streeter's, Keith's, and Van Allen's, that bands (as other amniotic and placental observed defects) and their so-called "effects" are, in fact, both consequences of a common cause.

3.3.3.5 Mice Disorganization Mutation

Several authors underlined that if the mechanical actions of amniotic bands could explain the presence of external damages, the same could not explain visceral anomalies frequently observed in the ABS [82]. Most of those authors agreed that bands would have to be the associated consequence of the same pathological process that affected the defective part of the fetus. Streeter's hypothesis matched this opinion and explained some of the visceral damages but not all of them.

Another point is the frequency of supernumerary appendages in the cleft edges and even partial duplications of anatomical structures and even supernumerary limbs in ectopic positions. Streeter gave a partial explanation for some of them in this sentence, already quoted above: "*When, by chance, the disruption wave produces a group of cells large enough to sustain limited further development, this development will be ectopic and incomplete*".

Bagg, in 1929 [83], was the first to report a series of inherited malformations on a strain of mice obtained by maternal X-ray exposition. The mode of transmission was a Mendelian recessive autosomal. Since it was before the discovery of DNA, the mutation was unknown. The observed anomalies include club foot, syndactyly, polydactyly, ectrodactyly, limb, kidney, and eye defects. The sequence leading to those defects seems to start with the extravasation of lymph, forming a "blister-like bleb" followed by a blood clot, then a hematoma.

More striking was Hummel's publication about a strain of mice presenting an array of pleomorphic malformations [84]. The transmission was determined to be related to a semi-dominant unit factor, lethal when homozygous and with incomplete penetrance in heterozygotes. She called the mutation disorganization in mice with the symbol Ds.

Ds is lethal when homozygous.

The statistic compiled from a series of 500 affected mice was as follows: *"Cranioschisis and exencephaly 53%; hamartomas (all nodules and papillae) 40%; anomalies of appendages 33%; eye defects, including malposition 21%; urogenital malformations 21%; pharyngeal defects 18%j gastroschisis 16%; curled, shortened and missing tail 15%; digestive tract anomalies 8%; and spina bifida 4%."*.

Among the multiple malformations that are met in the disorganization syndrome in mice, two points are worth to be mentioned here:

- Craniofacial malformations look very close to what we could observe as rare clefts in man;" *absence and reduction of mandibles, maxillae, and parts, separation of median nasal processes, separation of median and lateral nasal processes, cleft palate, microstomus, macrostomus, accessory mouth cavities with teeth."*
- The frequency of appendages, some very specific in shape or even differentiated into the ectopic limb or segment of limb, hamartoma.

The similarities between the manifestation of disorganization in mice mutation and some cases reported of association of craniofacial malformation with some specific additions. Such as appendages with unusual shapes did not escape many authors, and lately, several publications have come on this topic (Fig. 3.16).

Donnai, in 1989, was the first to evocate Ds for six patients with the features of ABS [85]. Purandare 2009 [86] sides with Donnai that most cases of ABS should be equivalent in man of Ds.

We found 13 publications evoking Ds as the hypothetic cause of birth defects. [87–98]. Among those authors, Crosby imagined a two-hit model to explain the high level of variability in expression [99].

Isidor, 2009, pointed out the superficial appendages as quite specific [100].

Several researchers have looked for the Ds homolog. White et al. in 1995, [101], out of the mapping of mouse and human genes, found that GATA 4 was a candidate gene for Ds.

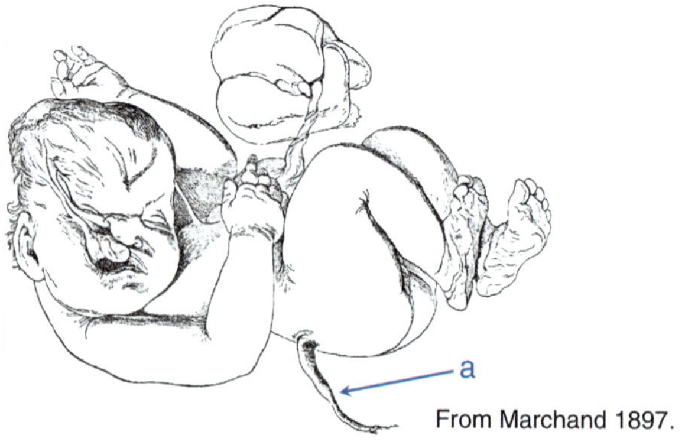

Fig. 3.16 Marchand's case of amniotic band syndrome, 1897. (**a**) The arrow points to an appendage specific of disorganization in mice

Huang assigned the human GATA4 gene 8p23.1 to p22 [102].

Kruszka, in 2015 [103], demonstrated, in a case very close to the Ds phenotype, that a mutation to the IQCK gene was responsible. Interestingly, even if the molecular pathway of this gene is not fully understood, it has a suspected role in the Ca^{2+}, which is known to interfere with the cytoskeleton and thus could induce a perturbation of NCCs motility.

3.4 Classification of Rare Clefts

The terms in use for describing birth defects, notably in the craniofacial area, have dramatically evolved and gained precision. When referring to Geoffroy de Saint Hilaire's treatise of teratology in 1837 [104], a publication considered the first comprehensive classification of teratologic conditions, the only citation found of a facial cleft is "hare lip".

If we look at Dick's report of a case in 1937 [105], we can read many terms that are no more in use today. The author uses the term "monster" to design an ABS; he used "cranial bone deficiency with a cerebral mass protrusion" to design an encephalocele; "eyeballs wide apart" for hypertelorism; "harelip" for cleft lip and "fissure of the cheek" for oblique facial cleft.

Several cases of rare clefts will be reported under the name of harelip as long as they concern the mouth. [71, 106–109]. Even after having replaced the ill-named "harelip" with the term "cleft lip," some keep cleft lip to name rare clefts [43].

Debout in 1862 [110] and Pelvet in 1864 [111] named "fissures horizontales" as a subtype of harelip, a series of macrostomia.

Van Duyse, a Belgian practitioner from Gent, was probably the first to use specific terms for the description of rare clefts. In 1882, he published two papers: on the first of August, "*Macrostomes congénitaux avec tumeurs préauriculaires et dermoïdes de l'oeil.(congenital macrostomia with pre-auricular appendages and ocular dermoids)*" [112], which describes Tessier's cleft 7 and craniofacial microsomia a long time before Goldenhar…

In October of the same year he published a second paper *"bride dermoide oculo-palpébrale et colobome partiel de la paupière avec remarques sur la génese de ces anomalies,(oculo-palpebral web and partial palpebral coloboma with remarks upon the origin of those anomalies)" [113].*

Then came the first systematic classification for some rare clefts involving the orbit, 1887 with Morian's publication.

3.4.1 Morian's Classification [114] (Fig. 3.17)

In his research, "*Ueber die schräge Gesichtsspalto. (about the oblique facial cleft)*" Morian from Berlin tells his disappointment that the term harelip or cleft lip would be the same applied to clefts that reach the orbit. Quoting Laroche's thesis [115],

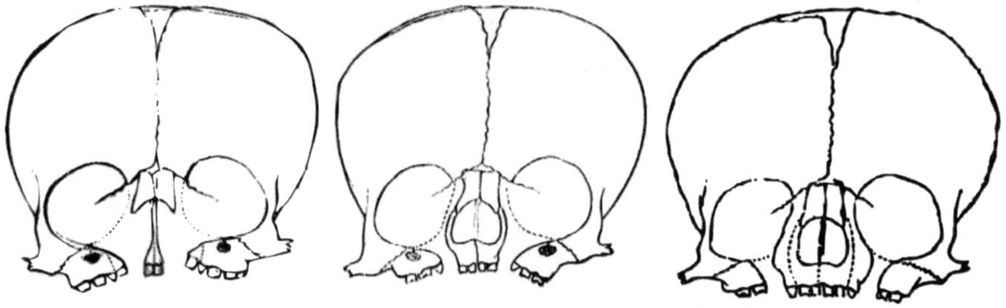

Fig. 1. Schema der I. Form. Fig. 2. Schema der II. Form. Fig. 3. Schema der III. Form.

From Morian

Fig. 3.17 Morian's classification

whom he praised for his attempt at giving a logical classification based on embryological considerations, he found the principles of his classification of facial clefts involving the orbit.

Reviewing seven personal observations and 29 cases found in the literature, he made the point that they could be sorted into three anatomical groups.

Morian's publication comprehensively describes those three types of deformities that are still accurate nowadays.

3.4.2 *Grünberg's Classification [116]*

In 1909, Erns Swalbe, editor of a book titled "Die Morphologie Der Missbildüngen Des Menschen Und Der Tiere" (The Morphology Of Malformations In Man And Animals), assigned the Chap. 4: "Die Gesichtsspalten und die zu ihnen in genetischer Beziehung stehenden anderweitigen Mißbildungen des Gesichts." (The facial clefts and other facial deformities genetically related to them), to Karl Grünberg, from Roskov. Grünberg, in this chapter, reported examples of all the known types of clefts and proposed a classification of his own. This classification was comprehensive and logical, and it is a pity that it was not widely spread then. It is worth to be reported hereafter.

1. Primary facial clefts (related to a fusional defect in facial primordia).
   - Midline clefts.
     - Nasal median cleft.
     - Upper lip median cleft.
     - Lower lip median cleft.

       Appendices: false upper lip cleft (arhinencephalia in which the premaxilla and nasal septum are missing).

- Lateral clefts.
  - Upper lip lateral clefts: usual cleft lip and palate and their combinations.
  - Oblique facial clefts.
  - Transverse cheek clefts (macrostomia).
- B secondary facial clefts (occurring after a, at first, normal formation of the facial primordia).
  - Lateral nasal clefts.
  - Oblique facial clefts.
  - Random facial clefts.
- C anomalies associated to facial clefts.
  - Aprosopie.
  - Proboscis lateralis.
  - Dermoid cysts and fistulae of the face.

3.4.3 Classification of the American Association for Cleft Palate Rehabilitation [117] (Fig. 3.18)

In 1962, in the United States, members of the American Association for Cleft Palate Rehabilitation gathered a committee under the presidency of Harkins who worked on classifying the cleft lip and palate. There was an understanding that interprofessional communication needed a standard nomenclature that made this measure mandatory.

Most of the nomenclature was devoted to the usual cleft lip and cleft palate and to comprehensively classifying its many clinical varieties. Also, they include some of the rare clefts that reached the oral aperture (Fig. 21 in Harkins's et al. publication), keeping, that way, some of the former habit of considering that all the clefts are organized around the oral cavity (Fig. 3.18).

Fig. 3.18 Classification of the American Association for cleft palate rehabilitation. (**a, b**) Naso-ocular clefts. (**c**) Oro-ocular clefts. (**e**) Oro-aural clefts

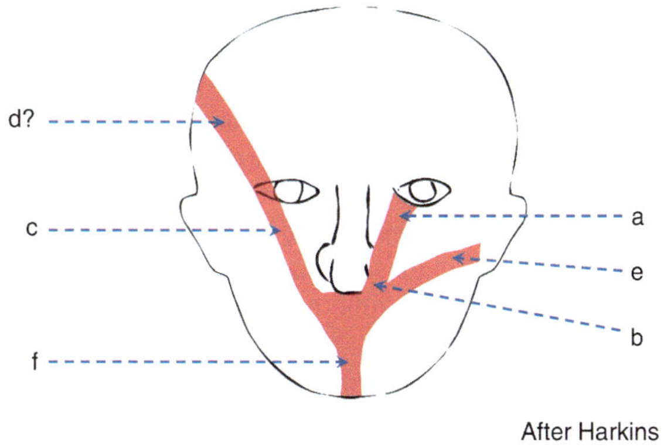

They named the clefts "*other than prepalatal and palatal*" rare.

- Naso-ocular.**a, b**
- Oro-ocular.**c**
  - Toward medial canthus.
  - Toward lateral canthus.
- Oro-aural.**e**

On the schematic drawing, an orbito-temporal could be seen **d** that did not appear in the text. Being based on the oral cavity, this classification misses a part of the craniofacial defects.

3.4.4 The Frontonasal Dysplasia and Its Subtypes

The name frontonasal dysplasia has been widely used since it was coined by Sedano [118] in 1970. From the beginning, Sedano has split this syndrome into several phenotypes.

Phenotype A: Ocular hypertelorism, broad nasal roots, median nasal groove with the absence of the nasal tip. True clefting of the midline is not present. This phenotype is similar to the Greig original cases of hypertelorism [119].

Phenotype B: Ocular hypertelorism, broad nasal root, deep median facial groove or true cleft affecting the nose or both the nose and the upper lip. The palate may also be cleft. Which is corresponding, as seen below, to Tessier's cleft 0–14.

Phenotype C: Ocular hypertelorism, broad nasal root, uni- or bilateral notching of the ala nasi, corresponding to Tessier's cleft 1–13.

Phenotype D: Combination of phenotypes B and C.

3.4.5 Tessier's Classification

Paul Tessier was training to be a surgeon in Nantes in the middle of his internship at the Hôtel Dieu, then the university hospital, when the American Nantes bombing totally destroyed it. Fortunately, he was at a picnic at the time and survived. He had to move since nothing was left in Nantes. He went to Paris and, at St Joseph Hospital, was introduced to cleft lip surgery by his mentor Georges Hue, a children's orthopedic surgeon.

He was a close friend of Dr. Hervouet, an ophthalmologist who later reached the position of head of the University Hospital department of ophthalmology in Nantes. Hervouet was at this time prominent in the French world of ophthalmology and referred all the cases of orbito-palpebral reparation to Tessier and gave him the position of surgical consultant in 1949 [120].

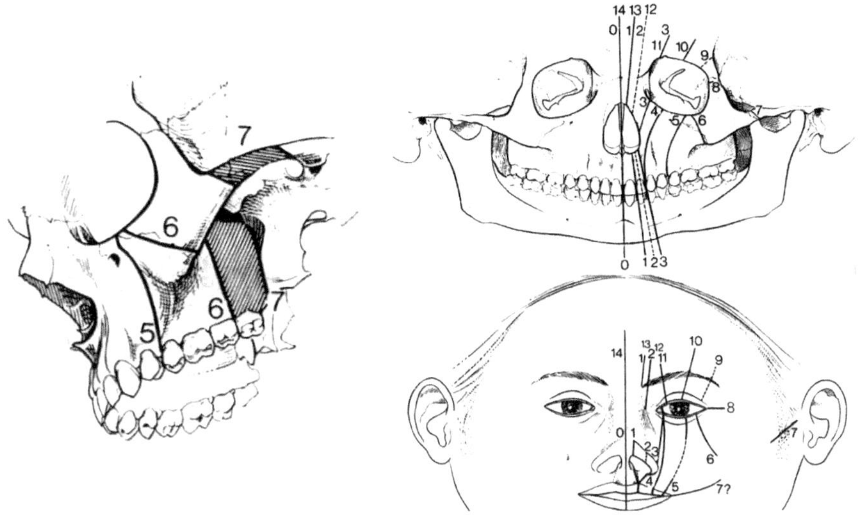

Fig. 3.19 Tessier's classification. With permission from Ms Tessier and Masson ed.

We could believe that the addition of those two fields of interest: cleft lip and oculo-palpebral malformation was the reason why he found the previous classifications incomplete.

He was stricken by Morian's publication, whose classification based on the spatial position around the orbit made sense to him. He proposed a classification completing Morian's one based on the relation with the orbit of axial defects. This classification was the first to include all the anatomical variety of craniofacial defects and even the most complex conditions by a combination of numbers when required.

Preceded by several publications on oblique clefts [121, 122] and hypertelorism [123–127], he published in 1976 *"Anatomical classification of facial, craniofacial and latero-facial clefts"* [128] (Fig. 3.19), a milestone in the history of plastic surgery, and in 1977 a more complete description in a chapter of the book *"Chirurgie Plastique Orbito-palpebrale"* [129] along with chapters on the others craniofacial malformations making this book the first book of craniofacial surgery.

This classification has been, nowadays, adopted worldwide in all the multidisciplinary teams of craniofacial surgery, and it will be the one that will be in use in this book.

Before moving on with this topic, we will insist on three points about Tessier's classification.

- The term cleft has to be understood as a very general term; most craniofacial pathologists start their clinical experience with cleft lip and palate, which are true defaults of fusion between parts of the facial primordia as understood by Vermeij-Keers [130] or a "*defect in apposition of structures along a junction*" as defined by De Myer [131]. The use of the term "cleft" by Tessier does not intend, as understood by many, to imply that those deformities are related to a default of fusion between embryonic structures. Very few of the rare clefts could be explained that way, and it is a characteristic of most rare clefts that their paths do not follow the embryonic lines of closure. Tessier's classification is free of any etiological hypothesis. It is solely a map of how the defects are organized along specific lines about the orbits.

- The term cleft and its number describe, as a whole, a defect including soft and hard tissues, knowing that all the components of the cleft could be found at any degree of severity. Thus, it is of utmost importance to the craniofacial pathologist to know the complete spectrum of rare clefts to be able when a symptom possibly related to a rare cleft is diagnosed to know where to look for even a very tenuous associated symptom belonging to the cleft spectrum; we see what we are looking at and just recognize what we know!
- Tessier performed his research at a time when only plain radiography and conventional noncomputerized frontal tomography were available. Even if he had, at this time, the larger series of rare clefts and do a throughout research of the literature, he had a limited number of cases. His anatomical descriptions were mostly based on clinical examinations, intraoperative dissections, and studies of dry skulls from anatomical museums. So, it left some room for improvements in his description of phenotypes, thanks to the studies of larger series of cases and the use of advanced medical imaging that was not available in 1976. Improving Tessier's classification does not mean a betrayal but the continuation of his work.

3.4.6 *Whitaker's Classification*

Whitaker, in 1981, proposed a general classification of craniofacial anomalies [132]. On behalf of the American Cleft Palate Association, he proposed to sort them between clefts, synostoses, atrophy, hypoplasia, neoplasia-hyperplasia, and unclassified.

For clefts, they proposed to use the Tessier classification. The only original contribution was the distinction between centric clefts: 0 to 4 and 11 to 14 and the acentric clefts: 4 to 8 and 9 to 10.

3.4.7 *Van der Meulen, Mazzola, and Stricker's classification [133] (Fig. 3.20)*

Those three authors tried something more ambitious than Tessier. They attempted to propose a general classification for craniofacial deformities based on embryological knowledge. Their mentor for embryological understanding was Vermeij-Keers, a Dutch anatomist and embryologist from Leiden [130].

Interestingly enough was their proposal to separate cerebro-cranial malformation from craniofacial ones. Then to call primary cleft a condition due to a default

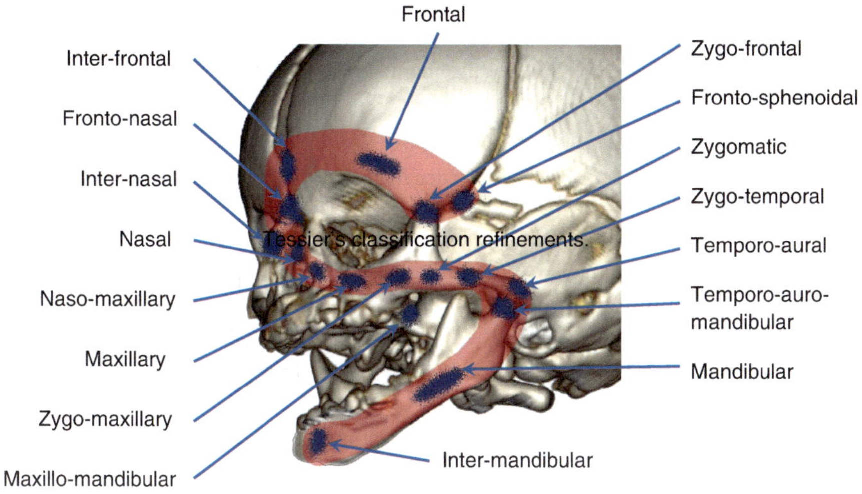

Fig. 3.20 Van der Meulen's classification

of fusion and secondary cleft a condition in which a dysplasia would occur after the normal fusion of embryonic parts. Then they differentiated this process, calling it dysplasia from dysostosis, another process frequently involved in craniofacial malformation.

Then they described a spatial disposition of dysplasia along an S-shaped path across the craniofacial skeleton in an attempt to include logically all the known craniofacial malformations, including, of course, the so-called rare clefts.

It was undoubtedly courageous and supposed to be built on the ground rock of science.

Unfortunately, it bore some difficulties. First, the opinion of Vermeij-Keers (P 129; L. 7 to 16 of reference [130] that the NCCs do not migrate has been proven a false opinion.

This opinion led the authors to miss many of the nowadays explanations of some of the rare clefts that do not match their classification.

Second, the nomenclature of the dysplasias encountered along the S was complex and confusing and lost the apparent simplicity of Tessier's number nomenclature that even does not need to be translated to be understood anywhere and in any language in the world.

3.4.8 A Last Tessier's Attempt at a Comprehensive Classification of Craniofacial Malformations

Around the same time as Van der Meulen et al. and Whitaker, Tessier tried to find a useful general classification of craniofacial malformations. He had already almost completed the redaction of a book on that purpose. Having put all the members of his team through the difficult task of collecting all over the world the skull of craniofacial malformations, analyzing again his cases and those that could be found in the literature, he decided to destroy the manuscript and throw it in a bin under the horrified look of his collaborators in 1982.

He gave his reasons in a public address in 2001 [134]:

> …I was finishing a book, completely forgotten for the only reason that this introduction to the 60 major craniofacial malformations was never published. Why? Because he was not grounded on known embryology or on a pathogenic hypothesis…

Forty years later, we have made some progress thanks to advanced medical imaging, cellular mechanisms of embryology are better known, and genetic regulation, as well as genetic dysregulations. New knowledge has brought a better understanding, but at the same time, those new bits of knowledge have introduced more complexity than we believed.

There is still no way today to propose a comprehensive classification of craniofacial malformations on a physiopathological ground. More and more cues come from the understanding of cellular and macromolecular genetics, and a general picture starts to emerge, which is very useful for biologists; but for surgeons, Tessier's classification keeps being the only one of interest since it draws attention to the anatomical axis along where the anomalies have to be looked for diagnosis and treatments.

Tessier's classification of rare clefts is widely used in craniofacial surgery, but it could be improved and made more precise in light of new knowledge.

3.4.9 Twenty-First-Century Tessier's classification (Fig. 3.21)

Considering that Tessier's classification was issued 50 years ago, since its original research, that progress has been made in medical imaging and in genetics, s considering that many cases have been published and that well-trained teams of craniofacial surgeons have carefully studied, operated on and followed up numerous cases, some gray aspects of this classification could be enlightened.

A first point has already been raised, even if partially by Whitaker [132], when he proposed to separate rare clefts into two groups: centric and acentric.

Tessier asserted that his classification bedrock was based on the orbit when clefts 0 to 2 and their cranial corresponding extension did not reach the orbit, as well as lateral clefts 6b, 6c, and 7.

As suggested by Whitaker [132], the distinction between centric and acentric is not a fancy thought but corresponds to a shift in the anatomical consequences and their treatment. Centric are inter-orbital and lead to hypertelorism. Acentric are not and do not.

But there is still a distinction to make between acentric involving the orbit and those that do not, and we could introduce the distinction between the clefts that reach the oral aperture and those that do not.

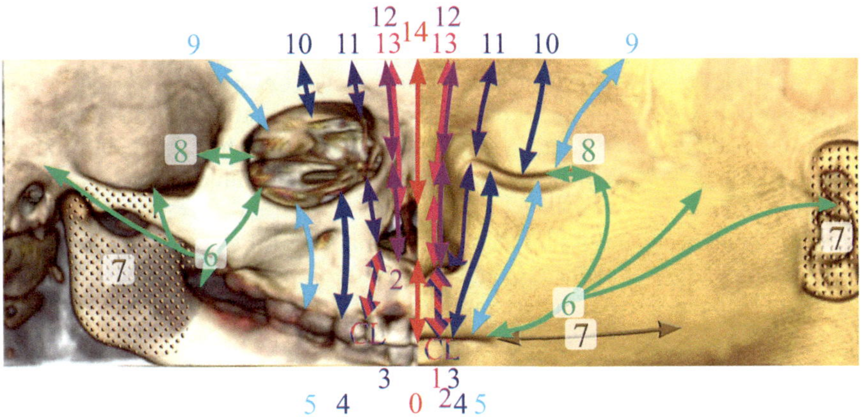

Fig. 3.21 Twenty-first-century Tessier's chart. Borders between 0-14 and 1-13 are into the nose. CL for cleft lip. Paths of 1-13 and 12 are almost the same. Cleft 6 has a trifurcated direction toward there subtypes (see corresponding chapter cleft 6). Skeletal component of cleft 7 as well as external ear are represented as tan doted areas to point out the craniofacial microsomia accompanying the cleft 7 macrostomia (see corresponding chapter cleft 6)

It will be discussed more in detail in the corresponding chapters, but we are inclined to relate the clefts to the facial aperture:

- Cleft 0 from the oral cavity toward the nasal aperture.
- Cleft 1 from the nostril toward the fronto-maxillary suture.
- Cleft 2 is a confusing appellation; Tessier himself, in his original paper, put it as the downward part of cleft 12 in an attempt at the systematization of his rule of 14 being the sum of upward and downward parts of rare clefts. Moreover, in another part of his paper, he quotes cleft 1, 2, and 3 as following the common path of the usual cleft lip [128] page 87 and further in the same paper (page 89, paragraph 3, line 18), he says: "*the identity of clefts 2,9 and 11 is not certain…*". Elsewhere in the same publication, about cleft 2, he said:" *Hemiatrophy of the nose, super-numerary nostrils and proboscis lateralis are probably different degrees of the same defect.*"

  Since nasoschisis, a real cleft, is already affected at cleft 1, we will name cleft 2 hemi-nasal aplasia or hypoplasia (hemi-arrhinia). It could be associated with proboscis lateralis or supernumerary nostril. In the 2009 publication "the arrhinia" [135], he admitted that the path of those malformations was similar to the path of the cleft 1–2," *but was of a different nature*" This point will be discussed in detail in the chapter Cleft 2–12.
- Cleft 3 starts from the nostril and reaches the orbit, the bridge between nasal and orbital clefts. Cleft 4 connects the oral aperture laterally to the location of the common cleft lip, with the orbit running through the maxillary medially to the infra-orbital foramen.
- Cleft 5 splits the upper lip more laterally, close to the commissure and goes through the maxillary laterally to the infra-orbital foramina.

- Cleft 6, considering only its skeletal part, was initially described by Tessier as a part of Treacher-Collins's syndrome (TCS) in combination with cleft 8 and possibly 7. However, what we know nowadays about TCS makes us remove it from the spectrum of rare clefts. In our research, cleft 6 could be described as a cleft of the malar and/or zygomatic arch with three distinct phenotypes, including a macrostomia. One of them, the 6a type, is associated with cleft 8 as its upward component.
- Cleft 7 had been confused with macrostomia, an error since macrostomia is a common feature of clefts 5, 6, and 7. Therefore, we propose to keep the name cleft 7 for macrostomia arising in the setting of craniofacial microsomia (CFM).
- Cleft 8, as seen above, has been considered a part of TCS. Therefore, we exclude as well TCS from our series of cleft 8. Cleft 8 splits the lateral canthus and the lateral orbital rim.
- Cleft 9 was theorized by Tessier since he has yet to meet a case. Also, its reality was later confirmed and, although very infrequent, is known as a lateral orbito-cranial cleft going across the superolateral orbital corner.
- Cleft 10, which is supposed to be the upward correspondent cleft of cleft 4 but is rarely associated with it, splits the upper palpebra and eyebrow. Its skeletal part concerns the frontal bone, the superior orbital rim and the orbital roof, yielding an encephalocele when present. It is frequently associated with a peak of the hairline.
- Cleft 11, Tessier said that the identity of cleft 11, which is supposed to spread between the paths of cleft 12 and 10, was not certain. However, our research did not find any specificity that could distinguish a cleft 11 from a cleft 10.
- Cleft 12, Tessier's description: *«is located medially to the medial canthus. The frontal process of the maxilla is flat (telecanthus). The cleft comes through the lateral mass of the ethmoid bone extending through the frontal bone (which is flattened). The frontal sinus is enlarged. Complete forms of this cleft, with encephalocele, have not been observed. On the soft tissues, there is a coloboma of the root of the eyebrow; N°12 is the cranial cleft corresponding with facial cleft no. 2.".* We will side with the opinion that the term cleft 12 describes the conditions where cleft 2 is associated with a cranial defect. This defect is either hypertelorism or an encephalocele.
- Cleft 13 is perfectly described without ambiguity and cleft 14 in Tessier's classification, and we will side with it.
- Cleft lip and palate. Tessier considers that clefts 1, 2, and 3 could have a part of their paths include the upper lip "*as a usual harelip*". Considering the number of clefts 1 and 2 as well as cleft 3 where the lip is intact, we will consider cleft lip and palate in the setting of rare cleft as an association to the rare cleft since the mechanism of cleft lip and palate (CLP) is well understood, unlike the mechanism of rare clefts. Therefore, the association of CLP, whose mechanism could be triggered by the defect involved in the rare cleft, is easily understandable.

3.5 Conclusion

Our research convinced us that understanding the mechanisms involved in the genesis of rare clefts will come from macromolecular genetics.

A better knowledge of the subtle paths of protein synthesis, the way they are affected by the genes, their mutations, and the epigenetics.

The study of rare clefts related to known mutations and transmitted as Mendelian inheritance, which are increasingly numerous, brings attention to nonhereditary conditions with close phenotypes. We could look in those patients for perturbation along the path to which the mutated gene of similarly affected patients belongs. Therefore, it is of utmost importance to be able to recognize the phenotype among large series of cases.

References

1. Hall BK. The neural crest in development and evolution. New York: Springer; 1999. https://doi.org/10.1007/978-1-4757-3064-7.
2. Haeckel E. The evolution of man, vol. 1. London: Watts & Co; 1910. p. 351.
3. Depew MJ, Simpson CA. 21st Century neontology and the comparative development of the vertebrate skull. Dev Dyn. 2006;235(5):1256–91. https://doi.org/10.1002/dvdy.20796.
4. Gans C, Northcutt RG. Neural crest and the origin of vertebrates: a new head. Science. 1983;220(4594):268–73. https://doi.org/10.1126/science.220.4594.268.
5. De Beer GR. The development of the vertebrate skull. Oxford: Clarendon Press; 1937. p. 550.
6. Dias MS, Walker ML. The Embryogenesis of Complex Dysraphic Malformations: A Disorder of Gastrulation? Pediatr Neurosurg. 1992;18(5–6):229–53. https://www.karger.com/Article/FullText/120670.
7. Langman J, Sadler TW. Langman's medical embryology. 6th ed. Baltimore: Williams and Wilkins; 1990. p. 409.
8. Agius E, Piccolo S, De Robertis EM. L'inducteur céphalique Cerberus est un inhibiteur multivalent extracellulaire. J Soc Biol. 1999;193(4–5):347–54. https://doi.org/10.1051/jbio/1999193040347.
9. Gur M, Edri T, Moody SA, Fainsod A. Retinoic acid is required for normal morphogenetic movements during gastrulation. Front Cell Dev Biol. 2022;10:857230. https://doi.org/10.3389/fcell.2022.857230/full.
10. Haworth KE, Healy C, Morgan P, Sharpe PT. Regionalisation of early head ectoderm is regulated by endoderm and prepatterns the orofacial epithelium. Development. 2004;131(19):4797–806. https://journals.biologists.com/dev/article/131/19/4797/42427/Regionalisation-of-early-head-ectoderm-is.
11. Le Douarin NM. The avian embryo as a model to study the development of the neural crest: a long and still ongoing story. Mech Dev. 2004;121(9):1089–102. https://linkinghub.elsevier.com/retrieve/pii/S0925477304001625.
12. His W. Untersuchungen über die erste Anlage des Wirbelthierleibes: die erste Entwickelung des Hühnchens im Ei [Internet]. Leipzig: F.C.W. Vogel; 1868. https://archive.org/details/b21993579/page/n288/mode/1up.
13. Kuriyama S, Mayor R. Molecular analysis of neural crest migration. Philos Trans R Soc B Biol Sci. 2008;363(1495):1349–62. https://doi.org/10.1098/rstb.2007.2252.
14. Abramyan J. Hedgehog signaling and embryonic craniofacial disorders. J Dev Biol. 2019;7(2):9. https://www.mdpi.com/2221-3759/7/2/9.

15. Saadi I, Alkuraya FS, Gisselbrecht SS, Goessling W, Cavallesco R, Turbe-Doan A, et al. Deficiency of the cytoskeletal protein SPECC1L leads to oblique facial clefting. Am J Hum Genet. 2011;89(1):44–55. https://linkinghub.elsevier.com/retrieve/pii/S0002929711002163.
16. Kulesa PM, Bailey CM, Kasemeier-Kulesa JC, McLennan R. Cranial neural crest migration: new rules for an old road. Dev Biol. 2010;344(2):543–54. https://linkinghub.elsevier.com/retrieve/pii/S001216061000240X.
17. Lim HYG, Plachta N. Cytoskeletal control of early mammalian development. Nat Rev Mol Cell Biol [Internet]. 2021;22(8):548–62. http://www.nature.com/articles/s41580-021-00363-9.
18. Blaue C, Kashef J, Franz CM. Cadherin-11 promotes neural crest cell spreading by reducing intracellular tension-mapping adhesion and mechanics in neural crest explants by atomic force microscopy. Semin Cell Dev Biol. 2018;73:95–106.
19. Andrieu C, Montigny A, Bibonne A, Despin-Guitard E, Alfandari D, Théveneau E. MMP14 is required for delamination of chick neural crest cells independently of its catalytic activity. Dev Camb Engl. 2020;147(7):dev183954.
20. McLennan R, Teddy JM, Kasemeier-Kulesa JC, Romine MH, Kulesa PM. Vascular endothelial growth factor (VEGF) regulates cranial neural crest migration in vivo. Dev Biol. 2010;339(1):114–25. https://linkinghub.elsevier.com/retrieve/pii/S0012160609014286.
21. Creuzet S, Schuler B, Couly G, Le Douarin NM. Reciprocal relationships between Fgf8 and neural crest cells in facial and forebrain development. Proc Natl Acad Sci. 2004;101(14):4843–7. https://doi.org/10.1073/pnas.0400869101.
22. Perris R, Perissinotto D. Role of the extracellular matrix during neural crest cell migration. Mech Dev. 2000;95(1):3–21. https://www.sciencedirect.com/science/article/pii/S0925477300003658.
23. Wedden SE. Morphogenesis of the head and face: discussion report. Dev Camb Engl. 1988;103(Suppl):61–2.
24. Thorogood P. Mechanisms of morphogenetic specification in skull development. In: Wolff JR, Sievers J, Berry M, eds. Mesenchymal-epithelial interactions in neural development. Springer Berlin Heidelberg; 1987:141–52. https://doi.org/10.1007/978-3-642-71837-3_12.
25. Sato T, Kurihara Y, Asai R, Kawamura Y, Tonami K, Uchijima Y, et al. An endothelin-1 switch specifies maxillomandibular identity. Proc Natl Acad Sci. 2008;105(48):18806–11. https://doi.org/10.1073/pnas.0807345105.
26. Compagnucci C, Fish JL, Schwark M, Tarabykin V, Depew MJ. Pax6 regulates craniofacial form through its control of an essential cephalic ectodermal patterning center. Genesis. 2011;49(4):307–25. https://doi.org/10.1002/dvg.20724.
27. Depew MJ, Simpson CA, Morasso M, Rubenstein JLR. Reassessing the Dlx code: the genetic regulation of branchial arch skeletal pattern and development. J Anat 2005 207(5):501–561. https://doi.org/10.1111/j.1469-7580.2005.00487.x
28. Hu D, Marcucio RS, Helms JA. A zone of frontonasal ectoderm regulates patterning and growth in the face. Development. 2003;130(9):1749–58. https://journals.biologists.com/dev/article/130/9/1749/52408/A-zone-of-frontonasal-ectoderm-regulates.
29. Griffin JN, Compagnucci C, Hu D, Fish J, Klein O, Marcucio R, et al. Fgf8 dosage determines midfacial integration and polarity within the nasal and optic capsules. Dev Biol. 2013;374(1):185–97. https://linkinghub.elsevier.com/retrieve/pii/S0012160612006331.
30. Le Douarin NM, Creuzet S, Couly G, Dupin E. Neural crest cell plasticity and its limits. Development. 2004;131(19):4637–50. https://journals.biologists.com/dev/article/131/19/4637/42419/Neural-crest-cell-plasticity-and-its-limits.
31. Young NM, Hu D, Lainoff AJ, Smith FJ, Diaz R, Tucker AS, et al. Embryonic bauplans and the developmental origins of facial diversity and constraint. Dev Camb Engl. 2014;141(5):1059–63. https://www.ncbi.nlm.nih.gov/pmc/articles/PMC3929406/.
32. Hu D, Young NM, Li X, Xu Y, Hallgrímsson B, Marcucio RS. A dynamic Shh expression pattern, regulated by SHH and BMP signaling, coordinates fusion of primordia in the amniote face. Dev Camb Engl. 2015;142(3):567–74.
33. Twigg SRF, Wilkie AOM. New insights into craniofacial malformations. Hum Mol Genet. 2015 24(R1):R50–R59. https://doi.org/10.1093/hmg/ddv228

34. Kurosaka H, Iulianella A, Williams T, Trainor PA. Disrupting hedgehog and WNT signaling interactions promotes cleft lip pathogenesis. J Clin Invest. 2014;124(4):1660–71. http://www.jci.org/articles/view/72688
35. Zaghloul NA, Brugmann SA. The emerging face of primary cilia. Genesis. 2011;49(4):231–46. https://www.ncbi.nlm.nih.gov/pmc/articles/PMC3118297/.
36. Huangfu D, Anderson KV. Cilia and hedgehog responsiveness in the mouse. Proc Natl Acad Sci U S A. 2005;102(32):11325–30.
37. Neugebauer JM, Amack JD, Peterson AG, Bisgrove BW, Yost HJ. FGF signalling during embryo development regulates cilia length in diverse epithelia. Nature. 2009;458(7238):651–4.
38. Strutt D. The planar polarity pathway. Curr Biol. 2008;18(19):R898–902. https://linkinghub.elsevier.com/retrieve/pii/S0960982208009640.
39. Zhang Z, Wlodarczyk BJ, Niederreither K, Venugopalan S, Florez S, Finnell RH, et al. Fuz regulates craniofacial development through tissue specific responses to signaling factors. PLoS One. 2011;6(9):e24608. https://doi.org/10.1371/journal.pone.0024608.
40. Liu B, Chen S, Johnson C, Helms JA. A ciliopathy with hydrocephalus, isolated craniosynostosis, hypertelorism, and clefting caused by deletion of Kif3a. Reprod Toxicol Elmsford N. 2014;48:88–97.
41. Poswillo D. The pathogenesis of the first and second branchial arch syndrome. Oral Surg Oral Med Oral Pathol. 1973;35(3):302–28. https://linkinghub.elsevier.com/retrieve/pii/0030422073900704.
42. Poswillo D. The aetiology and pathogenesis of craniofacial deformity. Dev Camb Engl. 1988;103(Suppl):207–12.
43. Braithwaite F, Watson J. A report on three unusual cleft lips. Br J Plast Surg. 1949;2(1):38–49. https://linkinghub.elsevier.com/retrieve/pii/S0007122649800075.
44. Ribatti D. Genetic and epigenetic mechanisms in the early development of the vascular system. J Anat. 2006;208(2):139–52. https://doi.org/10.1111/j.1469-7580.2006.00522.x.
45. Aghi M, Chiocca EA. Contribution of bone marrow-derived cells to blood vessels in ischemic tissues and tumors. Mol Ther. 2005;12(6):994–1005. https://www.cell.com/molecular-therapy-family/molecular-therapy/abstract/S1525-0016(05)01431-0.
46. Ausprunk DH, Folkman J. Migration and proliferation of endothelial cells in preformed and newly formed blood vessels during tumor angiogenesis. Microvasc Res. 1977;14(1):53–65. https://linkinghub.elsevier.com/retrieve/pii/0026286277901418.
47. Carmeliet P. Angiogenesis in health and disease. Nat Med. 2003;9(6):8.
48. Finley EB. The development of the subcutaneous vascular plexus in the head of the human embryo. In: Contribution to embryology. Washington: Carnegie Institution; 1922. p. 155–61. https://archive.org/details/contributionstoe14carn/page/n191/mode/2up.
49. Hochstetter F. Über die Vaskularisation der Haut des Schädeldaches menschlicher Embryonen. Wien: Komm. A. Hölder; 1917.
50. Marcelo KL, Goldie LC, Hirschi KK. Regulation of endothelial cell differentiation and specification. Circ Res. 2013;112(9):1272–87. https://doi.org/10.1161/CIRCRESAHA.113.300506.
51. Richman JM, Buchtová M, Boughner JC. Comparative ontogeny and phylogeny of the upper jaw skeleton in amniotes. 2006;235(Dev Dyn, 5):1230–43. https://doi.org/10.1002/dvdy.20716.
52. Frohman MA, Boyle M, Martin GR. Isolation of the mouse Hox-2.9 gene; analysis of embryonic expression suggests that positional information along the anterior-posterior axis is specified by mesoderm. Development. 1990;110(2):589–607.
53. Spranger J, Benirschke K, Hall JG, Lenz W, Lowry RB. Errors of morphogenesis: concepts and terms. J Pediatr. 1982;1:6.
54. Sulik KK, Cook CS, Webster WS. Teratogens and craniofacial malformations: relationships to cell death. Development. 1988;103(Supplement):213–32. https://journals.biologists.com/dev/article/103/Supplement/213/36094/Teratogens-and-craniofacial-malformations.
55. Panoutsopoulos AA, De Crescenzo AH, Lee A, Lu AM, Ross AP, Borodinsky LN, et al. Pak1ip1 loss-of-function leads to cell cycle arrest, loss of neural crest cells, and craniofacial abnormalities. Front Cell Dev Biol. 2020;8:510063.

56. van Boxtel AL, Pieterse B, Cenijn P, Kamstra JH, Brouwer A, van Wieringen W, et al. Dithiocarbamates induce craniofacial abnormalities and downregulate sox9a during zebrafish development. Toxicol Sci. 2010;117(1):209–17. https://doi.org/10.1093/toxsci/kfq169.
57. Obwegeser HL, Weber G, Freihofer HP, Sailer HF. Facial duplication—the unique case of Antonio. J Maxillofac Surg. 1978;6:179–98. https://linkinghub.elsevier.com/retrieve/pii/S0301050378800885.
58. Perea-Gomez A, Vella FDJ, Shawlot W, Oulad-Abdelghani M, Chazaud C, Meno C, et al. Nodal antagonists in the anterior visceral endoderm prevent the formation of multiple primitive streaks. Dev Cell. 2002;3(5):745–56. https://linkinghub.elsevier.com/retrieve/pii/S1534580702003210.
59. O'Rahilly R, Müller F. Bidirectional closure of the rostral neuropore in the human embryo: closure of rostral neuropore. Am J Anat. 1989;184(4):259–68. https://doi.org/10.1002/aja.1001840402.
60. Fong KSK, Adachi DAT, Chang SB, Lozanoff S. Midline craniofacial malformations with a lipomatous cephalocele are associated with insufficient closure of the neural tube in the tuft mouse. Birth Defects Res A Clin Mol Teratol. 2014;100(8):598–607. https://www.ncbi.nlm.nih.gov/pmc/articles/PMC4426337/.
61. Quaderi NA, Schweiger S, Gaudenz K, Franco B, Rugarli EI, Berger W, et al. Opitz G/BBB syndrome, a defect of midline development, is due to mutations in a new RING finger gene on Xp22. Nat Genet [Internet]. 1997;17(3):285–91. http://www.nature.com/articles/ng1197-285.
62. Calo E, Gu B, Bowen ME, Aryan F, Zalc A, Liang J, et al. Tissue-selective effects of nucleolar stress and rDNA damage in developmental disorders. Nature. 2018;554(7690):112–7. http://www.nature.com/articles/nature25449.
63. Gfrerer L, Shubinets V, Hoyos T, Kong Y, Nguyen C, Pietschmann P, et al. Functional analysis of SPECC1L in craniofacial development and oblique facial cleft pathogenesis. Plast Reconstr Surg. 2014;134(4):748–59. http://journals.lww.com/00006534-201410000-00032.
64. Twigg SRF, Versnel SL, Nürnberg G, Lees MM, Bhat M, Hammond P, et al. Frontorhiny, a distinctive presentation of frontonasal dysplasia caused by recessive mutations in the ALX3 homeobox gene. Am J Hum Genet. 2009;84(5):698–705. https://linkinghub.elsevier.com/retrieve/pii/S0002929709001517.
65. Uz E, Alanay Y, Aktas D, Vargel I, Gucer S, Tuncbilek G, et al. Disruption of ALX1 causes extreme microphthalmia and severe facial clefting: expanding the spectrum of autosomal-recessive ALX-related frontonasal dysplasia. Am J Hum Genet. 2010;86(5):789–96. https://linkinghub.elsevier.com/retrieve/pii/S000292971000203X.
66. Dee CT, Szymoniuk CR, Mills PED, Takahashi T. Defective neural crest migration revealed by a zebrafish model of Alx1-related frontonasal dysplasia. Hum Mol Genet. 2013;22(2):239–51.
67. Smith JD, Hing AV, Clarke CM, Johnson NM, Perez FA, Park SS, et al. Exome sequencing identifies a recurrent De novo ZSWIM6 mutation associated with acromelic frontonasal dysostosis. Am J Hum Genet. 2014;95(2):235–40. https://linkinghub.elsevier.com/retrieve/pii/S0002929714003176.
68. Twigg SRF, Ousager LB, Miller KA, Zhou Y, Elalaoui SC, Sefiani A, Bak GS, Hove H, Hansen LK, Fagerberg CR, Tajir M, Wilkie AOM. Acromelic frontonasal dysostosis and ZSWIM6 mutation: phenotypic spectrum and mosaicism. Clin Genet. 2016;90(3):270–5. https://doi.org/10.1111/cge.12721.
69. Lehalle D, Altunoglu U, Bruel AL, Arnaud E, Blanchet P, Choi JW, et al. Clinical delineation of a subtype of frontonasal dysplasia with creased nasal ridge and upper limb anomalies: report of six unrelated patients. Am J Med Genet A. 2017;173(12):3136–42. https://doi.org/10.1002/ajmg.a.38490.
70. Hufnagel RB, Zimmerman SL, Krueger LA, Bender PL, Ahmed ZM, Saal HM. A new frontonasal dysplasia syndrome associated with deletion of the SIX2 gene. Am J Med Genet A. 2016;170A(2):487–91. https://www.ncbi.nlm.nih.gov/pmc/articles/PMC8108007/

71. Ross W. A curious monster which lived for some time after birth. Trans Obstet Soc Lond. 1867;IX:31–2.
72. Chavane A. Malformation faciale (section par bride amniotique). Bull Société Anat Paris. 1890;5(4):137–41. https://gallica.bnf.fr/ark:/12148/bpt6k6327302h/f159.item#.
73. Marchand F. Missbildungen. In: Eulenburg A, editor. Real-encyclopädie der gesammten heilkunde: medicinisch-chirurgisches handworterbuch fu˝r praktische aerzte. Wien: Urban and Schwarzenberg; 1897. p. 423–596.
74. Opitz JM, Johnson DR, Gilbert-Barness EF. ADAM "sequence" part II: hypothesis and speculation. Am J Med Genet A. 2015;167(3):478–503. https://doi.org/10.1002/ajmg.a.36937.
75. Ballantyne JW. Spontaneous or congenital amputations. In: Manual of antenatal pathology and hygiene. Edinburgh: William Green & sons; 1902. p. 396–7. http://www.archive.org/details/manualofantenata00ballrich.
76. Jones KL, Smith DW, Hall BD, Hall JG, Ebbin AJ, Massoud H, et al. A pattern of craniofacial and limb defects secondary to aberrant tissue bands. J Pediatr. 1974;84(1):90–5. https://linkinghub.elsevier.com/retrieve/pii/S0022347674805597.
77. Higginbottom MC, Jones KL, Hall BD, Smith DW. The amniotic band disruption complex: timing of amniotic rupture and variable spectra of consequent defects. J Pediatr. 1979;95(4):544–9.
78. Torpin R. Amniochorionic mesoblastic fibrous strings and amnionic bands. Am J Obstet Gynecol. 1965;91(1):65–75. https://linkinghub.elsevier.com/retrieve/pii/0002937865905880.
79. Bamforth JS. Amniotic band sequence: Streeter's hypothesis reexamined. Am J Med Genet. 1992;44(3):280–7. https://doi.org/10.1002/ajmg.1320440304.
80. Keith A. Concerning the origin and nature of certain malformations of the face, head, and foot. Br J Surg. 2005;28(110):173–92. https://academic.oup.com/bjs/article/28/110/173/6222774.
81. Van Allen MI, Curry C, Gallagher L, Reynolds JF. Limb body wall complex: I. Pathogenesis. Am J Med Genet. 1987;28(3):529–48. https://doi.org/10.1002/ajmg.1320280302.
82. Hunter AGW, Carpenter BF, Opitz JM, Reynolds JF. Implications of malformations not due to amniotic bands in the amniotic band sequence. Am J Med Genet. 1986;24(4):691–700. https://doi.org/10.1002/ajmg.1320240414.
83. Bagg HJ. Hereditary abnormalities of the limbs, their origin and transmission. II. A morphological study with special reference to the etiology of club-feet, syndactylism, hypodactylism, and congenital amputation in the descendants of X-rayed mice. Am J Anat. 1929;43(2):167–219. https://doi.org/10.1002/aja.1000430203.
84. Hummel KP. The inheritance and expression of disorganization, an unusual mutation in the mouse. J Exp Zool. 1958;137(3):389–423. https://doi.org/10.1002/jez.1401370303.
85. Donnai D, Winter RM. Disorganisation: a model for 'early amnion rupture'? J Med Genet. 1989;26(7):421–5. https://doi.org/10.1136/jmg.26.7.421.
86. Purandare SM, Ernst L, Medne L, Huff D, Zackai EH. Developmental anomalies with features of disorganization (Ds) and amniotic band sequence (ABS): a report of four cases. Am J Med Genet A. 2009;149A(8):1740–8. https://doi.org/10.1002/ajmg.a.32716.
87. Lowry RB, Yong SL. Cleft lip and palate, sensorineural deafness, and sacral lipoma in two brothers: a possible example of the disorganisation mutant. J Med Genet. 1991;28(2):135–7. https://doi.org/10.1136/jmg.28.2.135.
88. Lin AE. Two additional patients representing the possible human homologue for the mouse mutant disorganisation (ds). J Med Genet. 1991;28(9):645–7. https://jmg.bmj.com/lookup/doi/10.1136/jmg.28.9.645.
89. Crosby JL, Varnum DS, Washburn LL, Nadeau JH. Disorganization is a completely dominant gain-of-function mouse mutation causing sporadic developmental defects. Mech Dev. 1992;37(3):121–6. https://linkinghub.elsevier.com/retrieve/pii/092547739290074T.
90. De Michelena MI, Stachurska A. Multiple anomalies possibly caused by a human homologue to the mouse disorganization (Ds) gene. Clin Dysmorphol. 1993;2(2):131–4. https://journals.lww.com/clindysmorphol/Abstract/1993/04000/Multiple_anomalies_possibly_caused_by_a_human.6.aspx.

91. Elliott AM, Chen MF, Azouz EM, Teebi AS. Developmental anomalies suggestive of the human homologue of the mouse mutant disorganization. Am J Med Genet. 1995;55(2):240–3. https://doi.org/10.1002/ajmg.1320550218.
92. Teebi AS, Elliott AM. Another case of the human homologue of the mouse mutant disorganization. Am J Med Genet. 1996;61(1):94.
93. Van Langen IM, Hennekam RCM. Another example of the human homologue of the mouse mutant disorganization? Clin Dysmorphol. 1994;3(4):361–2. https://journals.lww.com/clindysmorphol/Citation/1994/10000/Another_example_of_the_human_homologue_of_the.15.aspx.
94. Robin NH, Nadeau JH. Disorganization in mice and humans. Am J Med Genet. 2001;101(4):334–8. https://doi.org/10.1002/1096-8628(20010715)101:4<334::AID-AJMG1233>3.0.CO;2-7.
95. Korniszewski L, Skorka A, Donnai D. Disorganisation: a case with popliteal pterygia and placental-skin appendages. Clin Dysmorphol. 1999;8(4):277–81.
96. Delgado Luengo WN, Luisa Hernández Rodríguez M, Valbuena Pirela I, González Ferrer S, Estrada Corona P, Chacón Fonseca I, et al. Human disorganization complex, as a polytopic blastogenesis defect: a new case: human disorganization and blastogenesis defect. Am J Med Genet A. 2004;125A(2):181–5. https://doi.org/10.1002/ajmg.a.20307.
97. O'Driscoll M, Peckham C, Kerr B. Four limb syndactyly, constriction rings and skin tags; amniotic bands or disorganization-like syndrome. Clin Dysmorphol. 2008;17(4):255–8. https://journals.lww.com/clindysmorphol/Abstract/2008/10000/Four_limb_syndactyly,_constriction_rings_and_skin.4.aspx.
98. Vallejo OG, Benítez Sánchez Mdel C, Cánovas CS, Ontiveros JD, Ruiz Jiménez JI, Bermejo-Sánchez E, et al. Patient with disorganization syndrome: Surgical procedures, Pathology, and potential causes: patient with disorganization syndrome. Birth Defects Res A Clin Mol Teratol. 2013;97(12):781–5. https://doi.org/10.1002/bdra.23203.
99. Crosby JL, Varnum DS, Nadeau JH. Two-hit model for sporadic congenital anomalies in mice with the disorganization mutation. Am J Hum Genet. 1993;52(5):866–74.
100. Isidor B, Baujat G, Le Caignec C, Pichon O, Martin-Coignard D, Toutain A, et al. Congenital skin pedicles with or without amniotic band sequence: extending the human phenotype resembling mouse disorganization. Am J Med Genet A. 2009;149A(8):1734–9. https://doi.org/10.1002/ajmg.a.32796.
101. White RA, Dowler LL, Pasztor LM, Gatson LL, Adkison LR, Angeloni SV, et al. Assignment of the transcription factor GATA4 gene to human chromosome 8 and mouse chromosome 14: Gata4 is a candidate gene for ds (disorganization). Genomics. 1995;27(1):20–6. https://linkinghub.elsevier.com/retrieve/pii/S0888754385710038.
102. Huang WY, HHQ H, Liew CC. Assignment of the human GATA4 gene to 8p23.1-->p22 using fluorescence in situ hybridization analysis. Cytogenet Genome Res. 1996;72(2–3):217–8. https://www.karger.com/Article/FullText/134194.
103. Kruszka P, Uwineza A, Mutesa L, Martinez AF, Abe Y, Zackai EH, et al. Limb body wall complex, amniotic band sequence, or new syndrome caused by mutation in *IQ Motif containing K (IQCK)*? Mol Genet Genomic Med. 2015;3(5):424–32. https://doi.org/10.1002/mgg3.153.
104. Geoffroy Saint Hilaire I. Histoire générale et particuliére des anomalies de l'organisation chez l'homme et les animaux. Paris: Bailliére; 1837. https://ia800106.us.archive.org/17/items/BIUSante_35541/BIUSante_35541.pdf.
105. Dick W. Case of Hyperencephalous monstrosity. Lond Med Gaz. 1837;19:897–9. https://archive.org/details/londonmedicalgaz19londuoft/page/898/mode/2up.
106. Guersant. presentation de malade. Gaz Hôp Civ Mil Lancette Fr 1860 33 (30 pp112 et N° 31 pp 119(fig.)):112. http://www.biusante.parisdescartes.fr/histmed/medica/cote?90130x1860
107. Butcher H. Reports in operative surgery. Dublin Quaterly J Med Sci. 1860;XXIX:258.
108. Fergusson W. A system of practical surgery. 5th ed. London: John Churchill and sons; 1870. p. 812. http://www.archive.org/details/5thsystemofpract00ferguoft.

109. Dupuy LE. Anormalité congénitale du globe oculaire chez un fœtus atteint également d'hydrocéphalie, de bec-de-lièvre et de syndactylie des pieds et des mains. Bull Société Anat Paris. 1874:12–4.
110. Debout. Coup d'oeil sur une des formes les plus rares du bec de liévre, les fissures horizontales. Remarques et observations. Bull Général Thérapeutique Médicale Chir. 1862;(N 63):13–22. https://services.biusante.parisdescartes.fr/medica-pdf/main.php?key=cGFydGlhbHw5MDAxNHgxODYyeDYzfDEyfDIz.
111. Pelvet. Mémoire sur les fissures congénitales des joues; lu à la société de biologie. Gaz Médicale Paris. 2022;3(N 19):418–22. https://services.biusante.parisdescartes.fr/medica-pdf/pdf.php?key=cGFydGlhbHw5MDE4MngxODY0eDE5fDQxOHw0MjI&f=OTAxODJ4MTg2NHgxOS00MTgtNDIy&one=1.
112. Van Duyse. Macrostomes congénitaux avec tumeurs préauriculaires et dermoïdes de l'oeil. Ann Société Médecine Gand. 1882. Aout [cited 2020 Apr 2];36. https://archive.org/details/b2163774x
113. Duyse V. Bride dermoide oculo-palpébrale et colobome partiel de la paupière avec remarques sur la génese de ces anomalies. Ann Ocul. 1882;LXXXXVIII(3 & 4):101–32.
114. Morian R. Über die schräge Gesichtsspalte (about oblique facial clefts). Arch Klin Chir. 1887;35:245–88.
115. Laroche V. Essai d'anatomie pathologique sur les monstruosités ou vices de conformation primitifs de la face. [Paris]: thése de medecine,Faculté de Médecine de Paris; 1823.
116. Grünberg K. Die Gesichtsspalten und die zu ihnen in genetischer Beziehung stehenden anderweitigen Mißbildungen des Gesichts. In: Swalbe E, editor. Die morphologie der missbildüngen des menschen und der tiere [Internet]. Jena: von Gustav Fischer; 1909. p. 113–204. https://archive.org/details/b21506899_0002.
117. Harkins CS, Berlin A, Harding RL, Longacre JJ, Snodgrasse RM. A classification of cleft lip and cleft palate. Plast Reconstr Surg. 1962;29(1):31–9. http://journals.lww.com/00006534-196201000-00005.
118. Sedano HO, Michael Cohen M, Jirasek J, Gorlin RJ. Frontonasal dysplasia. J Pediatr. 1970;76(6):906–13. https://linkinghub.elsevier.com/retrieve/pii/S0022347670803742.
119. Greig DM. Hypertelorism. A hitherto undifferentiated congenital cranio-facial deformity. Edinb Med J. 1924;XXXI(X):560–93.
120. Richmond C. Paul Tessier. The Guardian. 2008. https://www.theguardian.com/science/2008/aug/28/medicalresearch.highereducation.
121. Tessier P. Complete and forme fruste vertical and oblique orbito-facial clefts (colobomas). Ann Chir Plast. 1969;14(4):301–11.
122. Tessier P. Colobomas: vertical and oblique complete facial clefts. Simultaneous operation of the eyelid, inner canthus, cheek nose and lip Orbitomaxillary bone graft. Panminerva Med. 1969b;11(3):95–101.
123. Tessier P, Guiot G, Rougerie J, Delbet JP, Pastoriza P. Hypertelorism: cranio-naso-orbito-facial and subethmoid osteotomy. Panminerva Med. 1969;11(3):102–16.
124. Orbital TP. Hypertelorism: I. Successive surgical attempts. Material and methods. Causes and mechanisms. Scand J Plast Reconstr Surg. 1972;6(2):135–55. https://doi.org/10.3109/02844317209036714.
125. Tessier P, Guiot G, Derome P. Orbital Hypertelorism: II. Definite treatment of orbital hypertelorism (OR.H.) by craniofacial or by extracranial osteotomies. Scand J Plast Reconstr Surg. 1973;7(1):39–58. https://doi.org/10.3109/02844317309072417.
126. Tessier P. Orbital hypertelorism. Fortschr Kiefer Gesichtschir. 1974;18:14–27.
127. Tessier P. Experiences in the treatment of orbital hypertelorism. Plast Reconstr Surg. 1974;53(1):1–18.
128. Tessier P. Anatomical classification of facial, cranio-facial and latero-facial clefts. J Maxillofac Surg. 1976;4:69–92. https://linkinghub.elsevier.com/retrieve/pii/S0301050376800136.

129. Nouvelle TP. Classification anatomique des fentes faciales cranio-faciales et latéro-latérales, leur répartition autour de l'orbite. In: Rougier J, Société française d'ophtalmologie, editors. Chirurgie plastique orbito-palpébrale. Paris, New York: Masson; 1977.
130. Vermeij-Keers C, Mazzola RF, Van der Meulen JC, Strickler M. Cerebro-craniofacial and craniofacial malformations: an embryological analysis. Cleft Palate J. 1983;20(2):128–45.
131. DeMyer W. Median facial malformations and their implications for brain malformations. Birth Defects Orig Artic Ser. 1975;11(7):155–81.
132. Whitaker LA, Pashayan H, Reichman J. A proposed new classification of craniofacial anomalies. Cleft Palate J. 1981;18(3):161–76.
133. van der Meulen JC, Mazzola R, Vermey-Keers C, Strieker M, Raphael B. A morphogenetic classification of craniofacial malformations. Plast Reconstr Surg. 1983;71(4):560–72. http://journals.lww.com/00006534-198304000-00022.
134. Tessier P. Introduction aux dysplasies oto-mandibulaires (D.O.M.) ou "Vingt ans après". Ann Chir Plast Esthet. 2001;46(5):381–4. https://linkinghub.elsevier.com/retrieve/pii/S029412600100053X.
135. Tessier P, Ciminello FS, Wolfe SA. The arrhinias. Scand J Plast Reconstr Surg Hand Surg [Internet]. 2009;43(4):177–96. https://doi.org/10.1080/02844310802517259.

Chapter 4
Cleft 0/14

Renato da Silva Freitas, Nivaldo Alonso, Philippe Pellerin, and Cristiano Tonello

Pearls

- Tessier cleft 0–14 (TC0–14) has a substantial clinical variation and different embryological explanations, and hypertelorism is only a clinical sign of many different congenital deformities.
- Surgical treatment will depend on the primary etiology of the deformity, and intracranial procedure will be crucial to approach most of them.
- Age will be chosen based on the size of the deformity and its functional impairment.
- It is essential to determine the differences between false and true median clefts. The surgical procedures may vary in the type of involvement of the facial structures.

R. da Silva Freitas (✉)
Plastic Surgery Unit, Hospital de Clínicas, Universidade Federal do Paraná, Curitiba, Brazil

Craniofacial Surgery, Assistance Center for Cleft Lip and Palate (CAIF), Hospital do Trabalhador, Curitiba, Brazil

N. Alonso
Plastic Surgery, Universidade de São Paulo, São Paulo, Brazil

Craniofacial Surgery, Hospital de Reabilitação Anomalias Craniofaciais Bauru USPUniversidade de São Paulo, Bauru, Brazil

P. Pellerin
Centre Hospitalier Régional Universitaire de Lille, Lille, France

C. Tonello
Curso de Medicina Bauru Faculdade de Odontologia Bauru Universidade de São Paulo, Bauru, Brazil

Hospital de Reabilitação Anomalias Craniofaciais Universidade de São Paulo, Bauru, Brazil

N. Alonso et al. (eds.), *Facial Reconstruction of Unusual Facial Clefts*, https://doi.org/10.1007/978-3-031-40926-4_4

4.1 Introduction

According to Tessier classification, the median 0–14 cleft (TC 0–14) is a median craniofacial dysraphia [1]. It may also be referred to as internasal dysplasia, median cleft face syndrome, frontonasal dysplasia, and holoprosencephaly (Figs. 4.1 and 4.2). There is a paucity of articles related to this unusual malformation, and those that exist are confined to clinical examination and surgical treatment of a small number of patients [2–7].

The developmental origin of Tessier cleft 0–14 (TC 0–14) is not clearly understood; however, it is known that midline facial defects can be traced to a time

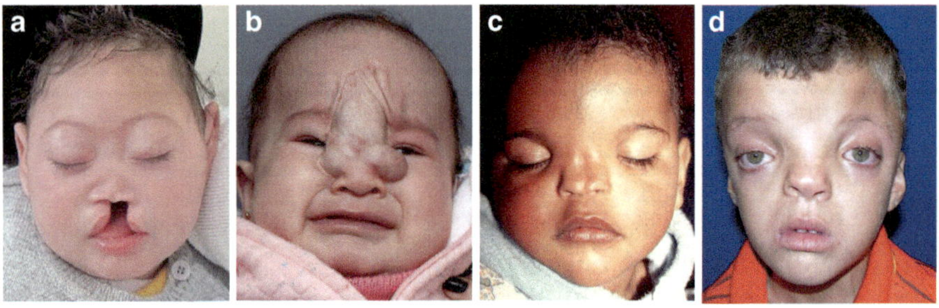

Fig. 4.1 Clinical features of TC 0–14. (**a**) Holoprosencephaly; (**b**) Encephalocele median cleft syndrome; (**c**) Facial duplication hypertelorism; (**d**) Syndromic hypertelorism frontonasal dysplasia

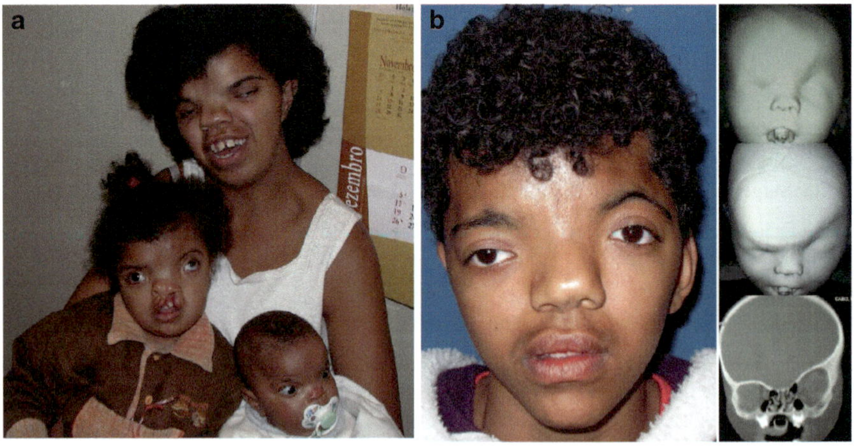

Fig. 4.2 Clinical variety of TC 0–14 syndromic hypertelorism. (**a**) Family with craniofrontonasal, dysplasia, X-linked inheritance gene EFNB1; (**b**) Wide hypertelorism, left plagiocephaly, unilateral coronal closing

corresponding to the third week of gestation. Currently, bilateral thickenings of the frontonasal process appear on the primitive forebrain. These elevations of the ectoderm become the lateral and medial nasal prominences. Fusion of the inferior medial nasal prominence, lateral prominence, and medial aspect of the maxillary process of the first visceral arch must occur for normal development of the upper lip. Fusion of the globular processes of His (from the medial nasal process) is responsible for forming the primary palate with the central dentoalveolar ridge and the central upper lip and philtrum [8, 9]. The TC 0–14 results from the failure of the two medial nasal processes to merge in the midline. An incomplete median cleft may occur as an isolated entity or as part of syndromes such as orofacial-digital syndrome and frontonasal dysplasia [10–12].

Because of the huge clinical variety, we use this table to understand better the TC 0–14 deformity where the clinical signs hypotelorism and hypertelorism can be part of the distribution of these patients. Midline defects may be grouped in four ways:

- Midline hypoplasia(holoprosencephaly), Fig. 4.3.
- True cleft or midline dysraphia, Fig. 4.4
- Duplication, Fig. 4.5
- Syndromic hypertelorism Fig. 4.2.

Based on this table, we evaluate the time and the type of procedure to be done [13] (Table 4.1).

The TC 0–14 involves the midline of the face and cranium. It includes the true or false median lip cleft, with or without associated hypertelorism or hypotelorism, respectively. The TC 0–14 is the most common of unusual craniofacial clefts and can be present either as a widening or duplication of the midline structures or as agenesis/hypoplasia of these structures. True median cleft lip begins as a median cleft upper lip, with a duplicated labial frenulum. The nose is often bifid, with a

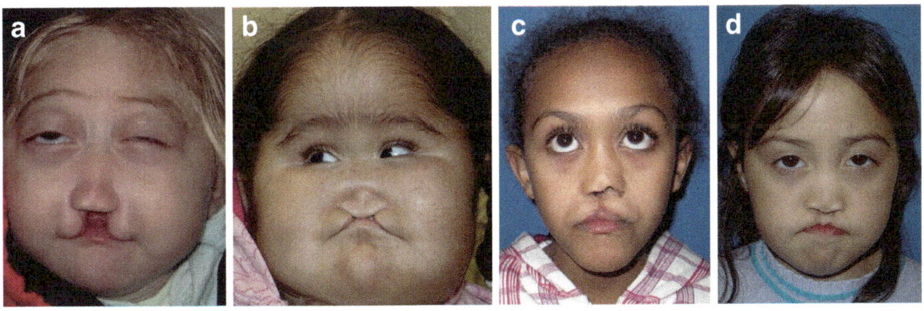

Fig. 4.3 Clinical variety of TC 0–14 holoprosencephaly–hypotelorism. (**a**) Semilobar holoprosencephaly. (**b**) Alobar holoprosencephaly with severe nasal deformity; (**c**) Lobar holoprosencephaly with cleft lip; (**d**) Lobar holoprosencephaly with bilateral cleft lip

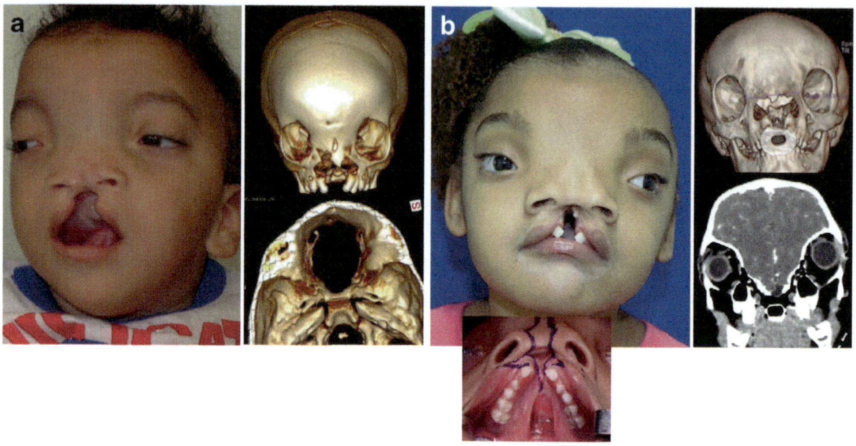

Fig. 4.4 Clinical variety of TC 0-14 dysraphia encephalocele hypertelorism. (**a**) Wide hypertelorism, nasal duplication, transsphenoidal encephalocele, median lip cleft, no cribriform plate; (**b**) Wide hypertelorism, nasal duplication, transsphenoidal encephalocele, median lip cleft, no cribriform plate

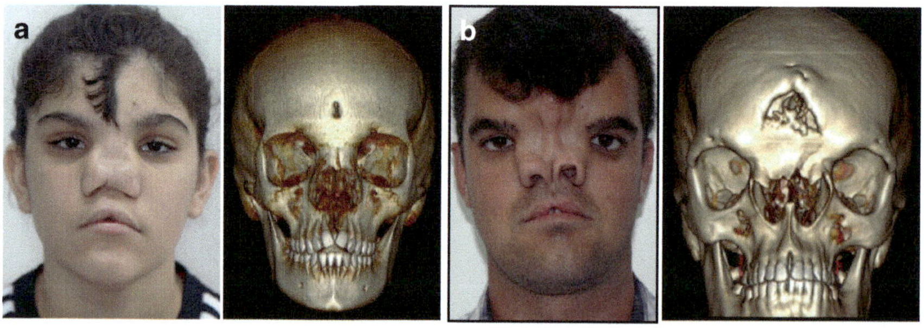

Fig. 4.5 Clinical variety of TC 0–14 duplication hypertelorism. (**a**) Mild hypertelorism, widow's peak, nasal duplication, median lip and alveolar cleft, wide crista galli; (**b**) Wide hypertelorism, nasal duplication, median lip and alveolar cleft, crista galli duplication

broad columella and a wide midline furrow. The nasal septum is thickened and often duplicated. A wide diastema of the upper central incisor teeth may be present. The nostrils may be asymmetric. The alar and upper nasal cartilages are hypoplastic and often displaced laterally. A thick subcutaneous fibromuscular band from the alar cartilage to the frontal bone can pull the columella upward and make the nose appear shorter.

Table 4.1 Rare craniofacial cleft 0–14 clinical distribution

Holoprosencephaly	Dysraphia median cleft syndrome	Duplication	Syndromic hypertelorism
Hypotelorism	Hypertelorism		
Nasal atresia	Encephalocele	Crista galli duplication	Frontorhiny syndrome Pai syndrome Opitz syndrome Fronto-orbito nasal dysplasia Craniofrontonasal syndrome
	Broadening		
	Choanal atresia		
	Bifid nose		
UCL	Midline cleft	Supernumerary organ	
BCL		Columella duplicated	Depending on syndrome
Midline cleft		Frenulum duplicated, mesiodens	

Other structures formed by the frontonasal process include the forehead, glabella, interorbital area, and prolabium, and may explain the association with midline cleft lip and hypertelorism. Cephalad, this deformity continues into the cranial base, where the enlarged ethmoid air cells, a low-lying cribriform plate, and hypertelorism are standard. Sometimes, a median encephalocele may accompany these other anomalies. The exact cause still is unknown, though studies demonstrate a possible relationship with certain teratogenic drugs [14]. Nearly all cases occur sporadically, with no evidence of a genetic basis. However, a few familial cases have been reported [12, 15, 16].

Alternatively, the false median cleft lip or hypotelorism type is characterized by an absence of philtrum and columella, premaxillary bone, nasal septum, and crista galli [9]. The cleft spans the entire height of the upper lip. The nasal septum is hypoplastic, vestigial, and unattached to the palate at any point. Holoprosencephaly represents a deficiency of midline tissue. A hypoplastic ethmoid bone accompanies but is not the reason for hypotelorism. Hypotelorism is more likely a response to reduced brain development. These findings should alert the possibility of severe brain malformations, as De Myer described, and be categorized into five groups of holoprosencephaly [17]. Cases of holoprosencephaly result from deficient anterior neural plate development, and severe cases are not compatible with life. It is unknown whether the malunion is due to alterations in the epithelial–mesenchymal interactions or some other factors [16].

4.2 Clinical Consideration

True Midline Cleft.

More accessible than a typical cleft lip, even a unilateral cleft lip, median cleft has some small particularity that must pay attention to obtain a good result. In many cases, a simple midline suture in three layers—mucosal, muscular, and cutaneous—may not be a great option.

From a surgical point of view, even microform clefts may be disfiguring. When treating TC0, the surgeon must determine if the cleft is true or false. In cases of true median clefts, a reconstruction of the Cupid's bow, labial philtrum, vermillion, and buccal mucosa must be carried out. When evaluating a patient with a true midline cleft, the surgeon should determine if there is horizontal excess tissue. Many patients have excess, and resection must be addressed to avoid a wide philtrum.

In some cases, the frenulum is too short and should be addressed. It is possible to release it from the maxilla, or a simple Z-plasty can be utilized to elongate it. Midline alveolar bone cleft may be presented and repercusses at the occlusal and facial appearance. Orthodontia is inappropriate when the osseous bridge is lost, taking the risk of losing the support of incisive medial teeth. Therefore, alveolar bone grafting was utilized for patients in mixed dentition—around 7 years of age. The iliac crest is the primary option for these patients, but the mental donor area should also be considered because the bone volume necessity is not so big. Even vertical discrepancies can be treated with the same protocol (Fig. 4.6).

The association of TC 0 and TC30 is possible, besides being rare. Patients may present an absence of lower and upper incisive teeth. Maxillary orthopedic

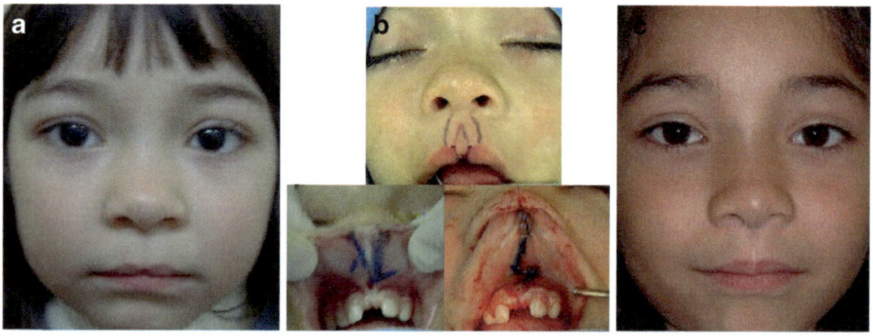

Fig. 4.6 Median lip cleft surgical treatment. (**a**) Median lip and alveolar cleft; (**b**) Skin markings and mucosal elongation with Z-plasty; (**c**) skin markings and mucosal elongation with Z-plasty; **c**: Late post-operative lip repair

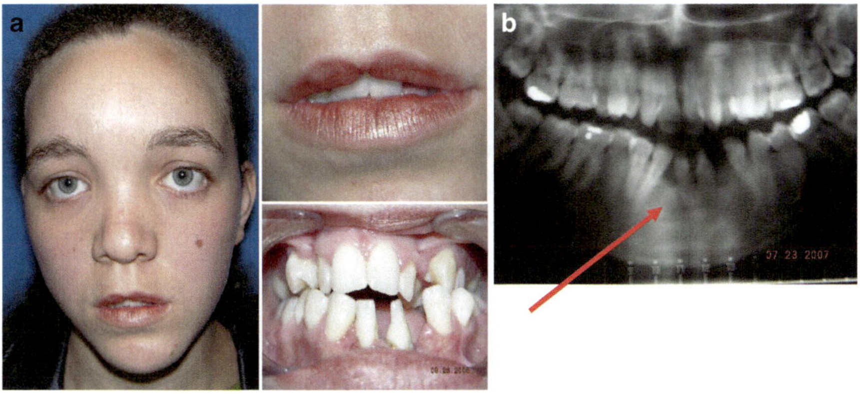

Fig. 4.7 Unusual association between TC 0 and TC 30. (**a**) Upper median cleft, absence of lower central incisors; (**b**) Panorex with absence of central incisors (red arrow)

treatment must be used to stimulate facial growth. Alveolar bone grafting will be necessary before (Fig. 4.7).

4.3 Pai Syndrome

Pai syndrome is a rare congenital disorder first described in 1987. The main clinical features are median cleft of the upper lip, intracranial lipoma, and cutaneous polyps. In literature, only a few cases of this syndrome have been described. Histopathology of the nasal tumor demonstrates fat hamartoma. In the same embryologic period, impaired mesodermal penetration and compensatory skin proliferation result in the median cleft (deficiency) and dermic mass formation (excess). This theory may answer an association of median cleft lip, nasal polypoid mass, and corpus callosum lipoma. Pai postulated no significance of genetic heritage. Nasal masses in infants are rare and must be diagnosed, excluding glioma, dermoid cysts, teratoma, hemangioma, and nasolacrimal cist. Lipoma of the corpus callosum is not symptomatic. However, it can be associated with convulsion, intracranial hypertension, dementia, and hemiparesis. Its resection is technically challenging due to the vascularization and proximity of great cerebral arteries [18, 19] (Fig. 4.8).

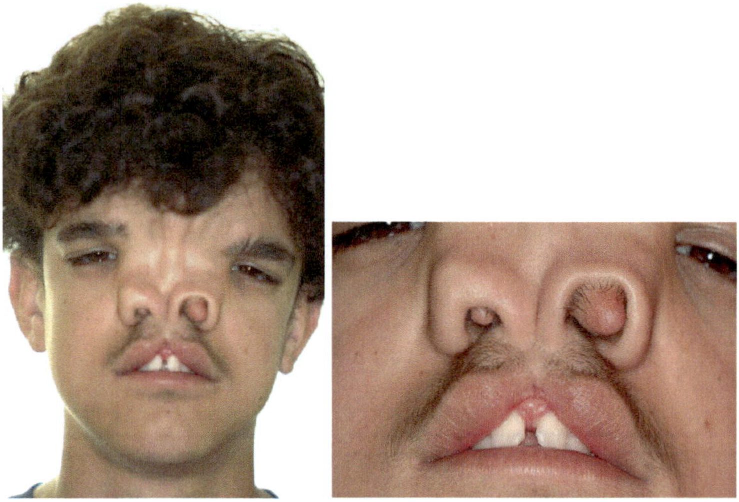

Fig. 4.8 Pai syndrome wide orbital hypertelorism. (**a**) Orbital hypertelorism, median cleft lip, cutaneous polyps, midline lipoma of central nervous system

4.4 Holoprosencephaly

Holoprosencephaly is a rare congenital brain malformation resulting from the incomplete separation of the two hemispheres. The incidence is 1 per 10,000–16,000 live births, the most common brain malformation. The early embryonic occurrence may be even higher but may not be detected due to most fetuses aborting in early gestation. The fundamental problem is a failure of the developing brain to divide into left and right halves (which usually occurs at the end of the fifth week of gestation). This results in variable loss of midline structures of the brain and faces and the fusion of lateral ventricles and the third ventricle. Environmental factors such as maternal diabetes mellitus, alcohol use, and retinoic acid have been implicated in the pathogenesis. As it has a mutation of several genes, including Sonic Hedgehog and ZIC2 (chromosome 13q32), the latter is also involved in syntelencephaly [20–22].

Generally, the diagnosis is evident at birth, with median cleft lip, absence of septum and columella, ocular hypotelorism, and solitary median maxillary central incisor. These children also have systemic problems, poor feeding, hypothalamic/pituitary dysfunction, and developmental delay. Other anomalies may occur, such as genital defects, polydactyly, vertebral defects, limb reduction defects, and transposition of the great arteries. The prognosis depends on the holoprosencephaly type, with almost all alobar and semilobar forms incompatible with extrauterine life. Patients born with holoprosencephaly and midline cleft lip have dire projections about their quality and long life. Therefore, the cleft team should understand that many will not be alive after the first year. Surgery must be discussed with parents and delayed until this date. Only patients with a lower grade of brain malformation will be healthy to undergo lip repair.

In the treatment of the false median cleft, where there is an absence of the tissue in the midline, such as premaxilla, prolabium, and septum, it is advisable to wait for the child's development up to 1–2 years of age for a corrective surgical procedure since most patients with severe holoprosencephaly do not survive past this age. Due to the absence of prolabium, these patients have only the lateral lip segments. And a simple lip adhesion in the midline will restore continuity and decrease parents' anxiety. Few surgeons have indicated a two-stage reconstruction and performed an Abbé flap to create the philtrum. This procedure must be associated with a temporary protective tracheostomy during the intermediary period between the two procedures. Also, we do not advocate the Abbé flap because this is a two-stage procedure and challenging for feeding. The use of the local flaps may simulate the columella. The absence of philtrum makes the surgeon utilizes Abbé flap in two stages. Technically, our approach is to bring the exact desire of the Cupid's bow and philtrum to create normal anatomy. It is essential to spend time making the donor area as less visible as possible [23] (Fig. 4.9).

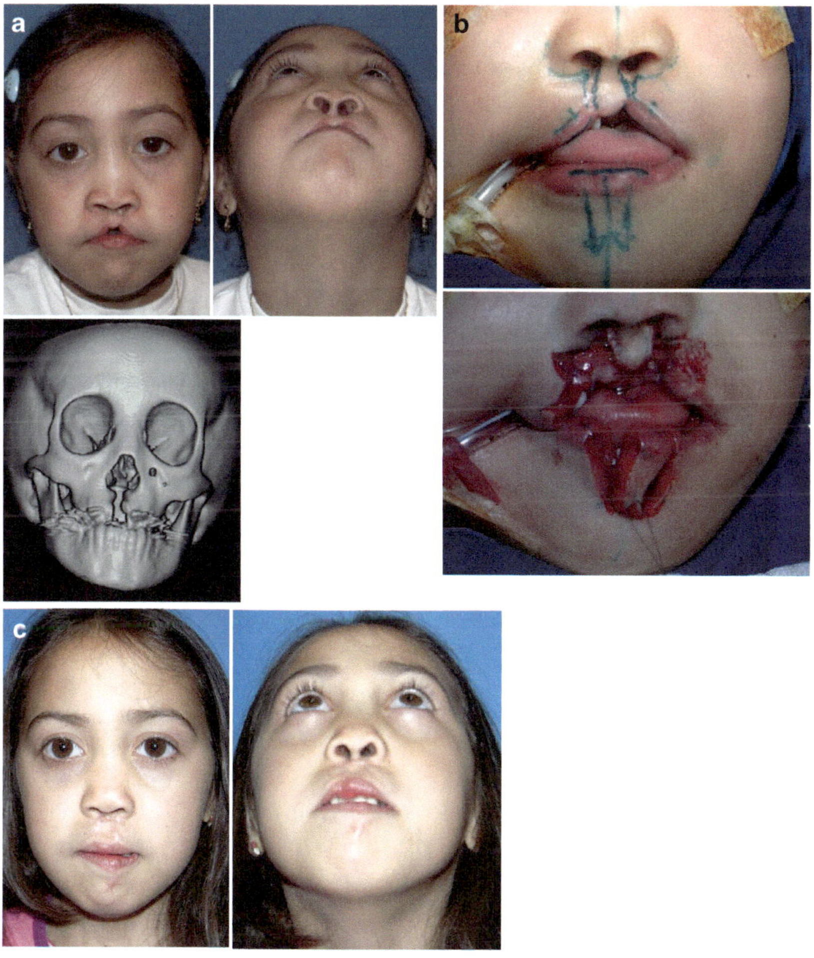

Fig. 4.9 Surgical treatment holoprosencephaly associated with false bilateral cleft lip. (**a**) Holoprosencephaly, median lip and alveolar cleft, absence of nasal septum, age 4 years old previously lip adhesion; (**b**) Lip repair with Abbe; (**c**) Post-operative of lip repair

4.5 Hypertelorism

Hypertelorism is a clinical symptom in a large spectrum of congenital craniofacial defects. Its diagnostic is done by clinical examination; measuring the inner canthal distance, the outer canthal distance, and the interpupillary distance is possible. It could be precisely measured by radiography. Standard curves of interorbital distance growth, which is mainly used, interorbital distance values were obtained from plain frontal radiography, the value calculated as the distance between the two lacrimal crests [24, 25]. Tessier has given a classification for adults in three levels of severity: grade I (30–34 mm), grade II (35–39 mm), and grade III (>40 mm). A grade III deformity involves gross facial disfigurement and requires surgical intervention [26, 27].In syndromic cases, hypertelorism can come with encephaloceles, craniosynostosis, and nasal deformities; the age for the procedure could be changed depending on the functional severity.

A rugose nose is not a common entity. The nasal malformation, including skin and bone cartilage structure, is often associated with hypertelorism. Few cases are published, and no consensus exists about the best technique. Simple median tissue resection would be necessary in a moment, but the exact moment is unclear. Our approach is to wait until nasal surgery is required because the median incision permits it to work on the dorsum and improve the nasal shape (Fig. 4.10).

4.5.1 Surgical Treatment for Hypertelorism

Many previous attempts to operate to approach the orbits and correct hypertelorism were made without success [28–31]. Based on their knowledge of the correction of secondary facial fractures, Converse et al. proposed an orbito-nasal

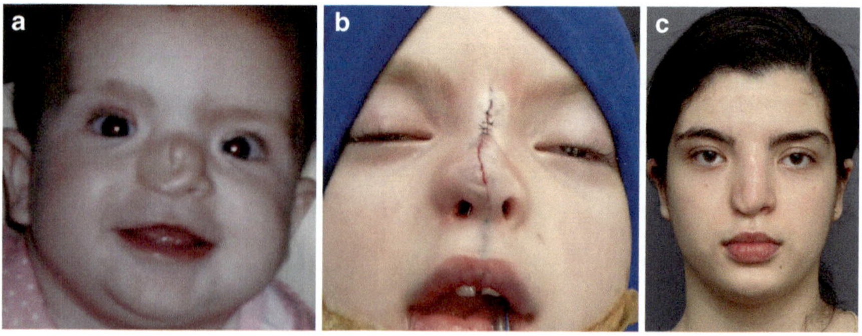

Fig. 4.10 Rugose nose surgical treatment. (**a**) Rugose nose with mild hypertelorism; (**b**) Early skin resection; (**c**) Late rhinoplasty with costal graft

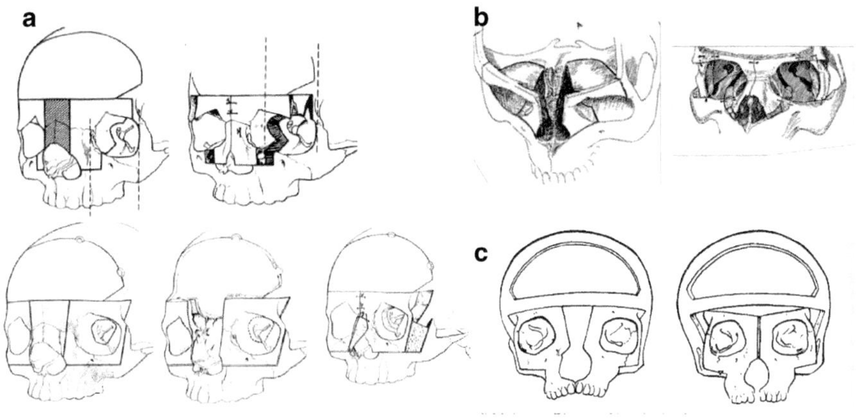

Fig. 4.11 Surgical treatment osteotomies for hyperteleorbitism correction. (**a**) Tessier's Technique 1972; (**b**) Converse 1970; (**c**) van der Meulen

osteotomy to approach this deformity without much success [32]. The first radical procedure Paul Tessier designed is the so-called "box osteotomy" because it moves the four orbital walls as a square box [26, 27]. The olfactory nerves would be sacrificed with the lateral mass of the ethmoid and the nasal septum after this initial radical resection; several proposals have been made to save the olfactory groove and olfaction by Converse et al. [32]. Hugo Obwegeser et al. were the first to perform a facial bipartition in July 1969, published in 1978 in a case of facial duplication (cleft TC 0–14) [33]. The other author who published about this procedure was Jacques Van der Meulen, 1979; he named it "medial faciotomy" [34] (Fig. 4.11).

In more severe cases of hypertelorism, when the nasal dorsum is affected, and the duplication of the septum occurs, resection of the excess skin of the nasal dorsum and the closing in the midline may be performed. Although some debate continues, the correction of hypertelorism is best delayed to approximately 8 years of age (Figs. 4.12, 4.13, and 4.14). More comprehensive techniques have been described to treat TC 0–14 patients. Ortiz-Monasterio and Taylor presented an extensive series of patients. They proposed a protocol for hypertelorism correction, managing the nose with resection of the dorsal nasal skin, reshaping cartilaginous structures, and performing osteotomies even in young child [3, 35]. Pellerin showed his experience in 38 patients and discussed indications of the osteotomies for the orbit and present advantages and problems between box osteotomies and facial bipartition and in his personal experience, the facial bipartition had advantages when compared to box osteotomies [13](Figs. 4.15 and 4.16). In our opinion majority of the patients, we perform box osteotomies, and only in patients with the inclination of the palatal plates with central diastema of the incisor we performed the facial bipartition. For patients with inner lateral orbital distance close to normal, we also used medial mobilization of naso-orbital structures.

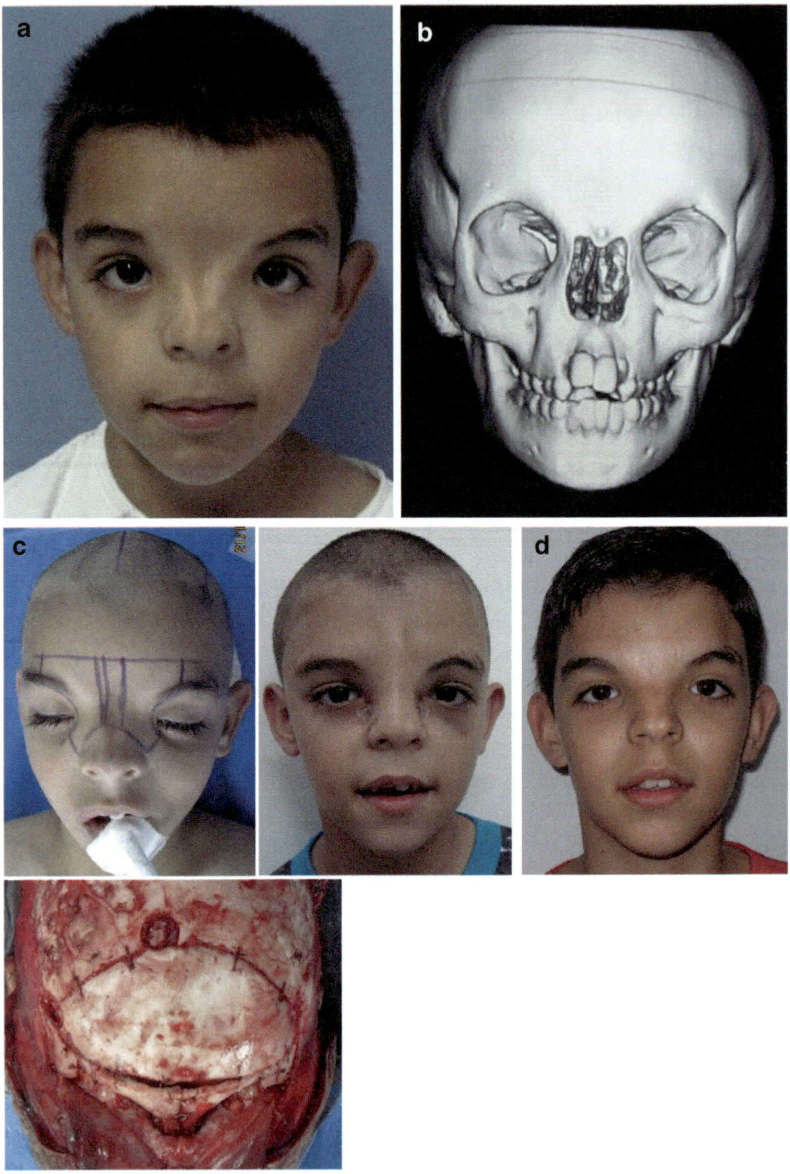

Fig. 4.12 Surgical treatment—correction of hypertelorism with medial naso-orbital osteotomies. (**a**) Mild hypertelorism, grade I, no median cleft; (**b**) CT duplication midline; (**c**) Marking the medial osteotomy, intraoperative ICD less than 15 mm, immediate PO; (**d**) 05 years late

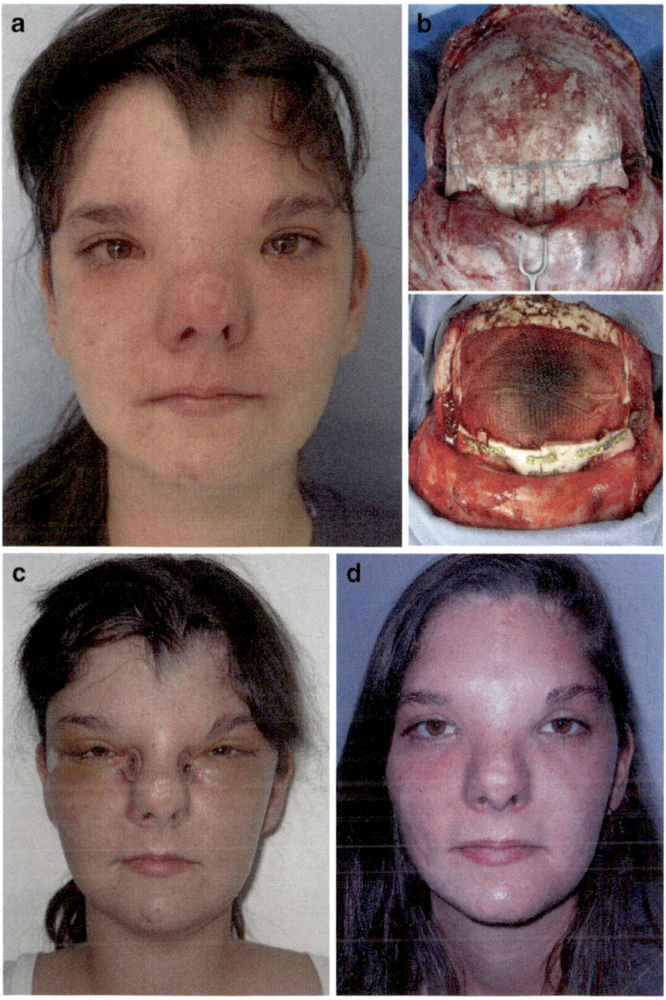

Fig. 4.13 Surgical treatment—correction of hypertelorism associated with rugose nose. (**a**) Grade II hypertelorism, widow's peak forehead; (**b**) Medial naso-orbital osteotomy, 15 mm resection; (**c**) Immediate PO; (**d**) Late result after resection of widow's peak 07 years late

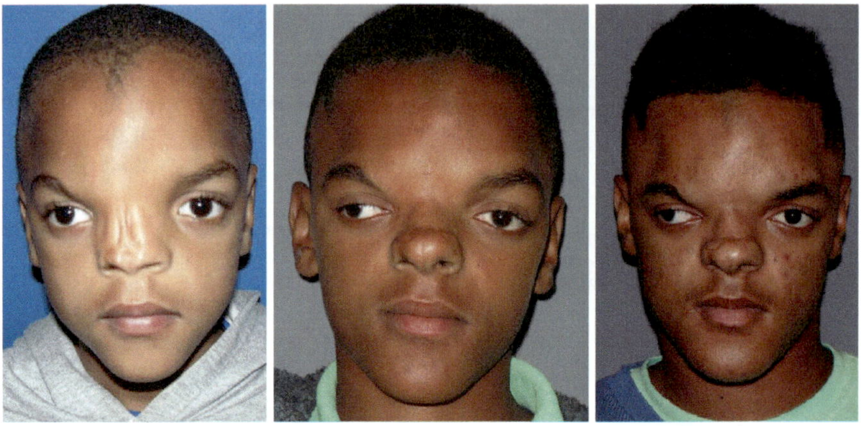

Fig. 4.14 Surgical treatment—correction of hypertelorism associated with wide rugose nose. Total orbital mobilization, skin resection, nasal reconstruction local flaps, bone graft for nose, mustard canthal flaps

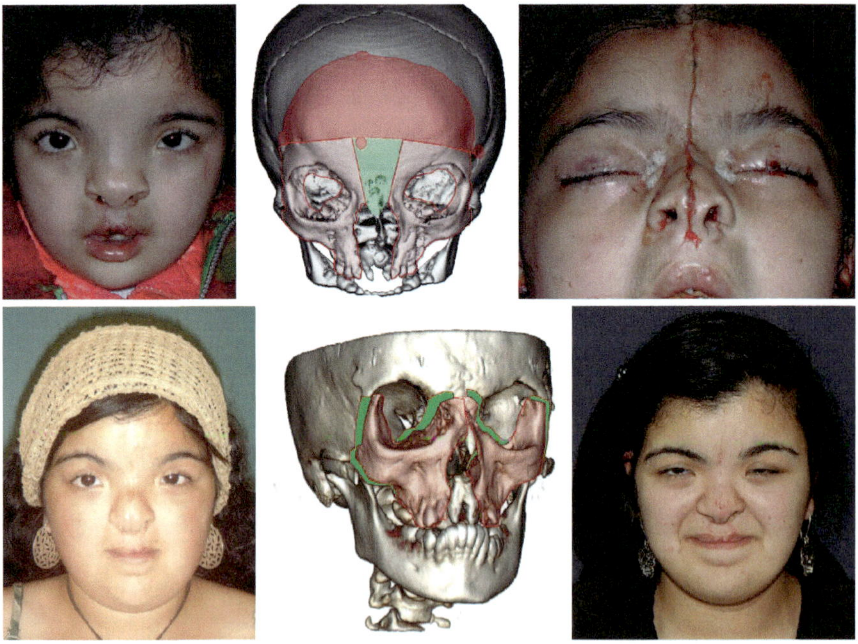

Fig. 4.15 Surgical treatment—correction of hypertelorism with facial bipartition twice

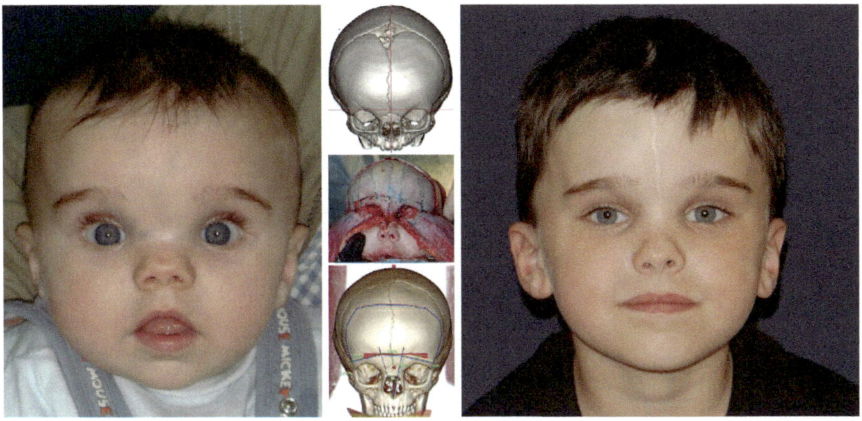

Fig. 4.16 Surgical treatment facial bipartition

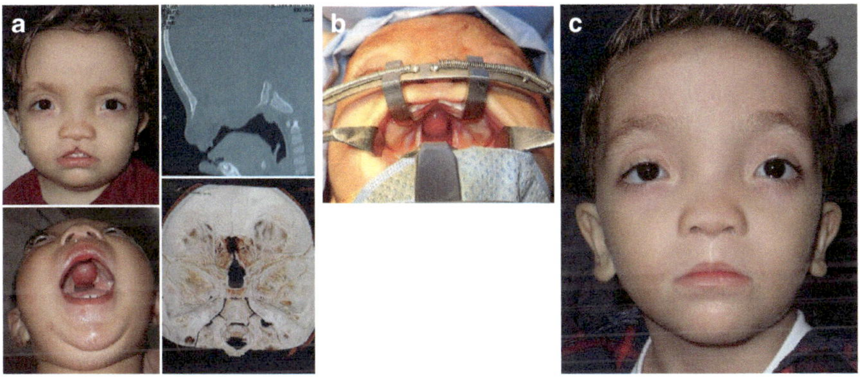

Fig. 4.17 Median lip cleft and encephalocele intraoral access for correction. (**a**) Median cleft lip associated with transsphenoidal encephalocele; (**b**) Intracranial and intraoral access; (**c**) Late result of the surgery

Encephalocele

Craniofacial TC 14 may be observed as an encephalocele, usually in the ethmoid area, protruding through the nose. However, it can be more posteriorly and invades the nasal and oral cavities. When the malformation is located more anterior, it is easier to repair. Our approach to anterior encephalocele is always made with facial bipartition; when the intraoral component is enormous, the access associated with transpalatal is done. In our series, we have 16 transsphenoidal encephaloceles associated with median cleft lip, with 3 of them without hypertelorisms (Figs. 4.17, 4.18, and 4.19).

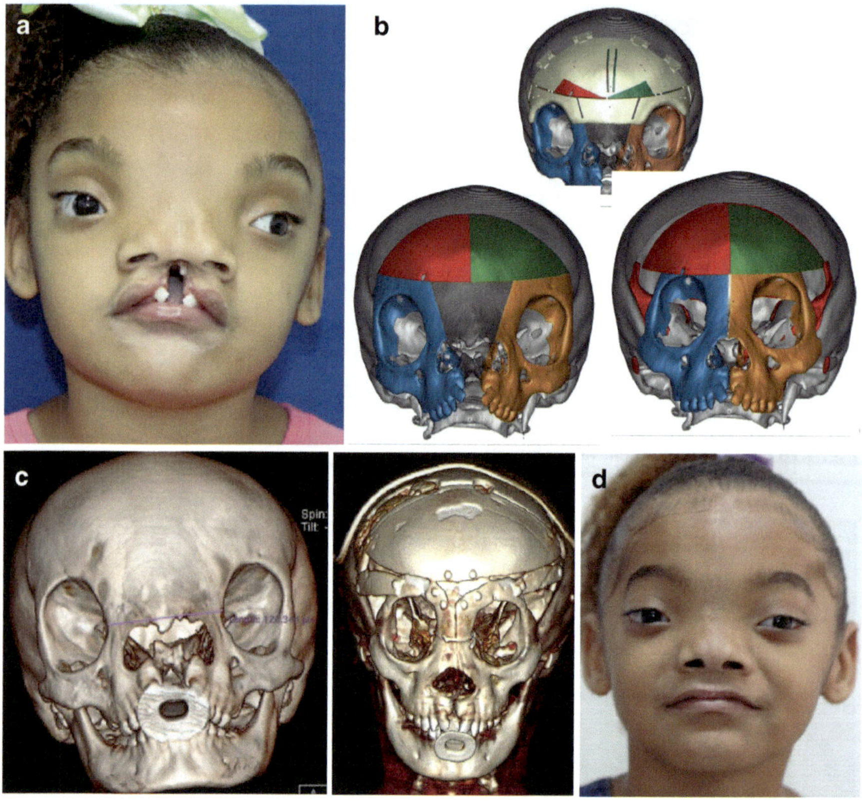

Fig. 4.18 Surgical treatment combined intracranial access and oral access for facial bipartition. (**a**) TC 0–14 with nasal encephalocele hypertelorism grade III 56 mm; (**b**) Surgical plannings with surgical guides; (**c**) Pre-CT and just after facial bipartition PO; (**d**) One year late PO

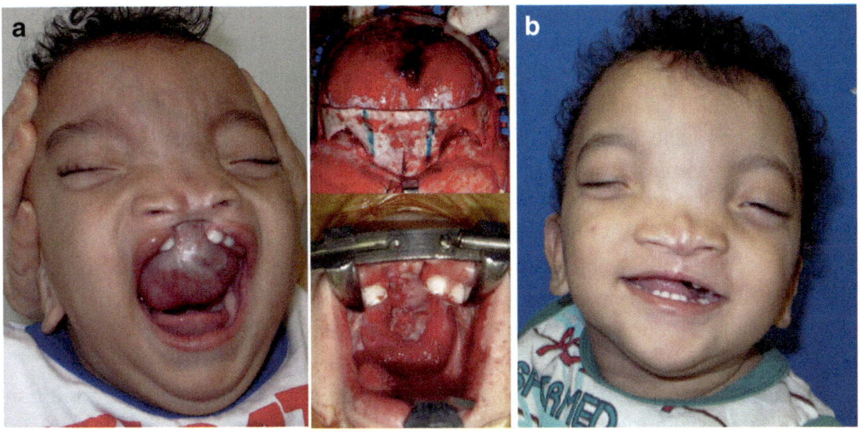

Fig. 4.19 Surgical treatment combined intracranial access and oral access for staged facial bipartition. (**a**) Combined surgical access to treatment of encephalocele naso-ethmoidal; (**b**) After encephalocele correction, second procedure hypertelorism correction

4.6 Clinical Cases

We have conducted a retrospective analysis of our extensive TC 0–14 cases series. The objective was to review the functional outcome and aesthetic results of the different techniques applied to each patient. Between 1997 and 2021, 238 TC 0–14 cases were evaluated and treated in three units: São Paulo, Curitiba, and Lille. The patients were divided into several groups:

- Holoprosencephaly (TC0–14)—31
- Hypertelorism (TC14)—90
- True median cleft (TC0)—32
- Craniofrontonasal dysplasia (TC0–14)—18
- Encephalocele (TC4)—47
- Bifid nose (TC0–14)—5
- Rugose nose (TC0–14)—9
- Pai syndrome (TC0–14)—6

In the treatment of the false median cleft, where there is an absence of the tissue in the midline, such as premaxilla, prolabium, and septum, it is advisable to wait for the child's development up to 1–2 years of age for a corrective surgical procedure since most patients with severe holoprosencephaly do not survive past this age. A simple closing of the lateral lip segments was the option for reconstructing the lip defect. The surgical procedure performed in the single patient with a false cleft lip was a mucosal Z-plasty, two lateral buccal incisions to proximate the segments together, muscle repair, and midline skin closure. A small flap of the skin from the inner lining of the nasal tip was harvested to recreate the columella. No cartilage or bone was used to give support. We do not advocate the Abbé flap because this is a two-stage procedure challenging for feeding and breathing in these patients. The use of the local flaps may simulate the columella. Thirty-two patients were noted to have an incomplete median cleft lip. All these patients underwent surgical treatment, using a Z-plasty of the mucosa, resection of excess tissues in the midline, muscle closure, and skin closure, performing a small V-Y flap in the base of the columella. The patient with Pai syndrome had a wide right nostril due to the intranasal tumor and underwent a resection of the tumor, associated with resection of the ala and a rotation of the vertical flap with the inferior pedicle to permit the inferior rotation of ala. In our series, 16 patients with median cleft lip had transsphenoidal encephalocele; not all but only 5 patients had orbital hypertelorism.

A bifid nose was seen, some associated alveolar median cleft and hypertelorism (TC 0–14), and rhinoplasty was performed, utilizing an external approach, resecting excess tissue in the midline with domal suturing and cartilage grafting. Patients with hypertelorism underwent correction of the interorbital distance with the box technique or using a C-shaped, depending on interorbital wideness. At the same procedure, resection of the excess tissue in the midline with a vertical incision and a small Z-plasty in the nasal base. Some other cases of associated hypertelorism had already undergone a previous rhinoplasty. A secondary rhinoplasty or three-stage nasal reconstruction was performed. Isolated median alveolar cleft was isolated or associated with TC 30 (median mandibular cleft) in very few patients (3 patients). They were treated with dental orthopedics with associated frenectomy and Z-plasty. Bone grafting was performed in cases where it was necessary and indicated by an orthodontist.

References

1. Tessier P. Anatomical classification of facial, cranio-facial and latero-facial clefts. J Maxillofac Surg [Internet]. 1976;4:69–92. https://linkinghub.elsevier.com/retrieve/pii/S0301050376800136.
2. Alonso N, Tonello C. Rare facial clefts. In: Hamdan U, Rogers-Vizena C, Vyas R, Sommerlad B, Low D, editors. Interdisciplinary cleft care global perspectives [internet]. San Diego CA: Plural Publishing; 2023. p. 689–701. http://www.pluralpublishing.com.
3. Monasterio FO, del Campo AF, Dimopulos A. Nasal clefts. Ann Plast Surg. 1987;18(5):377. http://journals.lww.com/00000637-198705000-00004.
4. Moore MH. Rare craniofacial clefts. J Craniofac Surg. 1996;7(6):408–11. http://journals.lww.com/00001665-199611000-00003.
5. Fearon JA. Rare craniofacial clefts: a surgical classification. J Craniofac Surg. 2008;19(1):110–2. http://journals.lww.com/00001665-200801000-00018.
6. Raposo-Amaral CE, Jarrahy R, Lim R, Alonso N. The rare facial cleft. In: Alonso N, Raposo-Amaral CE, editors. Cleft lip and palate treatment. Cham: Springer; 2018. p. 325–62. https://doi.org/10.1007/978-3-319-63290-2_21.
7. Alonso N, da Silva Freitas R. Craniofacial clefts and others related deformities. In: Plastic surgery indications and practice; 2009. p. 455–71.

8. Mazzola RF. Congenital malformations in the frontonasal area: their pathogenesis and classification. Clin Plast Surg. 1976;3(4):573–609.
9. Mazzola RF, Mazzola IC. Facial clefts and facial dysplasia: revisiting the classification. J Craniofac Surg. 2014;25(1):26–34. http://journals.lww.com/00001665-201401000-00009.
10. Guion-Almeida ML, Richieri-Costa A. Acrofrontofacionasal dysostosis: report of the third Brazilian family. Am J Med Genet. 2003;119A(2):238–41. https://doi.org/10.1002/ajmg.a.10444.
11. Guion-Almeida ML, Richieri-Costa A. Frontonasal dysplasia, severe neuropsychological delay, and midline central nervous system anomalies: report of 10 Brazilian male patients. Am J Med Genet A. 2009;149A(5):1006–11. https://doi.org/10.1002/ajmg.a.32717.
12. Guion-Almeida ML, Richieri-Costa A, Saavedra D, Cohen MM. Frontonasal dysplasia: analysis of 21 cases and literature review. Int J Oral Maxillofac Surg. 1996;25(2):91–7.
13. Pellerin P. Management of hypertelorism. J Pediatr Neurosci. 2022;17(Suppl 1):S4–13. https://www.ncbi.nlm.nih.gov/pmc/articles/PMC9648651/.
14. Edwards WC, Askew W, Weisskopf B. Median cleft face syndrome. Am J Ophthalmol. 1971;72(1):202–5. https://linkinghub.elsevier.com/retrieve/pii/0002939471916151.
15. Dube G, Jain S. Prevalence of true median cleft of upper lip as reflected from a small central Indian population: attempt to report and review the true median cleft of upper lip. J Maxillofac Oral Surg [Internet]. 2018;17(4):508–13. https://doi.org/10.1007/s12663-017-1072-1.
16. Hamzan MI, Sulaiman WAW. True median cleft lip—15 years of review and prevalence. Cleft Palate Craniofac J. 2020;57(8):1051–4. https://doi.org/10.1177/1055665620926346.
17. DeMyer W. The median cleft face syndrome: differential diagnosis of cranium bifidum occultum, hypertelorism, and median cleft nose, lip, and palate. Neurol Int. 1967;17(10):961–1. https://doi.org/10.1212/WNL.17.10.961.
18. Pai GS, Levkoff AH, Leithiser RE, Reynolds JF. Median cleft of the upper lip associated with lipomas of the central nervous system and cutaneous polyps. Am J Med Genet. 1987;26(4):921–4. https://doi.org/10.1002/ajmg.1320260421.
19. Coban YK, Boran C, Omeroglu SA, Okur E. Pai syndrome: an adult patient with bifid nose and frontal hairline marker. Cleft Palate Craniofac J. 2003;40(3):325–8.
20. Simon EM, Hevner RF, Pinter JD, Clegg NJ, Delgado M, Kinsman SL, et al. The middle interhemispheric variant of holoprosencephaly. AJNR Am J Neuroradiol. 2002;23(1):151–6. https://www.ncbi.nlm.nih.gov/pmc/articles/PMC7975493/
21. Takanashi J, Barkovich AJ, Clegg NJ, Delgado MR. Middle interhemispheric variant of holoprosencephaly associated with diffuse polymicrogyria. AJNR Am J Neuroradiol. 2003;24(3):394–7. https://www.ncbi.nlm.nih.gov/pmc/articles/PMC7973611/.
22. Winter TC, Kennedy AM, Woodward PJ. Holoprosencephaly: a survey of the entity, with embryology and fetal imaging. RadioGraphics. 2015;35(1):275–90. https://doi.org/10.1148/rg.351140040.
23. da Silva Freitas R, Alonso N, Shin JH, Busato L, Ono MCC, de Oliveria e Cruz GA. Surgical correction of Tessier number 0 cleft. J Craniofac Surg. 2008;19(5):1348–52. https://journals.lww.com/00001665-200809000-00022.
24. Gerald BE, Silverman FN. Normal and abnormal interorbital distances, with special reference to mongolism. Am J Roentgenol. 1965;95(1):154–61. https://doi.org/10.2214/ajr.95.1.154.
25. Feingold M, Bossert WH. Normal values for selected physical parameters: an aid to syndrome delineation. Birth Defects Orig Artic Ser. 1974;10(13):1–16.
26. Orbital TP. Hypertelorism: I. Successive surgical attempts. Material and methods. Causes and mechanisms. Scand J Plast Reconstr Surg. 1972;6(2):135–55. https://doi.org/10.3109/02844317209036714.
27. Tessier P, Guiot G, Derome P. Orbital hypertelorism: II. Definite treatment of Orbital Hypertelorism (OR.H.) by craniofacial or by extracranial osteotomies. Scand J Plast Reconstr Surg. 1973;7(1):39–58. https://doi.org/10.3109/02844317309072417.
28. Webster JP, Deming EG. The surgical treatment of the bifid nose. Plast Reconstr Surg. 1950;6(1):1. https://journals.lww.com/plasreconsurg/Citation/1950/07000/THE_SURGICAL_TREATMENT_OF_THE_BIFID_NOSE.1.aspx.

29. Murray JE, Swanson LT, Strand RD, Hricko GM. Evaluation of craniofacial surgery in the treatment of facial deformities. Ann Surg. 1975;182(3):240. https://journals.lww.com/annalsofsurgery/Abstract/1975/09000/Evaluation_of_Craniofacial_Surgery_in_the.7.aspx.
30. Schmid E. Surgical management of hypertelorism. Craniofacial Anom Pathog Repair. 1968:155–61.
31. Converse JM, Smith B. Naso-orbital fractures and traumatic deformities of the medial canthus. Plast Reconstr Surg. 1966;38(2):147. https://journals.lww.com/plasreconsurg/Citation/1966/08000/Naso_Orbital_Fractures_and_Traumatic_Deformities.11.aspx.
32. Converse JM, Ransohoff J, Mathews ES, Smith B, Molenaar A. Ocular hypertelorism and pseudohypertelorism advances in surgical treatment. Plast Reconstr Surg. 1970;45(1):1. https://journals.lww.com/plasreconsurg/Citation/1970/01000/OCULAR_HYPERTELORISM_AND_PSEUDOHYPERTELORISM.1.aspx.
33. Obwegeser HL, Weber G, Freihofer HP, Sailer HF. Facial duplication—the unique case of Antonio. J Maxillofac Surg. 1978;6:179–98. https://linkinghub.elsevier.com/retrieve/pii/S0301050378800885.
34. van der Meulen JC. Medial faciotomy. Br J Plast Surg. 1979;32(4):339–42. https://linkinghub.elsevier.com/retrieve/pii/000712267990095X.
35. Monasterio FO, Taylor JA. Major craniofacial clefts: case series and treatment philosophy. Plast Reconstr Surg. 2008;122(2):534–43. http://journals.lww.com/00006534-200808000-00027.

Chapter 5
Cleft 1/13

Philippe Pellerin, Nivaldo Alonso, Renato da Silva Freitas, and Cristiano Tonello

Pearls

Cleft 1–13 is one of the three interorbital rare clefts. Its consequences are hypertelorism and nasal anomalies. It runs from the nasal aperture toward the paramedian frontal area and the olfactive groove on the skull base. In its unilateral form it is asymmetric but confusingly symmetric when bilateral and easily confused with cleft 0–14.

Its path is identical to the cleft 2–12, the difference is between a clefting phenotype for cleft 1 versus a hypoplastic phenotype for cleft 2.

P. Pellerin (✉)
Centre Hospitalier Régional Universitaire de Lille, Lille, France

N. Alonso
Plastic Surgery, Universidade de São Paulo, São Paulo, Brazil

Craniofacial Surgery, Hospital de Reabilitação Anomalias Craniofaciais Bauru USPUniversidade de São Paulo, Bauru, Brazil

R. da Silva Freitas
Plastic Surgery Unit, Hospital de Clínicas, Universidade Federal do Paraná, Curitiba, Brazil

Craniofacial Surgery, Assistance Center for Cleft Lip and Palate (CAIF), Hospital do Trabalhador, Curitiba, Brazil

C. Tonello
Curso de Medicina Bauru Faculdade de Odontologia Bauru Universidade de São Paulo, Bauru, Brazil

Hospital de Reabilitação Anomalias Craniofaciais Universidade de São Paulo, Bauru, Brazil

N. Alonso et al. (eds.), *Facial Reconstruction of Unusual Facial Clefts*,
https://doi.org/10.1007/978-3-031-40926-4_5

5.1 Original Tessier's Classification (Fig. 5.1)

In his original paper, there is some confusing delimitation about the nasoschisis, which is the feature of cleft 1, the nasal cleft that one can find in the text as well as in the original drawing, and the cleft 2, which comes along almost the same path.

In the drawing (Figs. 5.1a, b); P71 reference [1]) (Fig. 5.1a), one can see that cleft 2 is drawn in a dotted line when other paths are drawn with plain lines.

When cleft 1 is precisely described, cleft 2 delineation is a bit confusing: "N°. 2 *looks similar to the preceding cleft. It is, however, slightly more lateral without being paranasal. On the soft tissues, this cleft comes through the nasal ala between the tail of the alar cartilage and the alar base and on the lip, it is manifested as a usual type harelip. On the skeleton, it comes through the lateral mass of the ethmoid (telorbitism). It is difficult to locate exactly on the frontal bone, whim is flattened while the frontal sinus is enlarged. Hemiatrophy of the nose, super-numerary nostrils and proboscis lateralis are probably different degrees of the same defect.*" At last, in the displayed illustration (Fig. 5.9a–e) of a nasal cleft 2, the nostril rim deformity is more related to a nasal hypoplasia with a vertical shrinking than to a cleft. Hence, we will keep the term cleft 1 to name the nasoschisis, cleft 2 will be reserved as hypothesized by Tessier for the arhinia, the proboscis, and the supernumerary nostril.

About Cleft 13 the description is more specific and does not leave place to doubt: *"Number thirteen No. 13 is the 'northbound' component of the paramedian craniofacial cleft no. 1. It is located between the nasal bone and the frontal process of the maxilla; it courses through the frontal bones (encephalocele) and along the olfactory groove."*

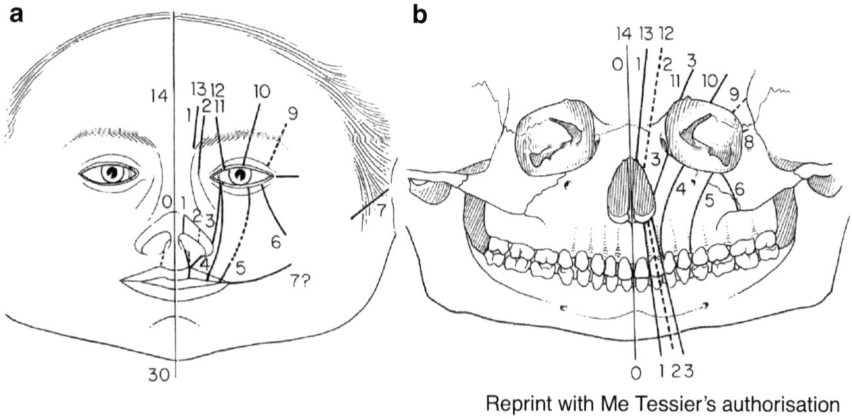

Fig. 5.1 Original Tessier's classification. (**a**) soft tissues tracks. (**b**) skeletal tracks

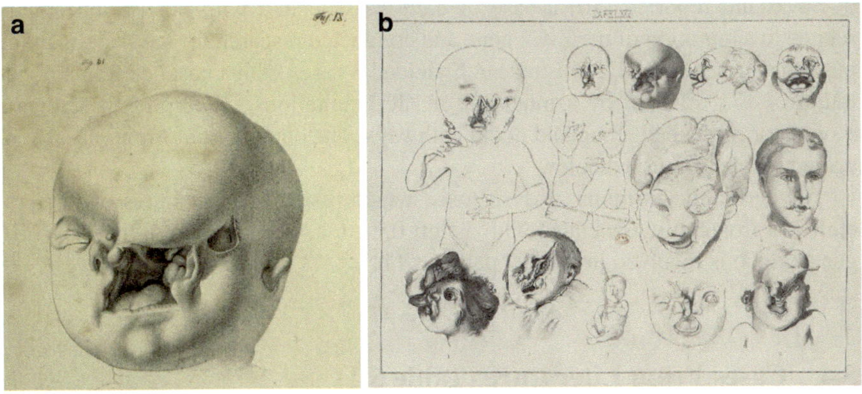

Fig. 5.2 The historical cases of cleft 1-13. (**a**) Leuckart -T.IX; Fig. 31. (**b**) Ahlfeld T. XXV; Fig. 1, 2, and 3

5.2 History (Fig. 5.2)

The first report of cleft 1–13 that we found is by Leuckart in 1840 [2]; his publication includes a detailed drawing of this malformation (Table IX; Fig. 31 of his book) which he said was found in the collections of the Zurich museum of anatomy. This illustration will later be reprinted in Förster's atlas [3] (Table XXV; Fig. 3) as well as two other cases (Table XXV; Figs. 1 and 2) assigned to Otto [4], those two cases being in the setting of amniotic band syndrome. Those three observations are, again, reported by Ahlfeld in his treatise in 1880 [5].

5.3 Etiology

From the "etiology, genetic and classification" chapter, we can understand that the fate of NCCs in the frontonasal process has many ways to be disturbed, leading to clefts 1–13.

It is striking that in a mouse strain with severe nasal clefting, a double mutation affecting Alx3/Alx4 has been found. The given mechanism is apoptotic [6]. Kayserili [7] reported four patients in two families with bilateral clefts 1–13 who had ALX4 gene mutation. We could hypothesize that the clefting in nasoschisis would be related to an excess of apoptosis of NCCs, whether in cleft 2–12, which follows a pretty similar path but is expressed as hypoplasia more than as cleft, would be related to a lack of migration. Ullah [8] interestingly found a splice variant in the ALX1 gene, responsible for a cleft 1–13 phenotype, when ALX1, 3, and 4 mutations use to yield medial cleft phenotypes. Meloni [9] also reported a novel ALX4 mutation with a cleft 1–13 phenotype.

Savastano reported [10] a case of cleft 1 associated with holoprosencephaly related to a mutation of the ZIC2 gene and conducted research for nasal clefts in the published cases of ZIC2. This research yielded 3 cases with a nasal cleft in a population of 171 affected by a mutation of ZIC2 mutations. ZIC2 protein acts as a modulator of the hedgehog and nodal pathways. The oculoauriculofrontonasal syndrome will be discussed below.

The acromelic frontonasal dysostosis, which displays the features of bilateral cleft 1–3 frequently associated with a cleft 0, is due to a mutation of the ZSWIM6 gene, which is involved in the HH pathway [11].

5.4 Cases From Literature (Table 5.1)

The research in literature with terms such as cleft 13, cleft 1, and nasoschisis does not bring many matches, so we had to comb through the 6486 matches for "nasal clefts" in PubMed. Single cases are seldom reported, and very few analyses of large series of rare clefts are available. Other cases were found during research through the 212 matches for the frontonasal keyword dysplasia. References of cases can be found in Table 5.1, third column.

5.4.1 Analyses of Large Series

Talking about large series, we found three: Ortiz Monasterio's one in Mexico, David's one in Australia, and Tessier's one in France.

The original Tessier's series used for his inaugural publication [1] was of 336 patients whom 76 were Treacher-Collins syndrome (TCS). Since we now remove TCS from the field of rare clefts, it left 260 genuine rare clefts. The number of clefts 1–13 is not specified.

Table 5.1 Literature series

Case Number	Author	Ref.	Sex	Side	Pictures	CT scan	Severity right side		Severity left side		Hypertelorism	Appendage	Associated facial cleft	Associated craniofacial malformation	Others association
							Soft tissue	Bone and cart	Soft tissue	Bone and cart					
1	Agrawal	[13]	m	l	y	n			a	abc	n	y	n		
2	Agrawal		f	l	n	n			a	abc	n	y	n		
3	Agrawal		F	r	y	n	a	a			n		n		
4	Altuntas	[14]	F	l	y	y			a		I		n	Choanal atresia	
5	Berndorfer	[15]		l	y	n			a	abc	n	y	n		
6	Berndorfer			l	y	n			abcd	abcd	III		n		
7	Bilen	[16]	m	r	y	y	a	a			n	n	n		
8	Bilgen	[17]	F	r	y	n	a	a			n	n	n		
9	Bütow	[18]		r	y	n	a	a			n	n	n		
10	Chaichoompol	[19]	f	r	y	n	ab	ab			n	y	UCL same side		
11	Ghareeb	[20]	m	r	y	n	abc	abc			n	n	n		
12	Fijałkowska	[21]	f	l									n		
12	Fijałkowska		f	l									n		
14	Fijałkowska		f	l									n		
15	Fijałkowska		m	l								y	n		
16	Fijałkowska		m	l								y	n		
17	Fijałkowska		f	r									n		
18	Fijałkowska		f	r									n		
19	Gargano	[22]	m	r	y	n	ab				n	n	n		
20	Reddy	[23]											n		
21	Reddy												n		

(continued)

Table 5.1 (continued)

Case Number	Author	Ref.	Sex	Side	Pictures	CT scan	Severity right side		Severity left side		Hypertelorism	Appendage	Associated facial cleft	Associated craniofacial malformation	Others association
							Soft tissue	Bone and cart	Soft tissue	Bone and cart					
22	Reddy												n		
23	Reddy												n		
24	Gupta	[24]	m	r	y	y	ab	ab			n	y	BCL	Microphthalmia colobomatous cyst	
25	Hallak	[25]	m	l	y	n			a		n		n	Supernumerary nostril	
26	Huang	[26]	m	l	y	y			abcd	abcd	III		n	Microphthalmia CFM	Chromosomal abnomaly
27	Jhamb	[27]	f	l	y	y			ab	ab	n	n	UCL same side		
28	Jian	[28]	m	l	y	n			a		n		UCL	Supernumerary nostril	Right
29	Jinka	[29]	f	r									n		
30	Jinka		f	l									n		
31	Jinka		m	l									n		
32	Jinka		f	l									n		
33	Jinka		m	r									n		
34	Jinka			l									n		
35	Jinka			l									n		
36	Jinka		f	l									n		
37	Jinka		f	l									n		
38	Jinka		m	l									n		
39	Jinka		m	b	n	n							n		

40	Jinka		m	r	n	n	abcd	abcd			y		n		
41	Kannan	[30]	m	r	y	n	a	a			n	n	n	N	N
42	Kobayashi	[31]	m	l	y	n			ab	ab	n	y	Cleft 0	Epignathus	
43	Boekhoff	[32]	m	l	y	n			ab	ab	n	n	n	Frontonasal encephalocele	N
44	Kurul	[33]	m	r	y	n	a	a			n	y	n	Supernumerary nostril	
45	Maes	[34]	m	l	y	n			abc	abc	n	n	n		N
46	Maisel	[35]	m	l	y	n			ab	ab	n	y	n		
47	Van der Meulen	[36]	m	r	y	y	abc	abc			n	n	UCL same side		
48-217	Monasterio	[37]													
218	Mullin	[38]	f	b	y	n	abcd	abcd	abcd	abcd	II	n	n		
219	Nayak	[39]	f	l	y	n			ab	ab	II	n	cleft 0		
220	Newman	[40]	f	l	y	n			a	a	n	y	n		
221	Newman		f	r	y	n	a	a			n	y	n		
222	Newman		f	[illegible]	y	n			ab	ab	n	n	n		
223	Newman		m	r	y	n	ab	ab			n	n	n		
224	Novaković	[41]	m	r	y	n	a	a			n	n	n		
225	Novaković		f	l	y	n			a	a	n	n	n		
226	Ohsaki	[42]	m	l	y	n			ab	ab	n	y	n		
227	Patel	[43]	f	l	y	n			a	a	n	y	n		
228	Reddy	[23]	f	l	y	n			ab	ab	n	y	n		
229	Ozek	[44]	f	r	y	y	abc	abc			I	y	UCL opposite side	Syndactyly	
230	Savastano	[10]	m	l	n	n			a	a	n	y	n	Holoprosencephaly	ZIC2 mutation
231-244	Rashid	[45]													

(continued)

Table 5.1 (continued)

Case Number	Author	Ref.	Sex	Side	Pictures	CT scan	Severity right side		Severity left side		Hypertelorism	Appendage	Associated facial cleft	Associated craniofacial malformation	Others association
							Soft tissue	Bone and cart	Soft tissue	Bone and cart					
245	Schweckendiek	[46]	m	r	y	n	ab	ab			n	y	n		
246	Shewmake	[47]	m	l	y	n			a	a	n	y	n		
247	Shewmake		m	r	y	n	abcd	abcd			I	y	n		
248	Smith	[11]	m	r	y	n	a	a			n	y	n		
249	Stupka	[48]	m	l	y	n	ab	ab			n	y	n		Miscarriage
250	Temel	[49]	f	l	y	n			a	a	n	n	n		
251	Temel		m	r	y	n	ab	ab			n	y	n		
252	Gupta	[24]	m	l	y	n			ab	ab	n	n	n		
253	Chapchay	[50]	f	r									n		
254	Chapchay		m	l									n		
255	Chapchay		f	r									n		
256	Chapchay		m	r								y	n		
257	Chapchay		m	r									n		
258-274	Li	[51]													
275	Mutav	[52]	m	l	y	n			a	a	n	n	n		
276-278	Thomson	[53]	f	l	y	n			a	a	n	n	n		
279	Tiwari	[54]	m	l	y	y			abcd	abcd	I	y	n		
280	Van der Meulen	[55]	f	r	y	y	abcd	abcd			III	n	n		
281	van der Meulen		m	r	y	y	abcd	abcd			II	n	BCLP-Cleft 10 right		
282	Addona	[56]	m	l	n	y			abcd	abcd	III	n	BCLP-Cleft 10 right	Exencephaly cerebral malformations	ABS syndactyly ectrodactyly

283	Karam	[57]		r	n	n	abcd	abcd					cleft 0	Epibulbar dermoid	
284	Becerra-Solano	[58]	f	r	y	n	abcd	abcd			III	n	Cleft3 homolateral	Hydrocephaly	ABS
285	Becerra-Solano		f	-	y	n	abcd	abcd			III	n	BCLP		ABS limb costovertebral
286	Becerra-Solano			b	y	n	abcd	abcd	abcd	abcd	III	n	BCLP	Exencephaly cerebral malformations	
287	Becerra-Solano		f	r	y	y	abcd	abcd			n	n	ucl same side		
288	Casey	[59]	m	l	y	n			abcd	abcd	II	n	ucl same side	CMF bilat epibulbar dermoid	
289	Edwards	[60]	f	b	y	n	abcd	abcd	abcd	abcd	III	n	n	Epibulbar dermoid	
290	Ergin	[61]	f	r	y	n			abcd	abcd	III	n	ucl opposite side	Mental retardation	
291	Fontaine	[62]	f	r	y	n	abcd	abcd			III	n	UCLP homolateral cleft 10 left	CMF bilat epibulbar dermoid	
292	Francesconi	[63]	f	r	y	n	ab	abcd			II		n		
293	Reddy	[23]	m	r	y	n	ab	abcd			II	y	n		
294	Guion-Almeida	[64]	m	l	y	n			ab	abcd	I	n	n		
295	Guion-Almeida		f	r	y	y			abc	abcd	III	n	UCLP homolateral cleft 4 cleft7	CMF epibulbar dermoid	

(continued)

Table 5.1 (continued)

Case Number	Author	Ref.	Sex	Side	Pictures	CT scan	Severity right side: Soft tissue	Severity right side: Bone and cart	Severity left side: Soft tissue	Severity left side: Bone and cart	Hypertelorism	Appendage	Associated facial cleft	Associated craniofacial malformation	Others association
296	Huang	[26]	m	l	y	y			ab	abcd	III	n	UCLP homolateral cleft 10 cleft 7	CMF microphthalmia	Duplication 1q31.1
297	Kasturi	[65]	m	r	y	n	a	abcd	a	abcd	I	n	n	Epibulbar dermoid	
298–301	Kayserili	[7]	m	b	y		a	abcd	a	abcd	II	n	n		ALX4 mutation
	Kayserili		m	b	y		a	abcd	a	abcd	II	n	n		ALX4 mutation
	Kayserili		m	b	y		a	abcd	a	abcd	II	n	n		ALX4 mutation
	Kayserili		m	b	y		a	abcd	a	abcd	II	n	n		ALX4 mutation
302	Khan	[66]	m	l	y	n			a	abcd	III	n	n	Frontal encephalocele	
303	Khan		m	b	y	n	a	abcd	a	abcd	II	n	n	Bilateral lipomeningocele	Familial (mother)304
304	Rüegg	[67]	m	b	y	y	a	abcd	a	abcd	III	y	cleft 0		
305	Rüegg		m	l	y	n			abc	abcd	III	n	n		
306	Rüegg		f	r	y	n	abc	abcd			III	n	n	Lipomeningocele	

307	Schwenzer	[68]	m	r	y	n	abc	abcd			II	n	BCLP	Bilateral microphthalmia	
308	Ferreira da silva	[69]	f	b	y	y	abc	abcd	abc	abcd	III	n	BCLP	Bilateral encephalocele limb bands	ABS
309	Heddie	[70]	f	ɔ	y	n	a	a	a	a	n	n	n	Microphthalmia bilateral	
310	Fontaine	[62]		r	y	n	abc	abcd			III	n	UCLP homolat-eral cleft 10 left	Microphthalmia	
311	Bello	[71]		b	y	y	abc	abcd	ab	abcd	III	n		Ear-shaped phe-notype	
312	Kapoor	[72]		ŀ	y	n	ab		a		I	n	UCLP homolat-eral	Microphthalmia bilateral	
313	Sharma	[73]		b	y	n	a	abcd	a	abcd	III	n	Cleft 0	Microphthalmia hair peak	Callosal agenesis
314	Warkany	[74]	f	b	y	n	a	abcd	a	abcd	III	n	Cleft 0	Hair peak	Callosal agenesis-limb defect
315	Warkany		f	b	y	n	a	abcd	a	abcd	III		Cleft 0	Hair peak	Callosal agenesis-limb defect
316	Schlund	[75]		b	y	y	a	abcd	a	abcd	III	n	Cleft 0	Hair peak	
317	Tunc	[76]	f	l	y	n			ab	abcd	III	n	UCLP homolat-eral	CFM hair peak	

(continued)

Table 5.1 (continued)

Case Number	Author	Ref.	Sex	Side	Pictures	CT scan	Severity right side		Severity left side		Hypertelorism	Appendage	Associated facial cleft	Associated craniofacial malformation	Others association
							Soft tissue	Bone and cart	Soft tissue	Bone and cart					
320	Meloni	[9]	m	b	y	y	a	ab	a	ab	II	n	Encephalocele occipital	Polymalformation	ALX4 mutation
321	Sunita Vegesna	[77]	f	b	y	n	a	abcd	a	abcd	III	n		Occipital defect-microphthalmia	
322	Kean	[78]	m	b	y	n		cd		cd	II	n			Corrugated nose
323	Lehalle	[79]		b				cd		cd	II	n			TENM3 mutation limb anomalies
324	Lehalle			b				cd		cd	I	n			Limb anomalies
325	Lehalle			b				cd		cd	II	n			Limb anomalies
326	Lehalle			b				cd		cd	II	n			Limb anomalies
327	Lehalle			b				cd		cd	III	n			Limb anomalies
328	Lehalle			b				cd		cd	III	n			Limb anomalies
329	Guion-almeida	[80]	m	b	y	n		cd		cd	II	n			Poland syndrome

330	Dubey	[81]	m	b	y	n	a	abcd	a	abcd	III	y	BCLP	Microphthalmia	Mental retardation
331	Balci	[82]	f	r	y	y	a	abcd			III			Frontal encephalocele	
332	Stevens	[83]	m	b	y	n		cd		cd	III	n			Chromosomal anomaly
333	Meguid	[84]	m	b	y	y	a	abcd	a	abcd	III	n		Frontal encephalocele callus lipoma	Fallot's tetralogy
334	Fryburg	[85]	m	b	y	n	a	abcd	a	abcd	III	n	Cleft0		Familial FND
335	Sedano	[86]	f	b	y	n	abc	abcd	abc	abcd	III	n	UCLP	Ear-shaped phenotype	
336	Heddie			b	y	n	a	abcd	a	abcd	III	n	Cleft0		
337	Lehalle	[87]		l	y	n			a	a	n	y			
338	Lehalle			l	y	n			ab	abcd	I	n			
339	Lehalle			r	y	n	a	a			I	n	Cleft10		
340	Lehalle			l	y	n			a	a	III	y	Cleft8	Epibulbar dermoid	
341	Lehalle			r	y	n	ab	ab			II	y	Cleft10		

Adelaide series of David in 1989 [12] was of 253 patients, including 33 TCS and 55 frontonasal encephaloceles, and 94 craniofacial microsomia (CFM), which lets 71 authentic rare clefts. This paper did not specify the relative number of clefts 1–13. Later, in 1996, Moore again analyzed the north-Adelaide series [88]; there were then 170 patients, totaling 488 clefts. 24 were cleft 1 and 25 clefts 13. They were compared in this paper with the Mexico series published in 1987, which reported the repartition of 345 clefts in 171 patients [37].

In the above publication, we found some confusion between cleft 2 and 1 when describing the defect.

In 2008, Monasterio published a more extensive series [89] of 495 patients, totalizing 826 clefts. TCS was included and CFM excluded. In this series, the number of clefts 1 was 81, and the number 13 was 81.

5.4.2 Analyses of Isolated Cases or Small Series

The cases in which a sufficient amount of data was available in the literature to be exploited are displayed in Table 5.1. When we merge the extensive series of Monasterio, David, Rashid, and Li with other reports of a single case or small series, we can say that at least 341 cleft 1–13 cases are known. We made our statistics for this study upon reports with helpful imaging. Thus, we used the data from 156 cases.

5.5 Our Clinical Series (Table 5.2)

We gathered the files of 50 cases for this study, which are reported in Table 5.2. As a whole, our description will be based on 206 descriptions of clefts 1–13.

Table 5.2 Clinical series

Patient #	Sex	Type	Side	Nasal tip	Nasal dorsum	Glabella	Hypertelorism	Associated cleft	Associated facial	Associated cranial	Other	Ct scan	MRI	Surgery
1	M	1-13	R	Clefted	Clefted	Enlarged	Mild	BCLP			None	Yes	No	Nose
2	f	1	R	Clefted	Normal	Normal	Absent			None	None	No	No	Nose
3	f	1	R	Clefted	Normal	Normal	Absent			None	None	No	No	Nose
4	m	1-13	R	Clefted	Clefted	Clefted	Severe	10r				No	No	
5	f	1-13	L	Clefted	Enlarged	Enlarged	Mild	UCL; 10r	Choanal atresia		None	Yes	No	Hypertelorism
6	m	1-13	L	Clefted	Clefted	Enlarged	Severe		CFM					
7	m	1	R	Clefted	Enlarged	Enlarged	Light	UCLr	CFM	None	None	No	No	
8	f	1-13	L	Clefted	Clefted	Clefted	Severe	UCLl				Yes		Hypertelorism
9	m	13	R	Normal	Normal	Enlarged	Mild	10l-7	CFM			No	No	
10	m	1	R	Clefted	Normal	Normal	Absent		CFM					Nose
11	m	1	R	Clefted	Normal	Normal	Absent					No	No	
12	m	13	Bil.=	Normal	Normal	Enlarged	Mild					Yes	No	
13	f	1-13	L	Clefted	Clefted	Clefted	Severe	10l	CFM			Yes	No	Hypertelorism
14	m	1	R	Clefted	Enlarged	Enlarged	Light							
15	m	1	R	Clefted	Normal	Normal	Absent							Nose
16	m	1-13	Bil.=	Normal	Enlarged	Enlarged	Mild					Yes	No	Hypertelorism
17	m	1	L	Clefted	Normal	Normal	Absent							Nose
18	f	1-13	R	Clefted	Clefted	Enlarged	Severe					Yes		Hypertelorism
19	m	13	bil.=	Normal	Enlarged	Enlarged	Severe					Yes		Hypertelorism
20	m	1-13	Bil.=	Clefted	Enlarged	Enlarged	Severe	BCLP	Choanal atresia			Yes		Hypertelorism
21	m	1	D	Clefted	Enlarged	Enlarged	Light					Yes		
22	m	1	D	Clefted	Clefted	Normal	Absent					Yes		Nose

(continued)

Table 5.2 (continued)

Patient #	Sex	Type	Side	Nasal tip	Nasal dorsum	Glabella	Hypertelorism	Associated cleft	Associated facial	Associated cranial	Other	Ct scan	MRI	Surgery
23	m	1-13	L	Enlarged	Enlarged	Enlarged	Severe		Choanal atresia-dermoid cyst-microphthalmia			Yes		Hypertelorism
24	f	1-13	L	Clefted	Enlarged	Enlarged	Mild	10l				No		
25	f	1-13	R	Clefted	Enlarged	Enlarged	Light					No		
26	m	1-13	R	Clefted	Enlarged	Enlarged	Absent					No	Yes	Nose
27	m	1-13	L	Clefted	Enlarged	Enlarged	Severe	10l-7l-0	CMF			Yes	No	
28	m	1-13	R	Clefted	Clefted	Enlarged	Severe	10r				Yes		
29	f	1-13	L	Clefted	Clefted	Enlarged	Severe	10l			None	Yes	No	Hypertelorism
30	f	1	R	Clefted	Normal	Normal	Absent	UCLr				No	No	Nose
31	m	13	R	Normal	Normal	Enlarged	Mild	7, 10	CFM					
32	m	1-13	L	Clefted	Normal	Enlarged	Light		Ethmoidal encephalocele					Encephalocele
33	f	1-13	L	Clefted	Clefted	Clefted	Severe			Appendage along path				
34		1		Clefted	Enlarged	Normal	Mild	3left-10 left						
35	f	1-13	R	Clefted	Enlarged	Enlarged	Severe			Hairline peak				
36	m	1	bil.=	Clefted	Normal	Normal	Light			Appendages				
37	m	1-13	L	Clefted	Enlarged	Enlarged	Mild			Hairline peak				
38	m	1	L	Clefted	Normal	Normal	Absent							

39	m	1	R	Clefted	Normal	Normal	Absent			Hamartoma nasal dorsum				
40	m	1	L	Clefted	Normal	Normal	Absent			Appendage				
41		1-13	bil.=	Clefted	Enlarged	Enlarged	Severe							
42	m	1-13	L	Clefted	Enlarged	Enlarged	Severe	10l-10r-9L	Ocular malformation					
43	f	1-13	L	Clefted	Enlarged	Enlarged	Light							
44	m	1-13	bil.=	Clefted	Enlarged	Enlarged	Severe	cleft 0						
45	f	1-13	bil.=	Clefted	Enlarged	Enlarged	Severe	cleft 0	Epibulbar dermoid					
46	m	1-13	R	Clefted	Enlarged	Enlarged	Mild		Frontal lipoma or encephalocele?					
47	f	1-13	L	Clefted	Clefted	Clefted	Severe							Ear-shaped phenotype
48	f	1-13	L	Clefted	Clefted	Enlarged	Mild							Ear-shaped phenotype
49	f	1-13	L	Clefted	Enlarged	Enlarged	Mild		CFM					Hypertelorism
50	f	1-13	bil.=	Clefted	Clefted	Enlarged	Severe	BCLP						

5.6 The Features of Cleft 1–13 (Fig. 5.3a, b)

5.6.1 The Soft Tissues in Cleft 1–13

For this research, we sort the cases according to the extent of the cleft (Fig. 5.3b): (**a**) between the tip and the alar lobule, (**b**) the dorsum up to the skeleton, (**c**) between the nasal bone and the medial orbital process of the maxillary (**d**) upward through the medial orbital process of the frontal bone toward the skull.

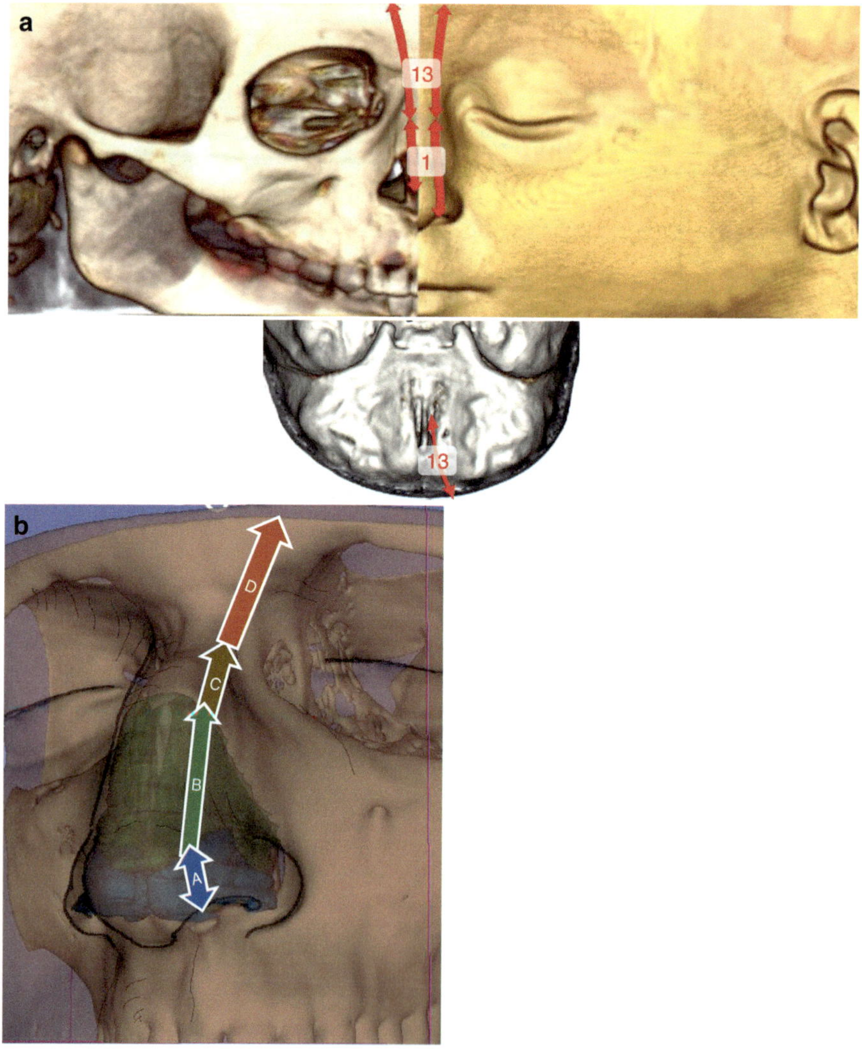

Fig. 5.3 (**a**) Proposed path for cleft 1-13. (**b**) Scoring the path of cleft 1-13. A, B, C, and D name the extent of the cleft

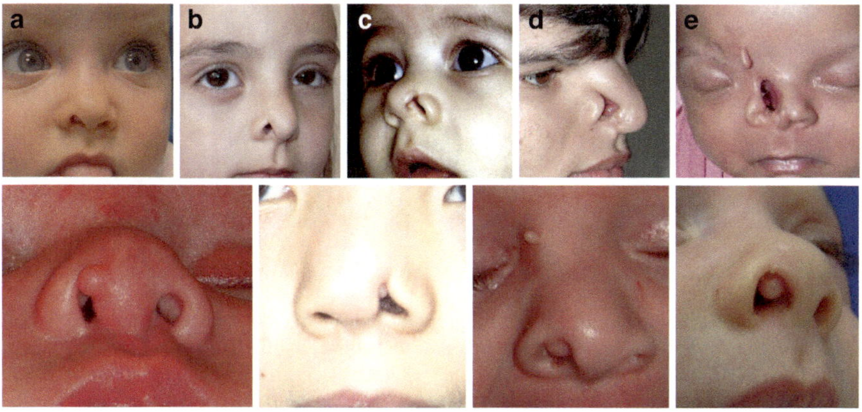

Fig. 5.4 Top: Examples of different severity of cleft 1. See the upward rotation of the alar lobule which shortens the lateral edge. (**a**) Minor notch associated with an appendage. (**b**) Light cleft 1. (**c**) Medium cleft 1. (**d**) Severe cleft associated with cleft 13. (**e**) Complete cleft 1. Bottom: Appendages associated with cleft 1

5.6.1.1 Cleft 1 (Fig. 5.4)

In the chapter on etiology and classification, we have asserted that the cleft lip would be considered an association with rare clefts and not a part of it. Thus, the cleft 1–13 path starts from the nostril. The nasal part of the cleft, alternatively called "nasoschisis", splits the alar rim through the soft triangle separating the alar lobule from the nasal tip. Then after it crosses the dorsum toward the frontonasal suture, this part of the path is cleft 1. The lateral edge of the cleft is always shortened. Thus, the alar lobule is displaced upward.

There is frequently an appendage associated with cleft 1; we found it 37 times out of 206, most of them in isolated cleft 1. Very few were observed in association with cleft 1–13. The only occurrences we found was a picture of a case reported by Monasterio [37] and another in Fig. 5.2b.

5.6.1.2 Cleft 13 (Fig. 5.5)

On the path of cleft 13, true cleft, which means skin disruption, does not occur further than onto the frontal bone; above, the teguments are enlarged, and the path is medial to the eyebrow, which is displaced laterally but left intact. A subcutaneous lipoma, although infrequent, could be observed isolated or associated with an encephalocele if there is a bone defect. The upper part of the path is frequently marked by a hairy peak of the hairline, which could reach as far as the tip of the nasal cleft. We once met a case in which cleft 13 was materialized by a linear subcutaneous defect (Fig. 5.6).

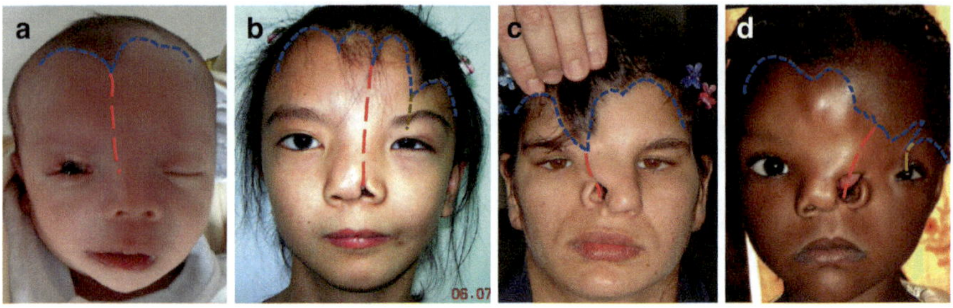

Fig. 5.5 (**a**) Peaks in the hairline. Blue dot line is the hair lie, red dot line is the cleft path, brown dot line is associated cleft. (**a**) Cleft 13 right associated with cleft 10. (**b**) Cleft 1-13 left associated with cleft 10 left. (**c**) Cleft 1-13 right. (**d**) Cleft 1-13 left associated with cleft 10 left

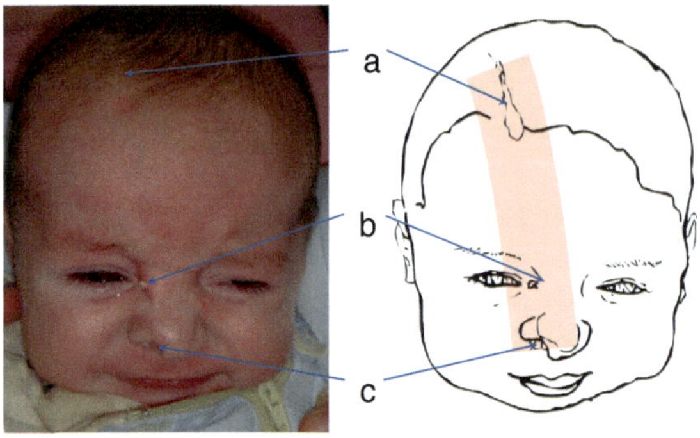

Fig. 5.6 Cleft 13 path materialized by a linear subcutaneous defect. Red band displays the course of the cleft. (**a**) Subcutaneous defect. (**b**) Appendage. (**c**) Nasal cleft and appendage

5.6.2 The Skeleton in Cleft 1–13 (Figs. 5.7 and 5.8)

Considering the cartilages of the nose, the dome of the alar cartilage is missing in cleft 1a, and the triangular cartilage is interrupted in cleft 1ab. In cleft 1abc, the skeletal course wounds between the nasal bone, medially and the ascending orbital process of the maxilla. The borderline between cleft 1 and 13 is the frontonasal suture, after which cleft 13 goes through the medial orbital process of the frontal bone.

The path on the frontal bone is oriented upward and laterally, sometimes leaving room for an encephalocele.

On the skull base, it runs through the olfactive groove, as said by Tessier, but we too noticed that the anterior part of the lateral ethmoidal mass is enlarged.

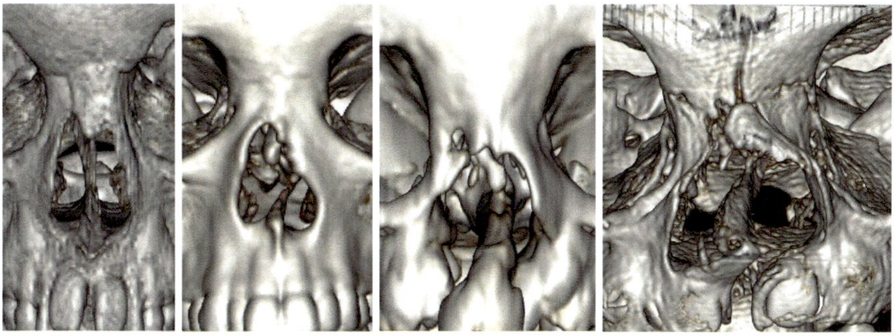

Fig. 5.7 The skeletal path of cleft 1

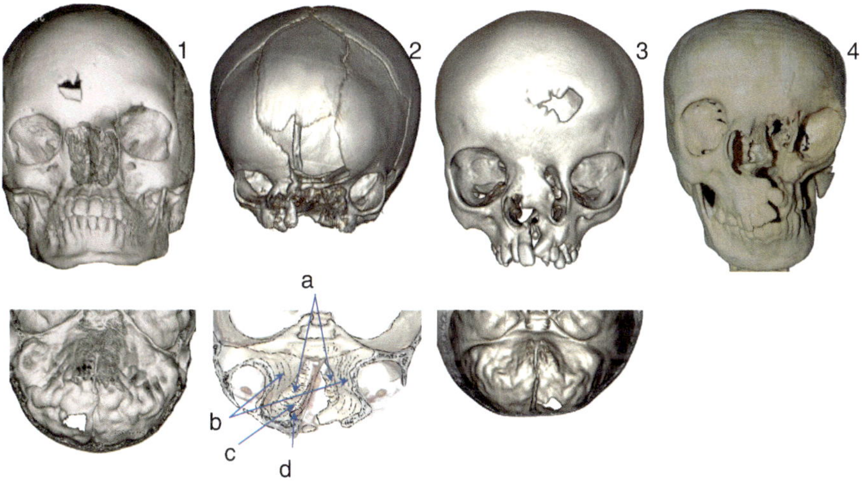

Fig. 5.8 The skeletal path of cleft 13. Skull base image belong to the above skull. 1 and 3 are pure cleft 1-13, 2 and 4 are associated with cleft lip. 3 is associated with a cleft 0. (a) Roof of the lateral mass of the ethmoid. (b) Orbital roof. (c) Cribriform area. (d) Crista galli

5.6.3 Hypertelorism in Cleft 1–13

Not surprisingly, hypertelorism was more frequent when the soft tissue cleft was more extensive, but it could be met even within the 1a group, and some patients with 1–13 abcd could be free of hypertelorism. Out of the 206 documented cases (DC) (literature plus our series cases), we recognized 18 grade I hypertelorism, 32 grade II, and 52 grade III. All the patients with bilateral cleft 13 had hypertelorism.

5.6.4 *Anomalies Associated with Cleft 1–13*

5.6.4.1 Association with Other Clefts

In the 206 DC series, 72 patients have associated clefts.

- Cleft 10 was the most frequent. It was encountered 15 times, 20% being a high rate; the coincidence would not be accidental but mostly related to a common mechanism and almost realizing a specific phenotype.
- Cleft 0 was associated 15 times. It has the same frequency, and its association with bilateral cleft 1–13 is a striking coincidence since 10 of the 15 cleft 0 were associated with severe bilateral cleft 1–13.
- Cleft 7 was found seven times in the setting of craniofacial microsomia (CFM).
- Usual cleft lips were present in 32 patients: 11 bilateral (BCL) and 21 unilateral (UCL). Amazingly, four patients had their cleft lip on the opposite side than the cleft 1–13. Remember that we consider cleft lip as an association and not a labial continuation of cleft 1.

5.6.4.2 Association with CFM

We found in the 206 DC 13 cases matching the requirements to be considered as being in the CFM setting but curiously, four more patients had dermoid epibulbar without other symptoms of CFM. As seen in other rare clefts, it is a frequent occurrence. We would believe that the description of oculoauriculofrontonasal dysplasia (OAFNS) corresponds to this association. OAFNS is named and found in literature: [76, 87, 90–92]. Although incompletely described, some pictures display features of cleft 1–13 and all the authors consider the nasal cleft as a major feature for the diagnosis. Till today, oculoauriculofrontonasal dysplasia stays a pure clinical appellation, which does not match a specific etiology. In spite of extensive exome sequencing, no candidate gene has been recognized. In consequence, we wonder if a specific appellation is worth and henceforth, we will name those cases as the association of cleft 1–13 with CMF.

5.6.4.3 Other Malformations

- We found in unilateral clefts 13 an abnormal ossification of the falx cerebri two times.
- ABS affected four patients in the literature but none of our clinical series.
- Three patients had choanal atresia.
- Eleven patients had microphthalmia.
- Nine patients had encephalocele.
- Two patients had exencephaly, and both had ABS.
- Eleven patients had limb anomalies.
- One case of holoprosencephaly (ZIC mutation).

5.7 Phenotypes of Clefts 1–13

Even if we agree with Tessier's statement: "*Other craniofacial clefts [...] manifest their degrees of completeness in highly variable ways. They may happen to be complete at one end and incomplete at the other; they may be complete at both ends (lip and eyelid) and incomplete in their intermediate segment*" when looking at our cases as well as to the pictures of published cases of literature when it comes to cleft 1–13, we distinguish four main phenotypes:

- Isolated cleft 1 (Fig. 5.9): they are pure nasoschisis, reaching the worst the frontonasal suture but staying below; most of the time, but with some rare exceptions (see above), intercanthal distance is average; frontal area and the hairline are normal. They are quoted in our research as 1a, 1ab, and 1abc. Out of the 154 (DC), 83 were this type, representing 56%. This has to be a bias due to the keywords used for the literature research since, in our clinical series alone, the ratio is 15 out of 47 (34%).
- Unilateral clefts 1–13 (Fig. 5.10): a total of 49 patients had a unilateral cleft 1–13, 26 to the right side and 23 to the left side.

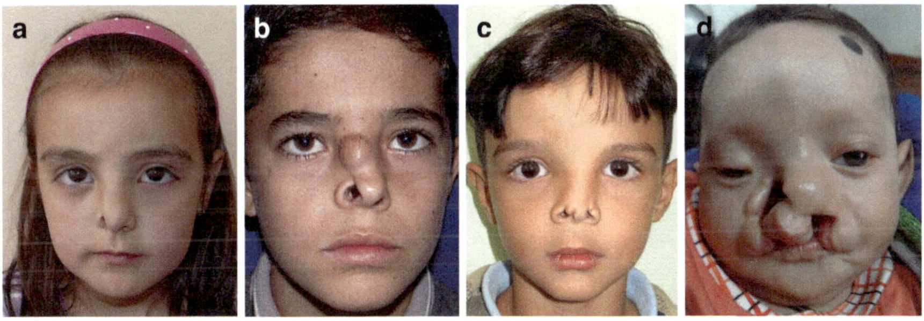

Fig. 5.9 Phenotypes of cleft 1. (**a**) Single right cleft 1. (**b**) Right cleft 1 and dorso-nasal hamartoma. (**c**) Bilateral cleft l and appendages. (**d**) Right cleft 1 associated with bilateral cleft lip

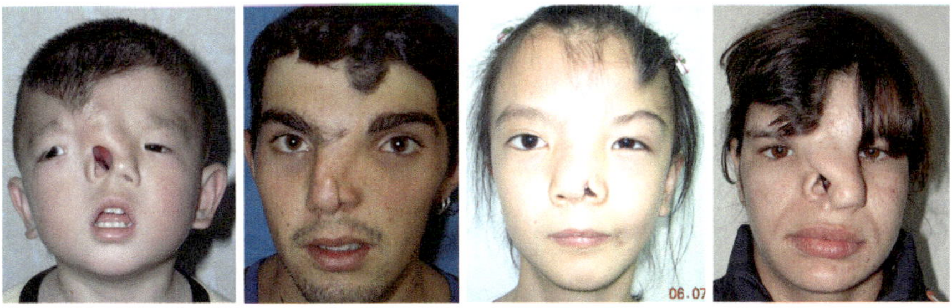

Fig. 5.10 Unilateral cleft 1-13. Four examples of unilateral cleft 1-13, each of them has a paramedian hairline peak. The two on the right have an associated cleft 10 (hairline peak and eyebrow anomaly

- Isolated cleft 13: they are pure orbital dystopia with paramedian frontal defect leaving intact the eyebrow. In our clinical series of 47, only 3 patients were in this condition, but we could not find such patients in the literature. Those cases are probably indexed with cleft 14 elsewhere.
- Bilateral cleft 1–13 (Fig. 5.11): the typical aspect of the frontonasal dysplasia in the acromelic frontonasal dysostosis syndrome due to a ZSWIM6 gene mutation.
- Bilateral symmetric cleft 13: this condition was found 16 times. The hypertelorism is constant, and this condition is easily confused with cleft 14.
- Corrugated nose (Fig. 5.12).

One of us (Nivaldo Alonso) has been struck by a particular phenotype of frontonasal dysplasia in which the hypertelorism was associated with vertical folds of skin of the nasal dorsum. He named it the "corrugated nose." We paid specific attention to this point during our research. We have 14 patients displaying this feature. We had high-resolution CT scans for 5 of them, which revealed that the skeletal defects were those of cleft 13: between the nasal bone and frontal process of the maxillary, then with a widening of the anterior part of the lateral mass of the ethmoidal bone, as described by Tessier. It is confusing that the frontal hairline presents a median

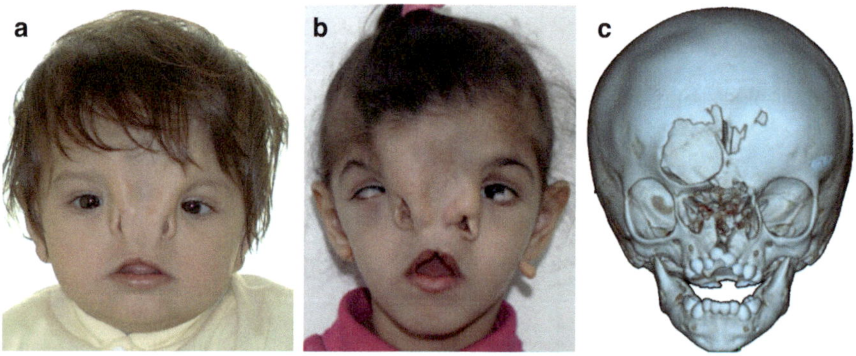

Fig. 5.11 Bilateral 1-13. (**a**) Pure bilateral cleft 1-13. (**b**) Bilateral cleft 1-13 associated with cleft 0. (**c**) CT scan of the patient b

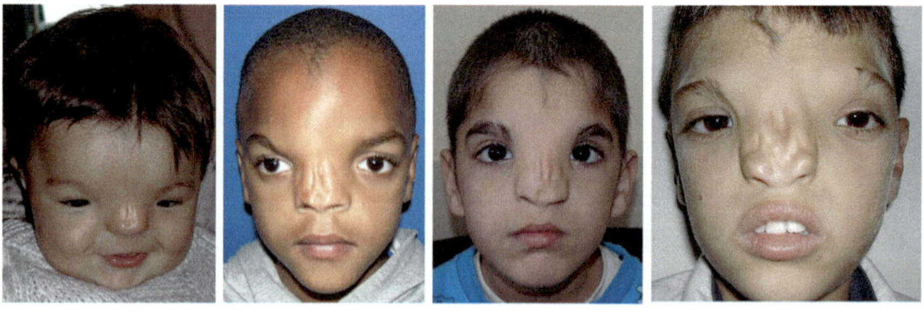

Fig. 5.12 Corrugated nose. Four examples of corrugated nose

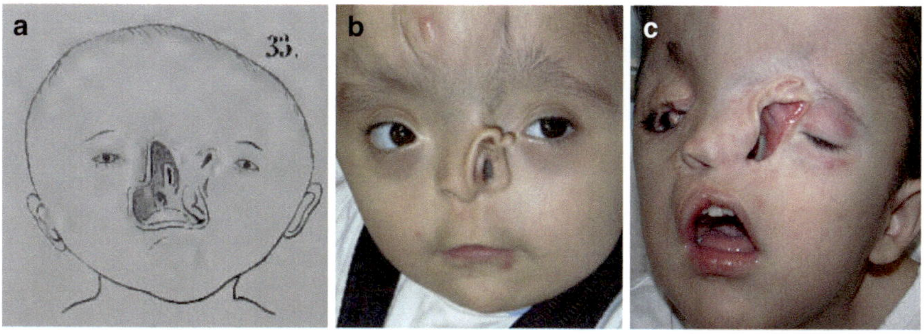

Fig. 5.13 Ear-shaped nose. (**a**) Otto's patient reported by Förster. (**b**, **c**) clinical examples

peak, when a bilateral paramedian would be expected. Lehalle [79] published a series of 6 patients displaying the features of a corrugated nose (*frontonasal dysplasia with creased nasal ridge*) associated with limb anomalies.

- Ear-shaped nose (Fig. 5.13): during our research about rare clefts affecting the nose, we came across a very unusual condition; the first cases reported were those by Otto [4], after then a case by Geoffroy de saint Hilaire [93], we found 8 more cases in modern literature [15, 58, 61, 68, 69, 89] most of them in the setting of ABS and we have two cases in our series, which, at first we found difficult to assign to one path. The features of this phenotype associate a vertical cleft along the path of cleft 1–13 without an alar remnant left in the lateral edge; the upper extremity is surrounded by a fold of skin that mimics the helix of an external ear.

Whatever the phenotype, any defect along the 1–13 path must lead to a careful examination looking for associated anomalies belonging to its spectrum.

5.8 Differential Diagnosis

As usual, the confusion with the neighboring clefts could be difficult for a precise diagnosis; it is especially true when there is a combination of several clefts in a close location.

5.8.1 Differential Diagnosis with Cleft 2–12 (Fig. 5.14)

As considered above in the very Tessier's description, there is a gray zone between clefts 2 and 1. This is as true as Reddy in a book chapter devoted to rare clefts [94] made the confusion, letting the chapter about cleft 1 without other illustration than an artist's drawing. Several authors reported cases of cleft 1 as cleft 2 like Tiwari [54], Ozek [44], and Altuntas [14].

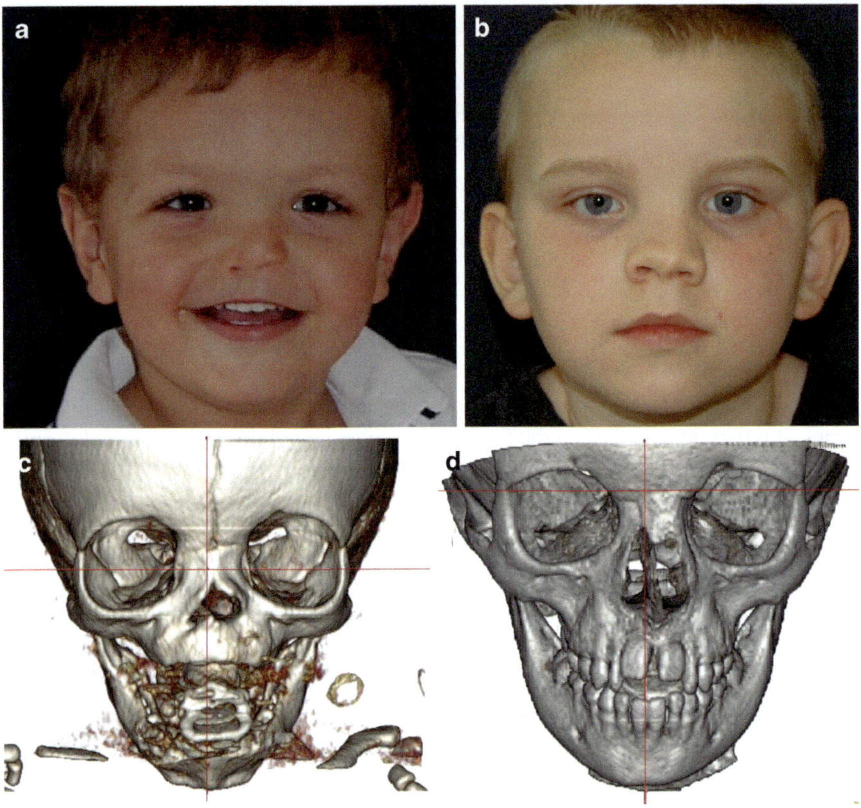

Fig. 5.14 Cleft 2-12 as a differential diagnosis. The clinical aspects are very close, the CT scan show the difference. (**a**, **c**) cleft 2. (**b**, **d**) cleft 1

There is no significant difference between the paths of those two clefts; Tessier wrote that the being of cleft 2 needs to be established. He said that the nasal anomalies of cleft 2 are more related to hypoplasia than cleft and that cleft 2 could come along with proboscis lateralis, supernumerary nostril. Thus, we will use cleft 2–12 to name conditions with hypoplasia ranging from light hypoplasia without notching to heminasal aplasia associated with hypertelorism. Partial nasal hypoplasia with a shrinking of the hypoplastic nose could be interpreted as the cleft of the nostril.

5.8.2 Differential Diagnosis with Cleft 0–14 (Fig. 5.15)

Since Sedano's appellation of frontonasal dysplasia (FND) for a set of malformations occurring in the naming area [86], there is confusion between FND and cleft 14. Sedano distinguished several phenotypes (that he called "facies"), a first in which there was a simple enlargement of the interorbital distance, a second in which

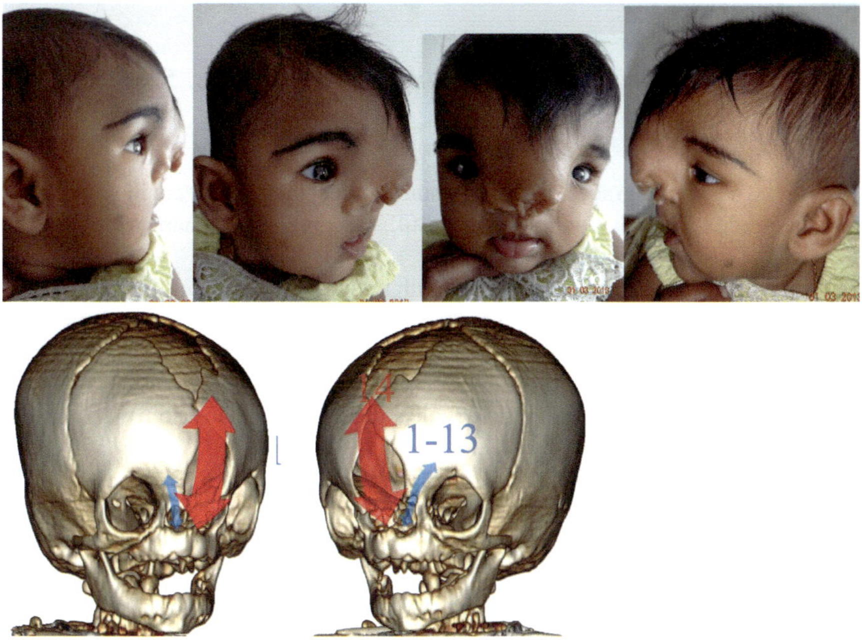

Fig. 5.15 Differential diagnosis. A case with cleft 1-13 associated with cleft 0 for which the diagnosis is very difficult

there is a median defect, a third where the defect is paramedian with a nostril defect, and a fourth that combines the facies of the second and third. According to Sedano, frontonasal dysplasia is not a synonym for cleft 0 and cleft 1–13 is part of the frontonasal dysplastic setting. Thus, it could be a difficult diagnosis when cleft 14 is associated with bilateral cleft 13.

5.8.2.1 In Unilateral Cleft 1–13

It is easy to differentiate unilateral cleft 13 from cleft 14 because of its paramedian situation, except when a cleft 0 is associated with cleft 1–13, a condition that occurred once in our series and four times in our literature review.

5.8.2.2 In Bilateral Cleft 1–13

Bilateral cleft 13 is frequently misdiagnosed as cleft 14 because of the confusion with frontonasal dysplasia discussed above. Bilateral cleft 1–13 are easier to recognize since there are notches of the nostril, but it is confusing. All the most when the bilateral cleft 13 is associated with a Cleft 14, which occurred in one of Rüegg's cases, [67], the same as Pittet's patient [95] and in one of our cases (Fig. 5.15).

5.9 Treatment

5.9.1 Hypertelorism Treatment in Clefts 1–13 Figs. 5.16, 5.17, and 5.18

In some cases with a grade I hypertelorism, an acceptable result could be obtained by addressing the nasal anomalies alone. Still, most of the time, narrowing the orbit is mandatory for a good correction.

Among the many technics proposed, with the progress of team surgery, the transcranial approach has grown very popular in groups of craniofacial surgeons.

We will discuss two procedures: the box-osteotomy and craniofacial bipartition.

Whenever there is an alveolar cleft or an occlusal anomaly such as an endomaxilly, facial bipartition will be the first choice since it will be able to fix at the same time the orbital and maxillary problems.

But the advantages of craniofacial bipartition are as we prefer, even in some cases without occlusal anomalies in young patients when the growth is not over since the occlusion could correct itself or with the help of orthodontics [96].

In bilateral cleft 13, there is no question about performing a bilateral procedure, but for unilateral cleft, the question is raised about performing a unilateral correction. Since we used the vestibular orientation to analyze the craniofacial deformities

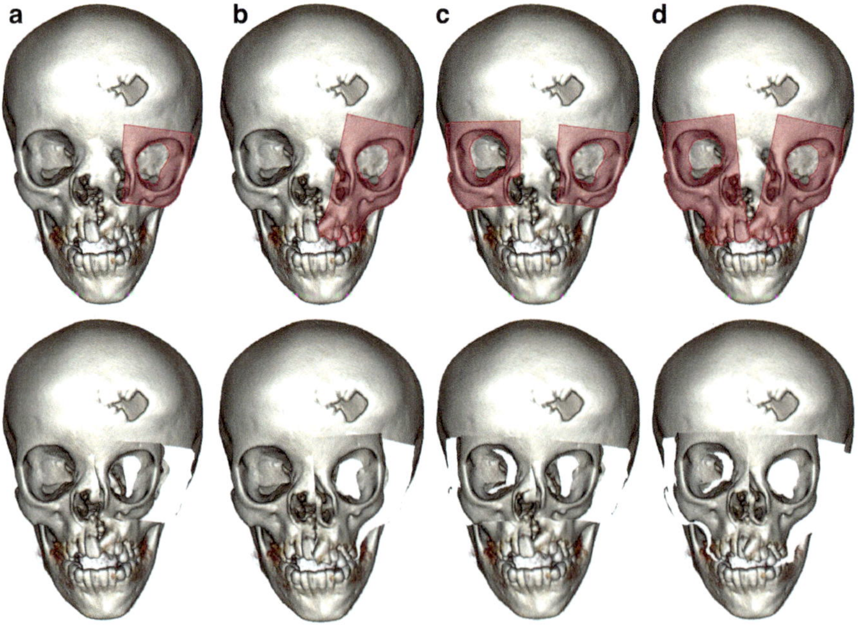

Fig. 5.16 The several ways to fix the hypertelorism. (**a**) Unilateral box-osteotomy. (**b**) Unilateral craniofacial osteotomy. (**c**) Bilateral box-osteotomy. (**d**) Facial bipartition.

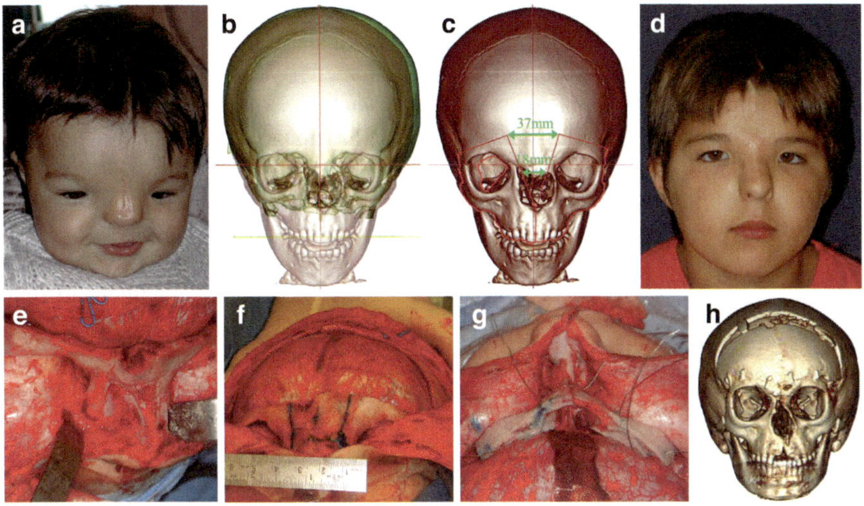

Fig. 5.17 Craniofacial bipartition for bilateral cleft 1-13. (**a**) Patient initial presentation. (**b**) Superposition of patient vestibular oriented scan (red) with a matching normal patient scan (green). (**c**) Preoperative planning. (**d**) Two years post-op. (**e**) Intraoperative view of the interorbital area. (**f**) Marking of the interorbital resection. (**g**) Two halves of the facial skeleton secured altogether. (**h**) Post-op. CT scan

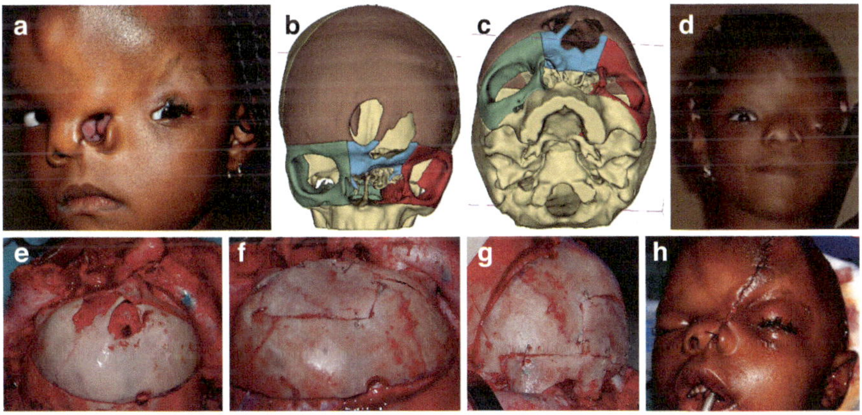

Fig. 5.18 Box osteotomy. (**a**) Initial presentation. (**b, c**) simulation with 3D slicer. (**d**) Two years postoperation. (**e**) Dissection before the osteotomy. (**f, g**) skeletal setting. (**h**) Aspect at the end of procedure

[97] and applied it to those patients, we learned that the contralateral orbit, even if seemingly standard, is displaced, so we now prefer a bilateral mobilization.

In our series of cleft 1–13, a typical bipartition was done three times; a bilateral box-osteotomy was done eight times, a unilateral box-osteotomy two times, and a unilateral craniofacial orbito-maxillary osteotomy one time.

Thanks to advanced medical imaging, precise preoperative planning can be done. We use two procedures. In the first procedure, we start by postprocessing the CT scan with the Horos software (https://horosproject.org/) to get an oriented and scaled volume rendering image of the skeleton, which is then exported as a JPEG file, scaled to the 1/1 ratio and superposed with the image of age matching normal patient (Fig. 5.17b, c).

The second procedure is a 3D simulation performed with the 3D slicer software (https://www.slicer.org/), which is very realistic (Fig. 5.18b, c).

5.9.2 *Nasal Repair in Cleft 1–13*

The technics of nasal reconstruction will differ depending on the presence or absence of associated hypertelorism.

5.9.2.1 Pure Cleft 1 Without Hypertelorism (Figs. 5.19 and 5.20)

Many technics have been described for repairing the isolated nasal cleft with diverse principles and variated drawings. They could be distinguished between z-plasty and rotation-advancement-plasty.

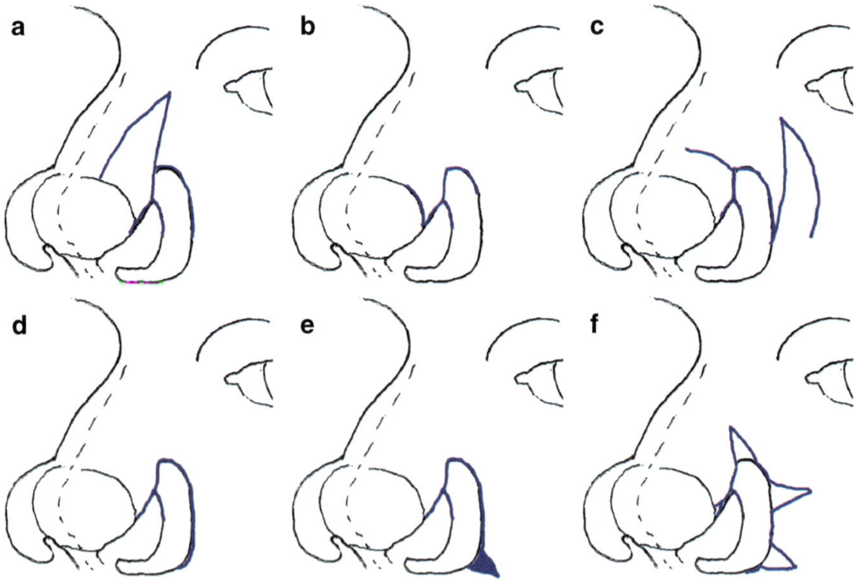

Fig. 5.19 Different designs for correction of the isolated nasal cleft. Z-plasty and rotation. (**a**) Maisels, Boekhoff/Denonvillier, Rashid, Mutaf, Kannan choice of z-plasty. (**b**) Bütow. (**c**) Bilgen. (**d**) Jinka. (**e**) Gupta. Monasterio. (**f**) Li

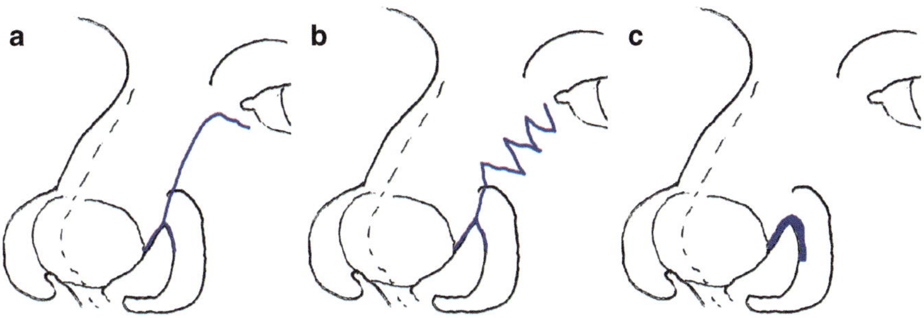

Fig. 5.20 Advancement and direct closure. (**a**) Reddy. (**b**) Temel. (**c**) Direct closure

Z-Plasty and Its Variations

Z-plasty is the more popular procedure; out of the DC, we found it 30 times, but they are only sometimes performed similarly, and the design could differ. The standard part of the design includes an incision along the alar crease to lengthen the lateral edge of the cleft. Still, the position of the triangular flap, which will fulfill the opening of this incision, differs according to the authors.

The vertical triangular flap from the dorsolateral part of the nose is proposed by Maisels [35]. Boekhoff [32] was the first to advocate the former Denonvillier's technic and give an eponym for this operation. This plasty for repairing the congenital alar cleft is a z-plasty in which the triangular flap is harvested vertically from the lateral side of the nose, as in Maisels's procedure. It is the technique Rashid uses for 13 cases [45]. Later, Mutaf claimed to have invented a new technic, which is precisely the same according to the photography of his case, [52]. Kannan [30] used the same technic.

Bütow designed a variation of the z-plasty in which the medial flap is harvested out of the tip of the nose instead of the dorsum.

Kobayashi [31] used the skin from an appendage as a flap to permit the alar rotation. It looks like Agrawal used a similar technique, but his drawing looks a bit confusing [13].

Bilgen [17] designs a vertical flap with a downward hinge out of the cheek.

Rotations Flaps

We found, of the documented cases, six references in which the rotation flap was advocated.

Denonvillier's publication, being misunderstood, was cited to support a different design of pure rotation by Jinka [29], about 13 cases.

Gupta [24] used the same technic of full-thickness rotation of the entire ala associated with Burrow's triangle of resection at its dorsal end.

Li [51] performed a pure rotation of the ala lobule outlined as a trifoliate flap by inserting three small triangular flaps in his drawing.

Advancement Flaps

Reddy [23] published a procedure in which he mobilizes the lateral nasal skin and the alar lobule, ending the upper incision into the inferior palpebra.

Temel [49], among several presented technics in his publication, used an advancement flap outlined by a series of W incisions.

Direct Closure

We found in the literature four examples of direct closure after a simple refreshment of the cleft edges: all four showed poor result.

Grafts

Attempts at solving small nasal clefts with a conchal cartilage graft have been made two times [27], but the result could have been better.

Our Comments About This Nasal Repair and Our Preferred Technic

Definitively we would abandon the ideas of direct closure and indirect correction by using conchal graft because of the poor results.

The analysis of all the cases supports evidence that the lateral edge of the cleft is shortened, thus pleading for bringing in the missing tissue. Thus, loaning those tissues from the lateral edge is not a good idea. So, we consider legitimate z-plasty as the so-called Denonvillier's one.

The Bütow technic respects this principle of taking from the medial edge to complete the lateral edge; our concern is that, from our observation, the medial edge is ever made of the tip of the nose and that there is never tissue left over to be used there. Harvesting out of the nasal tip does not respect the rule of anatomical units.

We did not personally use the pure rotation technic of the alar lobule as advocated by Jinka and Gupta, but the displayed results have seduced us. We would be keen to try it in a next incoming case of a minor form of alar rim cleft.

5.9.2.2 Our Preferred Technic (Figs. 5.21 and 5.22)

We prefer the Z-technic, in which a triangular flap comes out of the nasal dorsum: our first step is to outline the nasal anatomical units with marking devices, ink, or pen. The tissues of the nasal tip and alar lobule are recognized.

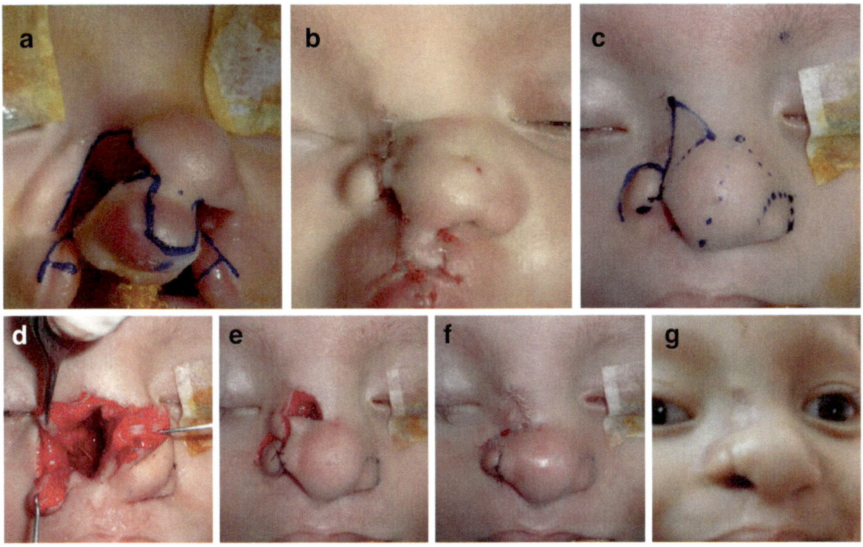

Fig. 5.21 Our preferred technic. Cleft 1 associated with bilateral cleft lip. (**a**) Initial condition. (**b**) Refreshment and straight-line closure. Persistent nasal notch. (**c**) Outlining of anatomical units and drawing z-plasty. (**d**) Full thickness flaps. (**e**) Positioning the alar rim. (**f**) Sutures. (**g**) Result

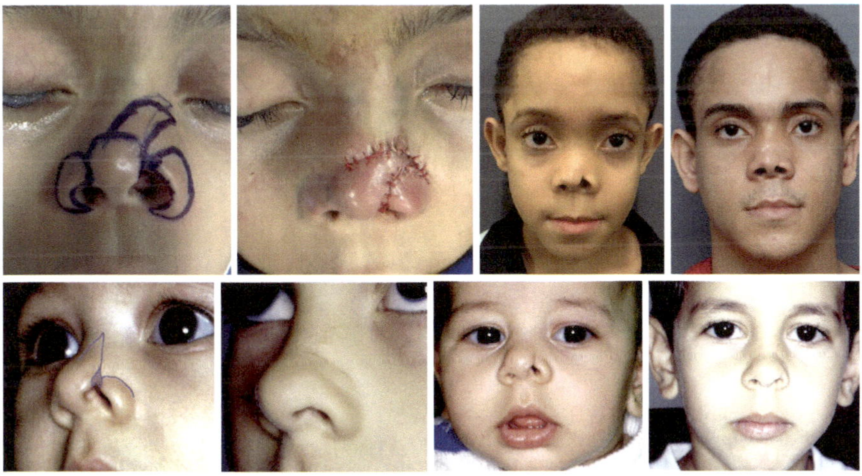

Fig. 5.22 Two clinical examples of isolated cleft 1 cured by Z-plasty

The medial streak of the z-plasty is drawn along the path of the cleft, its inferior end splits as an inverted Y in refreshing cuts to the edges, and its length is calculated proportionally to the discrepancy between the two edges of the cleft. The lateral streak of the z-plasty runs along the alar crease, and the medial crease length of the z-plasty is equal to the lateral and intermediate streaks.

The flaps are of total thickness; the transfixing incisions are performed with a surgical blade 11.

5.9.2.3 Cleft1–13 Associated with Hypertelorism

When the condition necessitates a combination of substantial orbital narrowing and nasal cleft repair, we have to combine the resection of interorbital skin excess with the repair of the nasal cleft defect. The design of incisions must combine those two intentions. Only Monasterio [89] and Van der Meulen [36] have published on this topic.

The main problem with this issue is using the interorbital skin in excess to repair the nasal defect. We do not believe doing a V-Y plasty in the frontal area is a good idea. Our opinion is that the lateral edge of the cleft is shortened and that a flap must be saved out of the skin of the enlarged interorbital area with a design close to the z-plasty used for simple cleft 1. In Monasterio's publication, the most interesting is his plea for the respect of aesthetic units, and we agree with this rule that the resulting scars of our procedures must be concealed whenever possible along the borders of facial aesthetic units. Figure 5.23 displays the drawings of a clever and inspiring solution he found for a severe bilateral cleft 1–13 case. Another solution like the one selected by Pittet [95] for a similar case that did not respect those principles brought a lesser result.

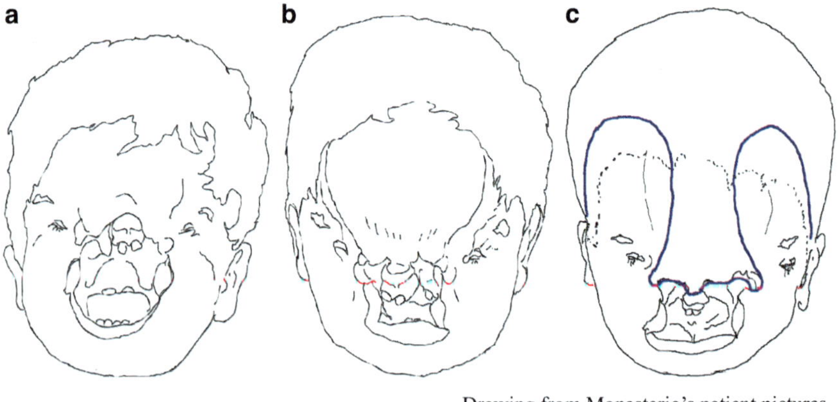

Drawing from Monasterio's patient pictures.

Fig. 5.23 Flap design in accordance with aesthetical units. Drawing after Monasterio's case published pictures. (**a**) Case of bilateral cleft 1-13 associated with bilateral microphthalmia. (**b**) Preliminary skin expansion in frontonasal area. (**c**) Incision allowing the approach for bipartition correction of the hypertelorism and nasal reconstruction

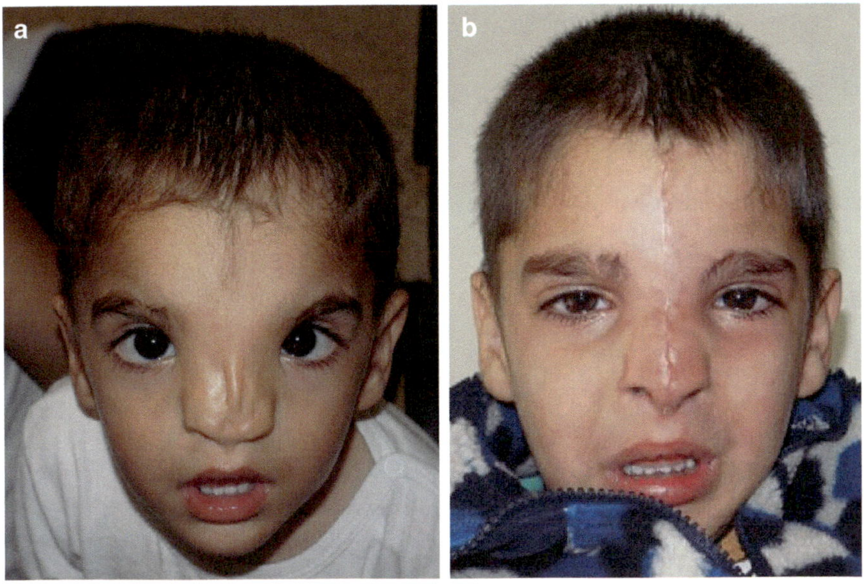

Fig. 5.24 Corrugated nose, result after a simple vertical skin resection. (**a**) Preoperative aspect. (**b**) Postoperative aspect. Courtesy Pr Youri Anastasov

5.9.2.4 Corrugated Nose

Vertical skin excision in the corrugated nose yields excellent results and even could avoid orbital mobilization in grade I hypertelorism (Fig. 5.24).

5.10 Author's Case (Fig. 5.25a–d)

This author's case is a girl with severe left cleft 1–13, bilateral cleft lip and palate, bilateral craniofacial microsomia, and vertebral malformations. The patient underwent a first craniofacial bipartition when she was 2 months old, and cutaneous repair of cleft 1 was performed according to a z-plasty drawing. When she reached 7 months, the bilateral cleft lip was repaired. By the age of 5 years, a new craniofacial bipartition was redone to fix the hypertelorism definitively. Contrary to box-osteotomy, redoing a craniofacial bipartition is not a big deal.

In the meantime, bilateral mandibular distraction has been done for obstructive apnea issues.

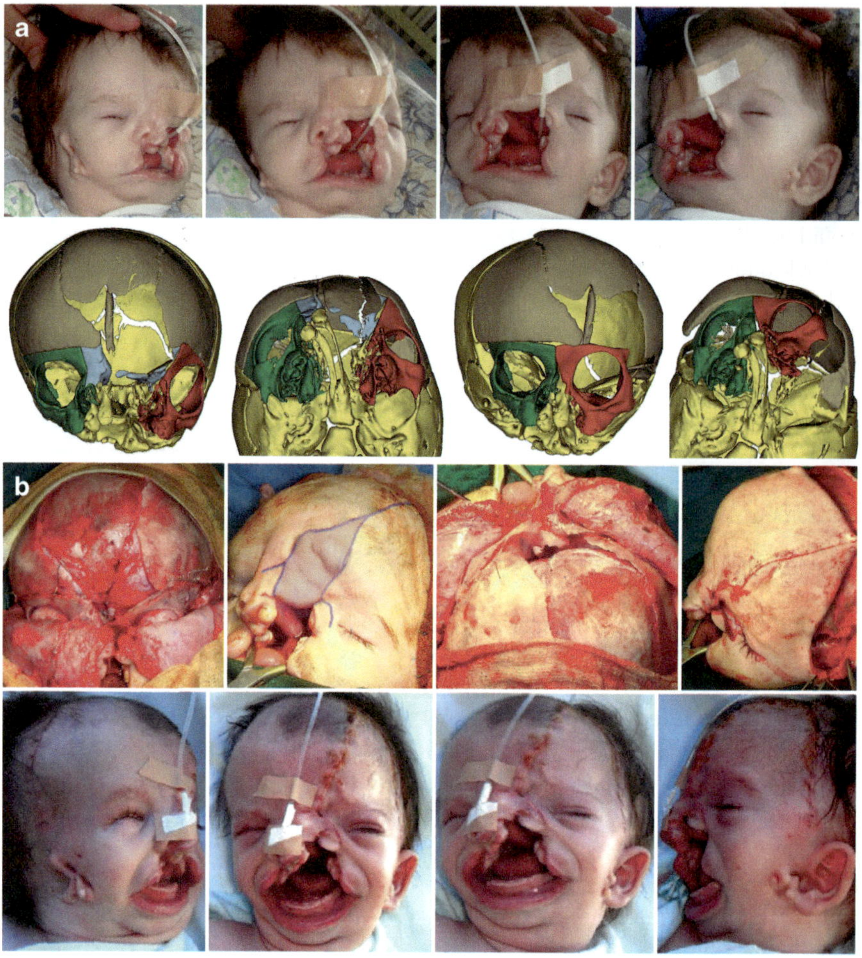

Fig. 5.25 Author's case. Patient with left cleft 1-13, BCLP, bilateral, vertebral malformations, craniofacial microsomia. (**a**) 2 months old: facial bipartition planning. (**b**) Intraoperative views and result. (**c**) 4 months old: bilateral cleft lip repair. (**d**) Iterative bipartition. (**e**) Immediate postoperative aspect

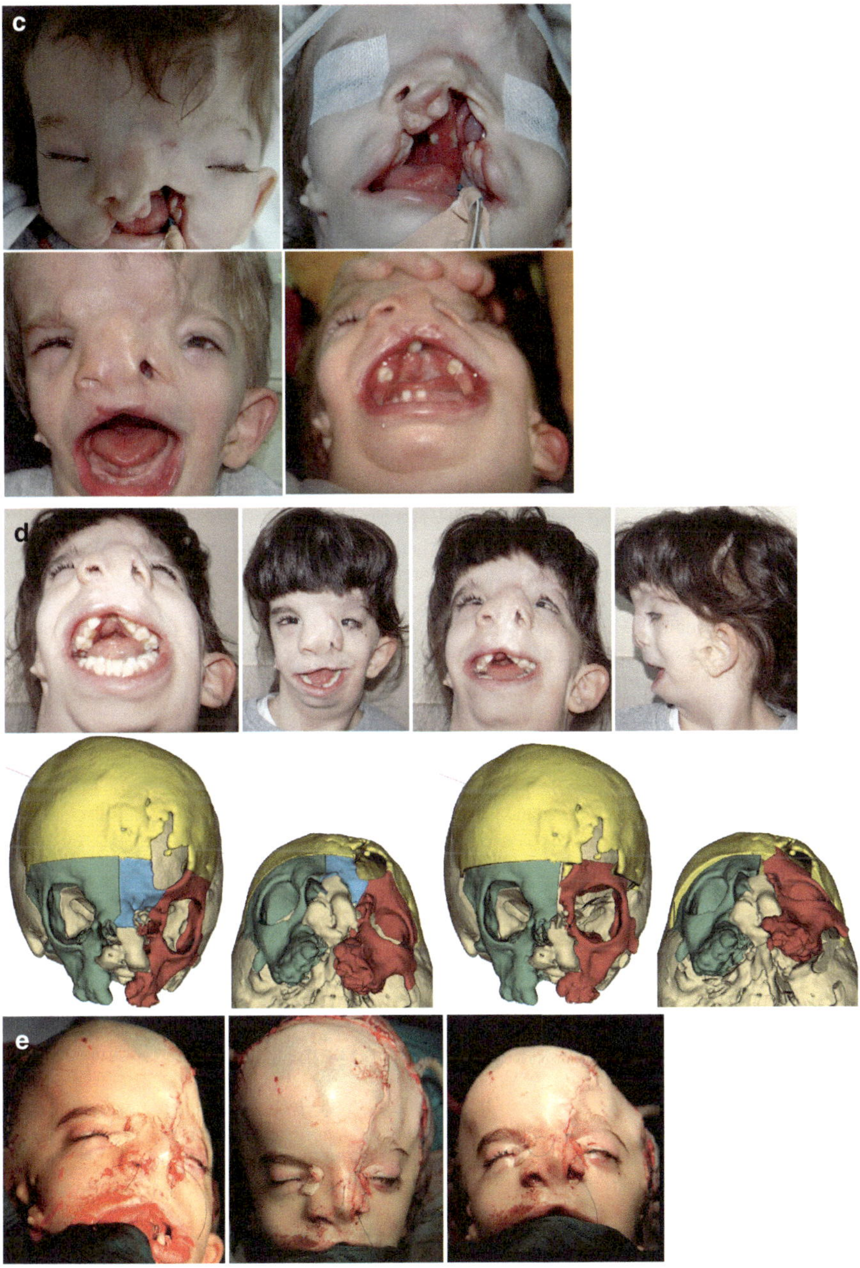

Fig. 5.25 (continued)

References

1. Tessier P. Anatomical classification of facial, cranio-facial and latero-facial clefts. J Maxillofac Surg. 1976;4:69–92. https://linkinghub.elsevier.com/retrieve/pii/S0301050376800136.
2. Leuckart FS. Untersuchungen über das Zwischenkieferbein des Menschen in seiner normalen und abnormen Metamorphose: ein Beitrag zur Entwickelungs-Geschichte des Menschen nebst Betrachtungen über das Zwischenkieferbein der Thiere [Internet]. Stuttgart: E. Schweizerbart's Verlagshandlung; 1840. p. 145. https://archive.org/details/b22413480/page/n143/mode/2up.
3. Förster A. Die Missbildungen des Menschen, systematisch dargestellt, text and atlas, vol. Text&Atlas. Jena; 1861. p. 168.
4. Wilhelm OA. Monstrorum sexcentorum descriptio anatomica. Vratislaviae [Breslau]: Sumptibus Ferdinandi Hirt; 1841. p. 335. https://wellcomecollection.org/works/akv5ftg7.
5. Ahlfeld F. Die Missbildungen des Menschen [Internet], vol. I. Leipzig: Fr. Wilh. Grunow; 1880. p. 163. http://www.biusante.parisdescartes.fr/histmed/medica/cote?44232x01.
6. Beverdam A, Brouwer A, Reijnen M, Korving J, Meijlink F. Severe nasal clefting and abnormal embryonic apoptosis in Alx3/Alx4 double mutant mice. Development. 2001;128(20):3975–86. https://journals.biologists.com/dev/article/128/20/3975/41482/Severe-nasal-clefting-and-abnormal-embryonic.
7. Kayserili H, Uz E, Niessen C, Vargel I, Alanay Y, Tuncbilek G, et al. ALX4 dysfunction disrupts craniofacial and epidermal development. Hum Mol Genet. 2009;18(22):4357–66. https://doi.org/10.1093/hmg/ddp391.
8. Ullah A, Kalsoom U-E, Umair M, John P, Ansar M, Basit S, et al. Exome sequencing revealed a novel splice site variant in the ALX1 gene underlying frontonasal dysplasia. Clin Genet. 2017;91(3):494–8. https://doi.org/10.1111/cge.12822.
9. Meloni VA, Moysés-Oliveira M, Melo MCC, Caneloi TP, Dantas AG, Soares MFF, et al. Novel homozygous *ALX4* mutation causing frontonasal dysplasia-2 in a patient with meningoencephalocele: letter to the editor. Clin Genet. 2015;88(6):593–6. https://doi.org/10.1111/cge.12595.
10. Savastano CP, Bernardi P, Seuánez HN, Moreira MÂM, Orioli IM. Rare nasal cleft in a patient with holoprosencephaly due to a mutation in the *ZIC2* gene. Birth Defects Res A Clin Mol Teratol. 2014;100(4):300–6. https://doi.org/10.1002/bdra.23216.
11. Smith JD, Hing AV, Clarke CM, Johnson NM, Perez FA, Park SS, et al. Exome sequencing identifies a recurrent De novo ZSWIM6 mutation associated with Acromelic frontonasal Dysostosis. Am J Hum Genet. 2014;95(2):235–40. https://linkinghub.elsevier.com/retrieve/pii/S0002929714003176.
12. David DJ, Moore MH, Cooter RD. Tessier clefts revisited with a third dimension. Cleft Palate J. 1989;26(3):163–84.
13. Agrawal K, Panda KN, Prasad S. Isolated Tessier No. 1 cleft of the nose. Ann Plast Surg. 1998;41(3):311–3. http://journals.lww.com/00000637-199809000-00016.
14. Altuntas A, Yılmaz MD, Kahveci OK, Dereköy S, Yücel A. Coexistence of choanal atresia and Tessier's facial cleft number 2. Int J Pediatr Otorhinolaryngol. 2004;68(8):1081–5. https://linkinghub.elsevier.com/retrieve/pii/S0165587604000813.
15. Über BA. Die Seitliche Nasenspalte. Acta Otolaryngol. 1962;55(1–6):163–74. https://doi.org/10.3109/00016486209127350.
16. Bilen BT, Kilin H. A congenital isolated alar cleft. J Craniofac Surg. 2006;17(3):602–4. http://journals.lww.com/00001665-200605000-00039.
17. Bilgen F, Ural A, Bekerecioğlu M. Isolated congenital cleft of the nose. J Craniofac Surg. 2018;29(8):e812–4. http://journals.lww.com/00001665-201811000-00110.
18. Bütow KW, Engelbrecht H. Tessier 2 nasal cleft: reconstruction with a resorbable sheet. Br J Oral Maxillofac Surg. 2014;52(1):93–4. https://doi.org/10.1016/j.bjoms.2013.05.148.
19. Suwantemee C. Facial cleft no 1. Plast Reconstr Surg. 1994;94(7):1055–9. http://journals.lww.com/00006534-199412000-00022.

20. Fawzy HAAR, Ghareeb F, Farghaly AS, Al Barah A, El Sheikh Y. Patterns and management of congenital nasal clefts. Menoufia Med J. 2015;28(1):99. http://www.mmj.eg.net/text.asp?2015/28/1/99/155960.
21. Fijałkowska M, Antoszewski B. Nose clefts: own experience of treatment with different types of congenital nasal anomalies. Eur J Plast Surg. 2016;39(6):409–14. https://doi.org/10.1007/s00238-016-1220-8.
22. Gargano F, Szymanski K, Bosman M, Podda S. Tessier 1-13 atypical craniofacial cleft. Eplasty. 2015;17(15: ic32):4.
23. Reddy SG, Reddy RR, Obwegeser J, Mommaerts MY. Options for the nasal repair of non-syndromic unilateral Tessier no. 2 and 3 facial clefts. Indian J Plast Surg. 2014;47(03):340–5. https://doi.org/10.4103/0970-0358.146588.
24. Gupta A, Gupta AK. Rotation advancement flap for isolated congenital alar rim defect: an effortless paradigm? Int J Pediatr Otorhinolaryngol. 2013;77(1):144–6. https://linkinghub.elsevier.com/retrieve/pii/S0165587612005411.
25. Hallak A, Jamjoom H, Hosseinzadeh T. Supernumerary nostrils: a case report and review. Aesthet Plast Surg. 2001a;25(3):241–3.
26. Shuang HX, Zhu B, Jiang HO, Fan WS, Qi ZZ, Xiao L, et al. A de novo 1.38Mb duplication of 1q31.1 in a boy with hemifacial microsomia, anophthalmia, anotia, macrostomia, and cleft lip and palate. Int J Pediatr Otorhinolaryngol. 2013;77(4):560–4. https://linkinghub.elsevier.com/retrieve/pii/S016558761200691X.
27. Jhamb A, Mohanty S. A chronicle of Tessier no. 0 and 1 facial cleft and its surgical management. J Maxillofac Oral Surg. 2009;8(2):178–80. https://doi.org/10.1007/s12663-009-0043-6.
28. Jian XC, Su HB, Chen XO. Triple nostrils associated with cleft lip and palate. Br J Plast Surg. 1995;48(1):53. https://linkinghub.elsevier.com/retrieve/pii/0007122695900330.
29. Jinka JR, Chekuri H, Annavarapu G. Isolated cleft of the ala nasi: A report of seven cases. Indian J Plast Surg. 2012;45(03):512–5. https://doi.org/10.4103/0970-0358.105962.
30. Kannan R, John R, Elangovan R. Isolated cleft of alar rim. Ann Maxillofac Surg. 2012;2(1):60–2.
31. Kobayashi S, Masuda T, Ohmori K. Repair of alar clefts, associated with nasal skin lumps and median clefts of the upper lip and alveolus. Br J Plast Surg. 1995;48(5):329–31. https://linkinghub.elsevier.com/retrieve/pii/000712269590073X.
32. Boekhoff E, Huffstadt AJC. Denonvilliers Z-plasty in the reconstruction of alar defects (1856). Chir Plast Berl. 1972;1:289–93.
33. Kurul S, Ozcan G, Cakalir C. Accessory nose associated with unilateral incomplete cleft lip. Eur Arch Otorhinolaryngol. 1995;252(1):61–2.
34. Maes J, Stark RB. Unusual cleft lip deformity. Plast Reconstr Surg. 1974;54(3):346. http://journals.lww.com/00006534-197409000-00015.
35. Maisels DO, Saad MN. The repair of notches of the alar margin. Br J Plast Surg. 1969;22(3–4):324–30. https://linkinghub.elsevier.com/retrieve/pii/S0007122669801347.
36. Van der Meulen JC, Moscona AR, Vaandrager JM, Hirshowitz B. Pathology and treatment of nasoschizis. Ann Plast Surg. 1982;8(6):474–85. http://journals.lww.com/00000637-198206000-00006.
37. Monasterio FO, del Campo AF, Dimopulos A. Nasal clefts. Ann Plast Surg. 1987;18(5):377. http://journals.lww.com/00000637-198705000-00004.
38. Mullin WR, Millard DR. Management of congenital bilateral cleft nose. Plast Reconstr Surg. 1985;75(2):253–7. http://journals.lww.com/00006534-198502000-00019.
39. Nayak BB, Lopamudra M. A rare case of a combination of Tessier cleft 0 and 3 in a 4-year-old child—A case report. Indian J Plast Surg. 2019;52(02):250–1. https://doi.org/10.1055/s-0039-1696791.
40. Newman MH, Burdi AR. Congenital alar field defects: clinical and embryological observations. Cleft Palate J. 1981;18(3):188–92.
41. Novaković M, Baralić I, Stepić N, Rajović M, Stojiljković V. Denonvilliers' advancement flap in congenital alar rim defects correction. Vojnosanit Pregl. 2009;66(5):403–6.

42. Ohsaki M, Iwahira Y, Maruyama Y. Pedunculated club-shaped swelling in the nostril. Plast Reconstr Surg. 1992;89(1):128–30.
43. Patel A, Knoll BI, Persing JA. A congenital cleft of the alar rim. Plast Reconstr Surg. 2009;123(2):67e–9e. http://journals.lww.com/00006534-200902000-00067.
44. Ozek C, Gundogan H, Bilkay U, Cankayali R, Guner U, Gurler T, et al. Rare craniofacial anomaly: Tessier No. 2 Cleft. J Craniofac Surg. 2001;12(4):355–61. http://journals.lww.com/00001665-200107000-00008.
45. Rashid M, Ul IMZ, Tamimy MS, Ul HE, Aman S, Aslam A. Rotation-transposition correction of nasal deformity in Tessier number 1 and 2 clefts. Cleft Palate Craniofac J. 2009;46(6):674–80. https://doi.org/10.1597/08-014.1.
46. Schweckendiek W. Nasal abnormalities in facial clefts. J Maxillofac Surg. 1976;4:141–9. https://linkinghub.elsevier.com/retrieve/pii/S0301050376800239.
47. Shewmake KB, Kawamoto HK. Congenital clefts of the nose: principles of surgical management. Cleft Palate Craniofac J. 1992;29(6):531–9. https://doi.org/10.1597/1545-1569_1992_029_0531_ccotnp_2.3.co_2.
48. Stupka W. The etiology of lateral nasal clefts. Am J Pathol. 1950;26(6):1085–95.
49. Temel M, Gunal E, Kahraman SS. Reconstruction of congenital isolated alar defect using mutaf triangular closure technique in pediatric patients. J Craniofac Surg. 2016;27(4):1087–9. https://journals.lww.com/00001665-201606000-00067.
50. Chapchay K, Zaga J, Billig A, Adler N, Margulis A. Surgical technique for nasal cleft repair. Ann Plast Surg. 2019;82(3):289–91. https://journals.lww.com/00000637-201903000-00008.
51. Li SY, Yu BF, Wei SY, Yin N, Yao ZJ, Wei J, et al. Designing a trifoliate flap for isolated congenital alar rim defect in pediatric patients. Plast Surg. 2021:229255032110196. https://doi.org/10.1177/22925503211019606.
52. Mutaf M, Günal E. A new technique for reconstruction of a congenital isolated alar defect. J Craniofac Surg. 2010;21(2):503–5. https://journals.lww.com/00001665-201003000-00050
53. Thomson HG. Isolated naso-ocular cleft: a one-stage repair. Plast Reconstr Surg. 1986;78(6):831–2. http://journals.lww.com/00006534-198678060-00034
54. Tiwari P, Bhatnagar SK, Kalra GS. Tessier number 2 cleft, a variation. J Cranio-Maxillofac Surg. 1991;19(8):346–7. https://linkinghub.elsevier.com/retrieve/pii/S1010518205802768.
55. van der Meulen JC, Roddi R, Gilbert PM, Vaandrager M. Median and paramedian orbito-facial clefts: value of the L-shaped incision in the surgical treatment of nasal deformities. Ann Chir Plast Esthet. 1994;38(3):253–9.
56. Addona T, Friedman A, Post A, Weiss N, Silver L, Taub PJ. Complete Calvarial agenesis in conjunction with a Tessier 1–13 facial cleft. Cleft Palate Craniofac J. 2012;49(4):484–7. https://doi.org/10.1597/08-232.
57. Allam KA, Lim AA, Elsherbiny A, Kawamoto HK. The Tessier number 3 cleft: A report of 10 cases and review of literature. J Plast Reconstr Aesthet Surg. 2014;67(8):1055–62. https://linkinghub.elsevier.com/retrieve/pii/S174868151400182X.
58. Becerra-Solano LE, Castañeda-Cisneros G, Corona-Rivera JR, Díaz-Rodríguez M, Figuera LE, López-Muñoz E, et al. Severe craniofacial involvement due to amniotic band sequence. Fetal Pediatr Pathol. 2018;37(1):27–37. https://doi.org/10.1080/15513815.2017.1392663.
59. Casey HD, Braddock SR, Haskins RC, Carey JC, Morales L. Frontonasal malformation and the Oculoauriculovertebral Spectrum: the Oculoauriculofrontonasal syndrome. Cleft Palate Craniofac J. 1996;33(6):519–23. https://doi.org/10.1597/1545-1569_1996_033_0519_fmatos_2.3.co_2.
60. Edwards WC, Askew W, Weisskopf B. Median cleft face syndrome. Am J Ophthalmol. 1971;72(1):202–5. https://linkinghub.elsevier.com/retrieve/pii/0002939471916151.
61. Ergin NO. Naso-ocular cleft: a case report. Plast Reconstr Surg. 1966;38(6):573–5. http://journals.lww.com/00006534-196638060-00014.
62. Fontaine G, Walbaum R, Poupard B, Bonte C, Dhellemmes P, Maquet E, et al. Fronto-nasal dysplasia (apropos of 4 cases). J Genet Hum. 1983;31(Suppl 5):351–65.

63. Francesconi G, Fortunato G. Median dysraphia of the face. Plast Reconstr Surg. 1969;43(5):481–91. http://journals.lww.com/00006534-196905000-00005.
64. Guion-Almeida ML, Richieri-Costa A, Saavedra D, Cohen MM. Frontonasal dysplasia: analysis of 21 cases and literature review. Int J Oral Maxillofac Surg. 1996;25(2):91–7. https://linkinghub.elsevier.com/retrieve/pii/S0901502796800488.
65. Kasturi N, Rajkumar J. Double limbal dermoid with Tessier's paramedian facial cleft. J Am Assoc Pediatr Ophthalmol Strabismus. 2018;22(5):395–7. https://linkinghub.elsevier.com/retrieve/pii/S1091853118300740.
66. Qureshi IL, Khan N, uz Z. Experience with frontonasal dysplasia of varying severity. J Pediatr Surg. 1996;31(7):885–9. https://linkinghub.elsevier.com/retrieve/pii/S0022346896904030.
67. Rüegg EM, Bartoli A, Rilliet B, Scolozzi P, Montandon D, Pittet-Cuénod B. Management of median and paramedian craniofacial clefts. J Plast Reconstr Aesthet Surg. 2019;72(4):676–84. https://linkinghub.elsevier.com/retrieve/pii/S174868151930018X.
68. Schwenzer N, Haßler W. Median craniofacial clefts. Mund-Kiefer-Gesichtschirurgie. 1998;2(Suppl 1):S16–9.
69. da Silva AJF, CSME S, SCR M. Amniotic band syndrome with double encephalocele: a case report. Surg Neurol Int. 2020;11:448. http://surgicalneurologyint.com/surgicalint-articles/amniotic-band-syndrome-with-double-encephalocele-a-case-report/.
70. Allam KA, Wan DC, Kawamoto HK, Bradley JP, Sedano HO, Saied S. The spectrum of median craniofacial dysplasia. Plast Reconstr Surg. 2011;127(2):812–21. http://journals.lww.com/00006534-201102000-00039.
71. Bello M, Garandawa H, Mustapha Z, Isa A, Tahir C, Ngamdu Y, et al. Frontonasal dysplasia Sequence: a case report. Niger J Paediatr. 2014;41(2):151. http://www.ajol.info/index.php/njp/article/view/101216.
72. Anand S, Kapoor A. Facial abnormality (frontonasal dysplasia sequence). Pediatr Oncall. 2014;11(4):125. https://www.pediatriconcall.com/pediatric-journal/view/fulltext-articles/847/I/0/231/0/0.
73. Sharma S, Sharma V, Bothra M. Frontonasal dysplasia (median cleft face syndrome). J Neurosci Rural Pract. 2012;3(1):65–7.
74. Warkany J, Bofinger MK, Benton C. Median facial cleft syndrome in half-sisters. Dilemmas in genetic counseling. Teratology. 1973;8(3):273–85. https://doi.org/10.1002/tera.1420080307.
75. Schlund M, Paré A, Joly A, Laure B. Computer-assisted surgery in facial bipartition surgery. J Oral Maxillofac Surg. 2018;76(5):1094.e1–7. https://linkinghub.elsevier.com/retrieve/pii/S0278239117315367.
76. Tunc T, Polat A, Altan B, Yapici AK, Saldir M, Sari S, et al. Oculoauriculofrontonasal dysplasia syndrome with additional clinical features. Cleft Palate Craniofac J. 2017;54(6):749–53. https://doi.org/10.1597/15-078.
77. Vegesna S, Gutthi L, Varanasi P, Gandhi TP. Frontonasal dysplasia with severe occipital lobe hypoplasia. Indian J Pediatr. 2014;81(10):1133–4. https://doi.org/10.1007/s12098-014-1429-0.
78. Kean J, Al-Busaidi SSM, Quaba AA. A case report of frontonasal dysplasia. Int J Pediatr Otorhinolaryngol. 2010;74(3):306–8. https://linkinghub.elsevier.com/retrieve/pii/S016558760900651X.
79. Lehalle D, Altunoglu U, Bruel AL, Arnaud E, Blanchet P, Choi JW, et al. Clinical delineation of a subtype of frontonasal dysplasia with creased nasal ridge and upper limb anomalies: report of six unrelated patients. Am J Med Genet A. 2017;173(12):3136–42. https://doi.org/10.1002/ajmg.a.38490.
80. Guion-Almeida ML, Silva Lopes V. Frontonasal dysplasia, Poland anomaly and unilateral hypoplasia of lower limb: report on a male patient. Clin Dysmorphol. 2003;12(4):233–6. http://journals.lww.com/00019605-200310000-00004.
81. Dubey SP, Garap JP. The syndrome of frontonasal dysplasia, spastic paraplegia, mental retardation and blindness: a case report with CT scan findings and review of literature. Int

J Pediatr Otorhinolaryngol. 2000;54(1):51–7. https://linkinghub.elsevier.com/retrieve/pii/S0165587600003414.
82. Balci S, Mavili ME, Son YA, Vargel I, Benli K, Erk Y. A female patient with frontonasal dysplasia sequence and frontonasal encephalocele. Ann Plast Surg. 1999;43(4):457–8. http://journals.lww.com/00000637-199910000-00023.
83. Stevens CA, Qumsiyeh MB. Syndromal frontonasal dysostosis in a child with a complex translocation involving chromosomes 3, 7, and 11. Am J Med Genet. 1995;55(4):494–7. https://doi.org/10.1002/ajmg.1320550420.
84. Meguid NA. Frontonasal dysplasia, lipoma of the corpus callosum and tetralogy of Fallot. Clin Genet. 2008;44(2):95–7. https://doi.org/10.1111/j.1399-0004.1993.tb03854.x.
85. Fryburg JS, Persing JA, Lin KY. Frontonasal dysplasia in two successive generations. Am J Med Genet. 1993;46(6):712–4. https://doi.org/10.1002/ajmg.1320460623.
86. Sedano HO, Michael Cohen M, Jirasek J, Gorlin RJ. Frontonasal dysplasia. J Pediatr. 1970;76(6):906–13. https://linkinghub.elsevier.com/retrieve/pii/S0022347670803742.
87. Lehalle D, Altunoglu U, Bruel A, Assoum M, Duffourd Y, Masurel A, et al. The oculoauriculofrontonasal syndrome: further clinical characterization and additional evidence suggesting a nontraditional mode of inheritance. Am J Med Genet A. 2018;176(12):2740–50. https://doi.org/10.1002/ajmg.a.40662.
88. Moore MH. Rare craniofacial clefts. J Craniofac Surg. 1996;7(6):408–11. http://journals.lww.com/00001665-199611000-00003.
89. Monasterio FO, Taylor JA. Major craniofacial clefts: case series and treatment philosophy. Plast Reconstr Surg. 2008;122(2):534–43. http://journals.lww.com/00006534-200808000-00027.
90. Adolphs N, Arnaud E, Haberl EJ, Graul-Neumann L, Schmidt G, Menneking H, et al. The oculo-auriculo-fronto-nasal syndrome (OAFNS)—description of a rare and complex craniofacial deformity and its interdisciplinary management before school age. J Cranio-Maxillofac Surg [Internet]. 2012;40(8):668–74. https://linkinghub.elsevier.com/retrieve/pii/S1010518211002666.
91. Evans KN, Gruss JS, Khanna PC, Cunningham ML, Cox TC, Hing AV. Oculoauriculofrontonasal syndrome: case series revealing new bony nasal anomalies in an old syndrome. Am J Med Genet A. 2013;161(6):1345–53. https://doi.org/10.1002/ajmg.a.35926.
92. Ito R, Osawa M, Yamamoto Y, Murao N, Hayashi T, Maeda T, et al. Oculo-Auriculo-Fronto-nasal syndrome with duane retraction syndrome and dysplastic bony structure in the midline of nose. J Craniofac Surg. 2019;30(6):e576–8.
93. Hilaire GS, I. Histoire générale et particuliére des anomalies de l'organisation chez l'homme et les animaux, vol. Atlas. Paris: Bailliére; 1837. https://ia800106.us.archive.org/17/items/BIUSante_35541/BIUSante_35541.pdf.
94. Gosla Reddy S, Acharya AP. Rare facial clefts. In: Bonanthaya K, Panneerselvam E, Manuel S, Kumar VV, Rai A, editors. Oral and maxillofacial surgery for the clinician. Singapore: Springer; 2021. p. 1735–68. https://doi.org/10.1007/978-981-15-1346-6_77.
95. Pittet B, Jaquinet A, Rilliet B, Montandon D. Simultaneous correction of major hypertelorism, frontal bone defect, nasal aplasia, and cleft of the upper lip (tessier 0–14). Plast Reconstr Surg. 2004;113(1):299–303. http://journals.lww.com/00006534-200401000-00042.
96. Pellerin P. About hypertelorism and its treatment. P Pediatr Neurosc. 2022;(17):4–1311. www.pediatricneurosciences.com.
97. Vinchon M, Pellerin P, Pertuzon B, Fénart R, Dhellemmes P. Vestibular orientation for craniofacial surgery: application to the management of unicoronal synostosis. Childs Nerv Syst. 2007;23(12):1403–9. https://doi.org/10.1007/s00381-007-0471-x.

Chapter 6
Cleft 2/12

Philippe Pellerin, Cristiano Tonello, Nivaldo Alonso, and Renato da Silva Freitas

Pearls
Cleft 2–12 has a path almost along the path of cleft 1–13. They are differentiated by nature: cleft 1–13 deserves the name nasoschisis since it is a true cleft, while cleft 2–12 deserves hemi-arhinia since it is an aplasia or hypoplasia.

6.1 Original Tessier's Classification

Tessier's description of cleft 2–12 [1] is ambiguous and will require clarification.

In the first part of his paper, he systematically describes cleft 2–12 between cleft 1–13 and cleft 3–11, writing: "*Number 2 looks similar to the preceding cleft. It is,*

P. Pellerin (✉)
Centre Hospitalier Régional Universitaire de Lille, Lille, France

C. Tonello
Curso de Medicina Bauru Faculdade de Odontologia Bauru Universidade de São Paulo, Bauru, Brazil

Hospital de Reabilitação Anomalias Craniofaciais Universidade de São Paulo, Bauru, Brazil

N. Alonso
Plastic Surgery, Universidade de São Paulo, São Paulo, Brazil

Craniofacial Surgery, Hospital de Reabilitação Anomalias Craniofaciais Bauru USPUniversidade de São Paulo, Bauru, Brazil

R. da Silva Freitas
Plastic Surgery Unit, Hospital de Clínicas, Universidade Federal do Paraná, Curitiba, Brazil

Craniofacial Surgery, Assistance Center for Cleft Lip and Palate (CAIF), Hospital do Trabalhador, Curitiba, Brazil

N. Alonso et al. (eds.), *Facial Reconstruction of Unusual Facial Clefts*,
https://doi.org/10.1007/978-3-031-40926-4_6

however, slightly more lateral without being paranasal. On the soft tissues, this cleft comes through the nasal ala between the tail of the alar cartilage and the alar base, and on the lip, it is manifested as a usual type harelip. On the skeleton, it comes through the lateral mass of the ethmoid (telorbitism). It is difficult to locate exactly on the frontal bone; whim is flattened while the frontal sinus is enlarged" then he casts, for illustration (Fig. 6.8), a patient who presents himself with a nasal hypoplasia, which is not a cleft in the meaning of nasoschisis.

Tessier then writes: "*Hemi-atrophy of the nose, super-numerary nostrils, and proboscis lateralis are probably different degrees of the same defect.*"

The use of the term "cleft" could be confusing, but we already know that in Tessier's mind, the signification of cleft is one of a malformation occurring along a determinate axis.

A last point in Tessier's research could be confusing: after having put hemi-arhinia, proboscis and supernumerary nostril as probable cleft 2, wondering if cleft 2 exists, in his 1977 paper [1], was published under his name in 2009, a paper about the arhinia [2] without naming cleft 2!

In it, it was stated that hemi-arhinia and total arhinia have the same topography as cleft 1–13 but have points of difference.

We have, above, in the cleft 1–13 chapter, pleaded to classify all the nasoschisis as cleft 1 since we could find neither in the literature nor in our cases significative differences in the locations of the clefts in relation to the nostril.

Thus, our final acceptance of the cleft 2 descriptions will be, according to the second part of the first Tessier's assessment in 1977: lateral nasal hypoplasia or aplasia (hemi-arhinia), possibly associated with proboscis lateralis or supernumerary nostril. Cleft 12, being the cranial counterpart of cleft 2, would manifest itself as hypertelorism or ethmoidal encephalocele.

6.2 History

Several authors [3] attribute the first description of the proboscis to Förster [4] advocating his description of a proboscis. Moreover, it was a case of cyclopia with a medial proboscis, a condition primarily distinct from the lateral proboscis (Fig. 6.1).

The first comprehensive description was from Selenkoff [5]. He reported the clinical and anatomical data of an adult male with a left proboscis lateralis associated with a hemi-arhinia. Selenkoff credited Geoffroy de Saint Hilaire for describing a similar hemi-arhinencephaly, but we could not find it in the original treatise [6] (Fig. 6.2);

Grünberg, in his extensive review in 1909 [7], reported several cases of cleft 2: a case of hemi-arhinia and cleft 3 from Hensen, a case of cleft 2–12 from Peters associated with a cleft 9 and an appendage on the edge of the cleft in the eyebrow, another cleft 2–12 from Lehman, two cases of proboscis lateralis: one from Kirchmayr, an association of proboscis lateralis and cleft lip and the Selenkoff's case.

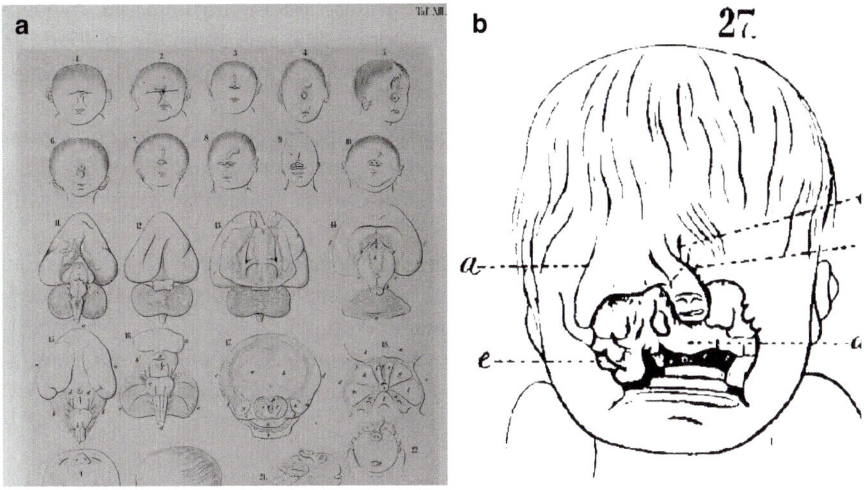

Fig. 6.1 Proboscis representations in Förster. (**a**) Plate XIII. (**b**) Fig. 27 in plate XXIV. All the figures of proboscis in Förster, are medial and associated with cyclopia. He did not give any example of proboscis lateralis

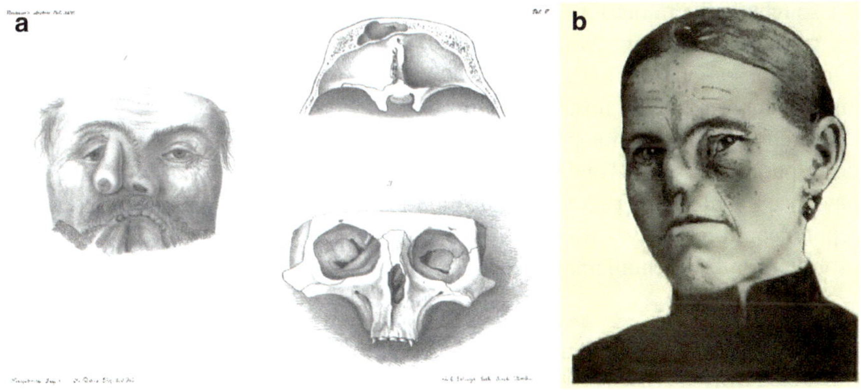

Fig. 6.2 Historical observations of cleft 2–12. (**a**) Illustrations of the Selenkoff's patient. (**b**) Hensen's patient in Grünberg

6.3 Etiology

Many authors have tried to explain those malformations on embryological bases; they are pure conjectures without any scientific proof. We will not try to follow this path.

Today the only scientific data come from macromolecular genetics.

Even if we do not have a complete understanding of the mechanisms involved, hereafter is what we know:

Bosma [8] 1981 published two cases of arhinia, microphthalmia, and hypogonadism with average intelligence. Thiele reported the same condition in 1996 [9]. This syndrome was later related in 2017 simultaneously by Gordon [10] and Shaw [11] to a mutation in SMCHD1.

The mutation yields a gain of gene function, which acts as an epigenetic repressor at an ATPase domain. The involved pathway concerns neural cells of the olfactive placode more than the neural crest cells most frequently concerned with craniofacial development.

Rahimov [12] reported cases of hemi-nasal aplasia related to GLI2 mutation; GLI2 is a transcription factor mediator of SHH signal transduction. SHH pathway plays an essential role in the biology of neural crest cells.

Amniotic band syndrome (ABS), frequently associated with rare clefts, is infrequently associated with cleft 2–12 since it occurs in only 2 patients out of the 151.

6.4 Cases from Literature (Table 6.1)

6.4.1 *General Review*

We sought the literature for relevant publications but considered only the references we could obtain a copy with the original illustrations. Otherwise, we looked for publications about hemi-arhinia with or without proboscis, isolated lateral proboscis, and supernumerary nostrils.

Cerebral malformations: cyclopia or cebocephalia, as the frequently alleged description of Föster [4] and holoprosencephaly in which proboscis could be found, have been excluded. From the publication to which we have access and to which reports could be analyzed, we garnered 102 cases of hemi-arhinia with or without proboscis and supernumerary nostril.

6.4.2 *Total Arhinia*

Since very recent research about total arhinia was published about a series of 101 cases by Shaw et al. [11] with a detailed analysis of symptoms, we have limited our review to publications about the surgical treatment of total arhinia.

Table 6.1 Cases from the literature. sex: f for female, m for male; side: r for right, l for left; hemi-arhinia, t for complete, p for partial; anywhere n is for no, y is for yes. CFM is for craniofacial microsomia. UCLP is for unilateral cleft lip; reconstr is for reconstruction. ins. proboscis is for the location of the proboscis attachment. 1/3 int. lid when the proboscis is in the medial part of the eyelid, 1/3 med.lid is when the proboscis is attached in the mid part of the eyelid, 1/3 lat.lid is when the proboscis is attached in the lateral part of the eyelid

Authors	Ref	Case #	Sex	Side	Hemi-arhinia	Proboscis	Ins. Proboscis	Supernumerary nostril	Hypertelorism	Encephalocele	Associated cleft	Associated craniofacial malformation	Associated general condition	Nasal treatment	Interorbital surgery	Miscellaneous
ABOU-ELHAMD	[13]	1	m	r	t	y	Inner canthus	n	n	n	n	n	n	n	n	
ABOU-ELHAMD	[13]	2	m	l	t	y	1/3int. Lid	n	light	n	n	n	n	n	n	
ABULEZZ	[14]	3	f	r	t	n		n	n	n	10 right	n	n	Hemi-rhinopoiesis	n	
ACARTURK	[15]	4	m	r	p	y	Inner canthus	n	n	n	n	n	n	Proboscis to the nose	n	
ACARTURK	[15]	5	f	r	t	y	Inner canthus	n	y	n	n	n	n	Proboscis to the nose	n	
AGARWAL	[16]	6	m	l	t	y	Inner canthus	n	light	n	Left UCLP, cleft3	n	n	Proboscis to the nose	n	
Ajike	[17]	7	f	l	n	y	1/3int. lid	n	medium	n	Left UCLP	n	n	Resection	n	
Akkuzu	[18]	8	f	b	p-t	n		n	n	n	n	Hypo-telorism-alobar holopros-encephalia		Resection	n	
AL-HELO	[19]	9		r	p	y	Inner canthus	n	Light	n	n			Resection	n	
BEG	[20]	10	m	r	t	n		n	Medium	n	cleft10 cleft0	Right microph-thalmia		n	n	

(continued)

Table 6.1 (continued)

Authors	Ref	Case #	Sex	Side	Hemi-arhinia	Proboscis	Ins. Pro-boscis	Supernu-merary nostril	Hyper-telorism	Enceph-alocele	Associ-ated cleft	Associated craniofa-cial mal-formation	Associated general condition	Nasal treat-ment	Inter-orbital sur-gery	Miscel-laneous
BELET	[21]	11	m	r	t	y	Inner canthus	n	Medium	n	cleft3	Right microph-thalmia			n	
BELET & al	[22]	12	m	r	t	y	1/3int. Lid	n	Medium	n	Right UCLP				n	
BHANDARI	[23]	13	f	r	t	n		n	n	n	n			In and out rhinopoiesis	n	
BINNS	[24]	14	m	l	t		1/3int. Lid	n	Medium	n	Cleft3			Proboscis adhesion	n	
BOAHENE	[3]	15	m	r	t	y	1/3int. Lid	n	Medium	y	Cleft 3-11				n	
BOTHRA	[25]	16	f	l	t	y	Inner canthus	n	light	n	Cleft 4left-uclp right			Proboscis adhesion	n	
ALI	[26]	17	m	l	t	n		n	Light	n	Left UCLP	Left microph-thalmia		Lachrymal	n	
BRYANT	[27]	18	f	l	y	y	Inner canthus	n	Medium	n	n			Excision-rhinopoiesis	n	Eye-brow peak
CHAISRI-SAWADISUK	[28]	19	m	r	p	y	Inner canthus	n	n	y	n			Excision-graft	n	
CHAUHAN	[29]	20	f	r	t	y	Inner canthus	n	n	n	n			Proboscis adhesion	n	
CHEN	[30]	21	m	b	n	n		y	n	n				Resection	n	

COESSENS	[31]	22	m	r	p	n		y	Light	n	n			Resection	n	Aborted probos-cis
COESSENS	[31]	23	f	r	p	y	Inner canthus	n	Light	n				Proboscis adhesion	n	
D'ASSUMPCAO	[32]	24	f	l	t	y		n		n	Cleft3			Proboscis adhesion	n	
DAVID	[33]	25	f	r	t	y		n			Cleft3			Proboscis adhesion	n	
DAS	[34]	26	m	b	t	y	Inner canthus	n	Severe				ABS		n	
ERICH	[35]	27	f	l	y	n		y	Medium		n			Resection	n	
BELL TAWSE	[36]	28	f	r	p	n		y	Medium		n			Resection	n	
EROGLU	[37]	29	m	r	y	y	Inner canthus	n	Light		ucl			Proboscis to the nose	n	Eye-brow peak
EROGLU	[37]	30	m	r	t	y	Inner canthus	n	Medium	n	Cleft3			Proboscis to the nose		
GHAREEB	[38]	31	m	l	t	n		n	Light	n		Microph-thalmia		I/2 rhinopoi-esis	n	Eye-brow peak
FISHER H	[39]	32	m	r	t	y	1/3int. Lid	n	n	n	n			Excision-rhinopoiesis		
FISHER H	[40]	33	m	r	p	n		n	n	n	n	Low globular appendage		1/2 rhinopoi-esis	n	Eye-brow peak
FISHER M	[40]	34	f	l	t	n		n	Light		Cleft3	CFM		Island flap	n	
FRANKLIN BISHOP	[41]	35		l	t	y	Inner canthus	n	n					Proboscis to the nose	n	

(continued)

Table 6.1 (continued)

Authors	Ref	Case #	Sex	Side	Hemi-arhinia	Proboscis	Ins. Proboscis	Supernumerary nostril	Hypertelorism	Encephalocele	Associated cleft	Associated craniofacial malformation	Associated general condition	Nasal treatment	Interorbital surgery	Miscellaneous
BIBER	[42]	36		r	t	n	1/3int. Lid	n	Light					Proboscis adhesion	n	
GALIE	[43]	37	m	r	t	y	Inner canthus	n	n	n				Proboscis adhesion	n	
GHIEH	[44]	38	f	l	t	y	1/3med. Lid	n	Medium	n	cleft10	Iris coloboma				Eyebrow peak
GUERRRERO	[45]	39	m	l	p	y	1/3int. Lid	n	Light	n		Iris coloboma microphthalmia				
HASSANI	[46]	40	f	l	t	y	Inner canthus	n	Light	n				Proboscis adhesion		
HOROZ	[47]	41	f	l	t	y	Inner canthus	n	n	n	Right UCLP			Proboscis to the nose		
HOROZ	[47]	42	m	l	t	n		n	Medium	n	BCLP			Hemi-rhinopoiedis		Eyebrow peak
JIAN	[48]	43	m	l	n	n		y	n	n	Right UCLP					
JOST	[49]	44	f	l	p	y	Inner canthus	n	n	n						
JOST	[49]	45	m	r	p	y	Inner canthus	y	n	n						Aborted proboscis
BOO-CHAI	[50]	46	f	l	p	y	Attached/nose	n	n	n	BCLP	Left microphthalmia				

KIRKPATRICK	[51]	47	m	r	t	y	Inner canthus	n	Light	n	Cleft3					
KUKREJA	[52]	48	f	l	t	n		n	Severe	n		Left microph-thalmia				
LELLI	[53]	49	f	l	p	y	Inner canthus	n	n	n				Migrating proboscis		
BAJARANG	[54]	50	m	r	p	y	Inner canthus	n	n	n				Proboscis adhesion		
MAHINDRA	[55]	51	f	l	t	y	Inner canthus	n	n	n	Cleft3-cleft0	Missing premaxilla				
MARTIN	[56]	52		l	t	y	1/3med. Lid	n	Severe	Frontal	Cleft10	Hydro-cephaly				
MATHUR	[57]	53	m	l	t	y	Inner canthus	n						Resection		
McLaren	[58]	54	f	l	p	y	Inner canthus	n	n		UCLP					
MEEKER	[59]	55	m	l	t	y	1/3int. Lid	n	n	n		Dupli-cation eyeball lid anomalies		Resection		
MLADINA	[60]	56	m	r	t	y	Inner canthus	n	n	n		Pit upper-lip muco-coele		Resection		
MOTOHASHI	[61]	57	f	r	t	n		n	light	n		Pit upper lip		Hemi-rhinopoiesis	n	
NAGASE	[62]	58	f	r	t	n		n	Light	n				3 flaps-scalping		Eye-brow peak
NAKAMURA	[63]	59	m	r	p	y		y	n	n				Local plasty		

(continued)

Table 6.1 (continued)

Authors	Ref	Case #	Sex	Side	Hemi-arhinia	Proboscis	Ins. Pro-boscis	Supernu-merary nostril	Hyper-telorism	Enceph-alocele	Associ-ated cleft	Associated craniofa-cial mal-formation	Associated general condition	Nasal treat-ment	Inter-orbital sur-gery	Miscel-laneous
SAH	[64]	60	m	l	n	n		y	n			Dermoid cyst right		Resection		
ASLANABADI	[65]	61	f	l	p			y	n	n			Esopha-geal atresia anal imper-foration			
NUMANOGLU	[66]	62	m	b	p			b					Esopha-geal atresia ductus arteriosus			
ONIZUKA	[67]	63	m	l	p	n		y	n					Resection		
KINGSLY	[68]	64	m	l	p	y	1/3int. Lid	n	Light	n	UCLP			Proboscis adhesion		
KINGSLY	[68]	65	m	l	t	n		n	Medium	n		Microph-thalmia		Hemi-rhinopoiedis		Eye-brow peak
OZEK	[69]	66	m	r	n	n		n	Severe	n					Box oste-otomy	
POED	[70]	67	m	l	t	y	Inner canthus	n	n			Microph-thalmia orbital cyst				Labial pit
POWAR	[71]	68	m	b	t	y		n	Severe							

RAO	[72]	69	f	r	p	y	1/3int. Lid	n	Medium	n	Cleft 3-Cleft 11					
RAPOSO	[73]	70	m	r	p	n		n	Light	n	Cleft3	Microph-thalmia				
RAWAT	[74]	71	f	r	p	n		y	n							
REDDY	[75]	72	f	l	p	n		y	n							
RONTAL	[76]	73		r	t	y	Inner canthus	n	n	n						
ROSEN	[77]	74	m	b	t	y	1/3med. Lid	n	n	n		Microph-thalmia-eye malforma-tion				
SAHU	[78]	75		l	n	y	1/3int. Lid	n	n	n		Iris malfor-mation				
KAUR	[79]	76	m	l	t	y	1/3med. Lid	n	Light	n	Cleft 3-Cleft 11	Laterona-sal hamar-toma	Meningeal angioma-tosa			
SARSMAZ	[80]	77	m	b	t	y	1/3med. Lid	n	Severe	Frontal		Microph-thalmia interhemi-spheric cyst	Meningeal angioma-tosa			
GITLIN		78		b	t	y	1/3med. Lid	n	Light			Interhemi-spheric brain	Meningeal angioma-tosa			
GOVILA	[81]	79	m	l	p	y	1/3int. Lid	n	n			Microph-thalmia		Resection		

(continued)

Table 6.1 (continued)

Authors	Ref	Case #	Sex	Side	Hemi-arhinia	Proboscis	Ins. Proboscis	Supernumerary nostril	Hypertelorism	Encephalocele	Associated cleft	Associated craniofacial malformation	Associated general condition	Nasal treatment	Inter-orbital surgery	Miscellaneous
SELENKOFF	[5]	80	m	r	t	y	1/3int. Lid	n	n	n						Eye-brow peak
SHAYE	[82]	81	f	r	p	y	i Nner canthus	n	Light	n				Resection		
SINGH	[83]	82	m	r	t	y	1/3int. Lid	n	light	n		Pit upper lip		Proboscis to the nose		Eye-brow peak
SKEVAS	[84]	83	f	l	p	y	Inner canthus	n	n	n				Resection		
STANEK	[85]	84	f	b	t	y	1/3med. Lid	n	severe	n	Cleft0		Disorga-nization in mice			
TAKCI	[86]	85	f	l	p	n		n	Light	n						
TAMBWEKAR	[87]	86	m	r	n	n		y	n		Cleft3					
THORNE	[88]	87	f	l	p	y	Inner canthus	n	n	n	n	Cheek skin tag				
UDAGAWA	[89]	88	m	l	t	n		n	light	n	UCLP right	Corpus callosum defect		Hemi-rhinopoiedis		
URUGLU	[90]	89	f	r	p	y	Latero nasal	y	Medium	n				V-Y	Box oste-otomy	
VAID	[91]	90	f	l	t	y	Inner canthus	n	n	n						

VERMA	[92]	91		l	t	y	Inner canthus	n	Medium	n						
VERMA	[92]	92		r	p	y	Inner canthus	n	n	n				Resection		
UMEDA	[93]	93	f	b				y	Light	n	UCLP right					
WILKINSON	[94]	94		l	t	y	Latero nasal	y	n	n						
WILLIAMS	[95]	95		r	p			y	n							
XU	[96]	96	m	l	p			y								
JAGANNATHAN	[97]	97		r	p			y	n	n	Cleft3 conro-lateral					
SHEN	[98]	98	f	r	p			y	n	n						
YILDIRIM	[99]	99	m	l	t	y	1/3int. Lid	n	medium	n		Microph-thalmia, lipoma, arach. Cyst				
METHA	[100]	100	f	l	t	y	inner canthus	n	n	n	Cleft3					
YOO	[101]	101	m	r	p	n		n		n						
ZBAR	[102]	102	m	l				y	n	n						

6.4.3 *Supernumerary Nostril*

In 2021 [98], in thorough research, Shen found 59 reported cases other than his own patient, which makes 60. Since three more cases have been published [103, 104]. Tessier's series of 51 patients published in 2009 is not included in our statistics since there was no detailed data on each case.

6.5 Our Clinical Series (Table 6.2)

Sao Paulo's and Lille's merged series of clefts 2–12 totalize 49 patients.

Unilateral nasal hypoplasia was found 43 times: total arhinia 31, partial arhinia 12.

Laterality was balanced: right side 26, left side 23.

The sex ratio was 1,13 in the clinical series (1,24 in the literature plus clinical series).

Proboscis lateralis were present seven times.

There were four patients with a supernumerary nostril.

The statistics in this chapter will rely upon the merged data of our 49 patients and 102 cases from the literature, which makes a total of 151.

Table 6.2 Our clinical series. sex: f for female, m for male; side: r for right, l for left; hemi-arhinia, t for complete, p for partial; anywhere n is for no, y is for yes. CFM is for craniofacial microsomia, UCLP is for unilateral cleft lip; reconstr is for reconstruction. ins. proboscis is for the location of the proboscis attachment. 1/3 int. lid when the proboscis is in the medial part of the eyelid, 1/3 med.lid is when the proboscis is attached in the mid part of the eyelid, 1/3 lat. lid is when the proboscis is attached in the lateral part of the eyelid

			Cleft 2				Cleft 12							
Case #	Sex	Side	Hemi-arhinia	Proboscis	Ins. Proboscis	Supernumerary nostril	Hypertelorism	Encephalocele	Associated cleft	Associated craniofacial malformation	Associated general condition	Nasal treatment	Inter-orbital surgery	Miscellaneous
1	f	r	t	n		n	n	n	Left UCLP	Lacrimal system/int canthal displ	n	Nasal reconstr	n	n
2	m	r	t	n		n	Medium	n	UCLP	CFM	Genito urinary problems	Nasal reconstr + orthognatic surgery	n	y
3	m	l	t	n		n	Medium	n	Left UCLP	CFM microphthalmia	n			
4	m	l	t	y	Inner canthus	n	Severe	n	n	n	n		y	n
5	m	r	p	n		n	n	n	n	Single nasal cavity	n	Nasal reconstr	n	n
6	m	l	t	n		n	n	n	Right UCL	CFM microphthalmia	n			
7	m	r	t	n		n	Severe	Frontal	n	Microphthalmia	n		y	Hairline peak
8	f	r	p	n		y	Medium	Frontal	n	Parietal encephalocele	n	Nostril reconstr	n	Mental retard
9	f	r	t	n		n	Severe	n	n	Microphthalmia	n	Nasal reconstr	n	n
10	m	l	n	n		n	n	n	n	No nostril left side	n	Nasal reconstr	n	n
11	m	r	t	n		n	Severe	n	Right UCLP	CFM microphthalmia	n			
12	f	l	p	n		n	n	n	Left UCLP	Microphthalmia	n	Nasal reconstr + orthognatic surgery	Frontofacial advance	n
13	m	l	t	n		n	Medium	n	UCLP	Microphthalmia	BOSMA S	Orthognathic surgery	n	

(continued)

Table 6.2 (continued)

Case #	Sex	Side	Cleft 2 Hemi-arhinia	Cleft 2 Proboscis	Cleft 2 Ins. Proboscis	Cleft 2 Supernumerary nostril	Cleft 12 Hyper-telorism	Cleft 12 Enceph-alocele	Associated cleft	Associated craniofacial malformation	Associated general condition	Nasal treatment	Inter-orbital surgery	Miscel-laneous
14	f	l	t	y	Latero-nasal	n	n	n	UCLP	n	n	n	n	n
15	m	r	t	n		n	n	Eth-moidal	n	Microphthalmia	Horizontal nistagmo	Nasal reconstr + encephalo-cele corr	n	Eyebrow peak-labial fistula
16	f	bil	t	n		n	n	n	n	Bil anophthamy + microblephary	n	Nasal reconstr	n	n
17	m	bil	t	n		n	n	n	n	n	n	n	n	
18	m	bil	t	n		n	n	n	n	Bil anophthamy + microblephary	Mental retard	n	n	n
19	f	bil	t	n		n	n	n	n	Lacrimal system/int canthal displ	BOSMA S	Nasal reconstr	n	Mental retard + genital problems
20	f	bil	t	n		n	n	n	n	Lacrimal system/int canthal displ	n	Nasal reconstr	n	Mental retard
21	m	bil	t	n		n	n	n	n	Anophthalmy + microblephary	n	n	n	Mental retard
22	m	l	t	y	Inner can-thus	n	n	n	n	Cleft3	n	Nasal reconstr	n	n
23	f	bil	t	n		n	n	n	n	Lacrimal system/int canthal displ	n	n	n	n
24	f	l	p	n		n	n	n	n	n	n	n	n	n
25	f	l	p	n		n	Medium	n	n	Lacrimal system/int canthal displ + nasal bone	y upper arm malforma-tion	n	n	n
26	f	n	t	n		n	n	n	Median lip cleft/palate	Holoprosoencephaly	y	n	n	n

27	m	n	y	n		n	y	n	Right eyelid	Hydrocephaly	ABS	Nasal reconstr	y	y
28	m	r	n	n		y	n	n	cleft 3+4	Lacrimal system/int canthal displ	n	Nasal reconstr	n	n
29	f	bil	n	n	n	n	n	n	Congenital ectropium bil	Abnormal cranial morphology	Frazer syndrome	Eyelid reconstruction	n	
30	f	l	t	n		n	Medium	n		Cutis aplasia microphthalmia	Inner ear malformation	Nasal reconstr		
31	f	l	p	y	Inner canthus	n	n	n						
32	f	l	p	n		n	Light	n						
33	m	l	p	n		y	Medium			Microphthalmia		SN/nose	Unilat. Box osteotomy	
34	f	r	t	y	Inner canthus	n	n	n	n	Cleft3				Left mucocele
35	m	l	t	n		n	Medium	n		CMF		Nasal reconstr	Box osteotomy	
36	m	r	p	n		n	Light	n	UCLP					
37	f	r	p	n		n	n	n		Fren.dupic.; Ear tags; hairline peak		Rhinoplasty		
38	f	l	p	n		n	n	n				Alae-rim plasty		
39	m	r	p	n		n	Light	n						
40	f	l	t	y	1/3int. Lid	n	Medium	n	Cleft 3			Resec. Nasal reconstr		

(continued)

Table 6.2 (continued)

Case #	Sex	Side	Cleft 2				Cleft 12		Associated cleft	Associated craniofacial malformation	Associated general condition	Nasal treatment	Inter-orbital surgery	Miscellaneous
			Hemi-arhinia	Proboscis	Ins. Proboscis	Supernumerary nostril	Hyper-telorism	Enceph-alocele						
41	m	l	t	n		n	n	n		CMF; microphthalmia				
42	f	l	t	y	Inner canthus	n	n	n		Labial fistulae to the nose				
43	m	bil	t	n		n	Light	n		Irian coloboma		Nasal reconstr		
44	m	r	n	n		y	n	n						
45	f	l	n	n		n	Medium	Eth-moidal	UCLP	Arachnoidal cyst				
46	f	l	p	n		n	n	n				Alar-rim plasty		
47	m	l	t	n		n	n					Nasal reconstr		
48	m	r	t	n		n	Medium		UCLP opposite	CFM microtia canthal dystopia		Nasal reconstr		Nasal fistula
49	f	r	t	n		n	Severe		Cleft 3					
50	f	l	n	n		n	medium							
51	m	r	p	n		n	Light			Frontal osseous defect				
52	m	l	p	n		n	Medium							
53	f	l	p	y	Latero-nasal	n	Light		Cleft 3					

6.6 Phenotypes and Their Spectrum

Even if they belong to the same track, we could describe four main phenotypes, which all have in common the hypoplasia of the nasal tract.

- Hemi-arhinia and proboscis.
- Hemi-arhinia without proboscis.
- Supernumerary nostril.
- Total arhinia.

6.6.1 Hemi-Arhinia with Proboscis Lateralis

Rontal [76] gave a general description of all the anomalies found associated with proboscis: Table 6.1; and Sahu [78], a more specific analysis, out of 108 cases of reported cases of proboscis, of ophthalmologic symptoms. Boo-Chai was the first to propose a classification for proboscis lateralis syndrome, [105].

Sakamoto [106] proposed a new classification but included holoprosencephaly, which we exclude from the cleft 2–12 spectrum.

We garnered 72 cases of proboscis whose data were available.

Amazingly there is a considerable divergence in percentages of proboscis with hemi-nasal involvement in the literature and our series. In the literature, 63% of cleft 2–12 have a proboscis, when it is 16% in our series. We hypothesize that there is a bias in the interest in the publication of striking and easily recognized conditions such as proboscis. Thus, it yields more publications than hemi-nasal hypo or arhinia. The same bias is undoubtedly the reason for a similar divergence for supernumerary nostrils, represented in 21% of the literature cases and only 9% of our cases.

6.6.1.1 Proboscis Anatomy

Anatomy of the Proboscis Itself (Fig. 6.3)

The term "proboscis" comes from the Greek name of the elephant trump: προβοσκίδα and is used to name any of various elongated or extensible tubular processes. The first description of proboscis was associated with cyclopia and located medially above the unique orbit and eyeball, which is the condition reported by Föster [107]. The proboscis lateralis, to the contrary, as suggested by the term "lateralis", is paramedian, as reported by Selenkoff.

The proboscis has the shape of a cylinder appendage, where the distal flattened end is marked by a pit, which could be the opening of a medial inner canal. In its complete form, it could be catheterized up to its proximal attachment, usually osseous. Selenkoff, in his inaugural case, describes the inner lining as "a smooth mucous membrane", few histological studies have been performed since most of the authors

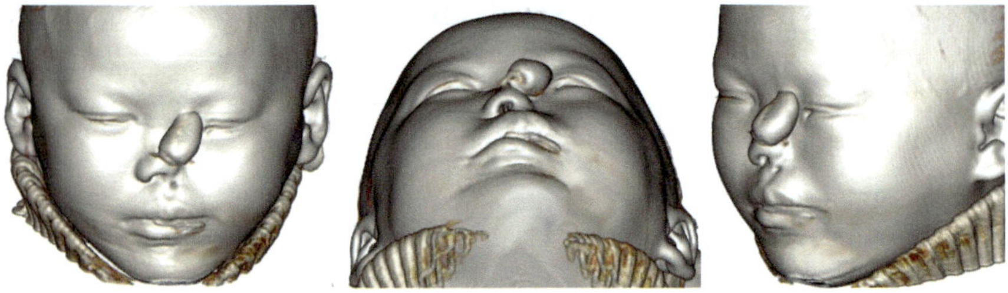

Fig. 6.3 The typical proboscis with hemi-arhinia: long proboscis with a canal, inserted at the inner canthus

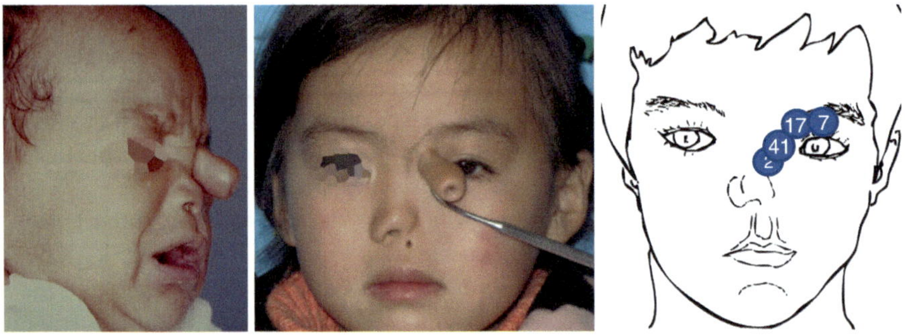

Fig. 6.4 The insertions of the proboscis. Blue circles indicate the location of the insertion. Numbers are those of cases at the location

use the proboscis to repair the missing nostril. Thorne [88] described squamous and ciliated respiratory epithelium lining a tract extending the whole length of the proboscis, with a blind end at a small osseous prominence.

The Bishop's [41] and Guerrero's [45] patients' proboscis were fully examined, and histologists found a surrounding layer of skin with normal adnexa, a central tract lined with respiratory epithelium and its glandular adnexa; the stromal was mainly composed of fibro adipose tissue containing muscles, cartilage, vessels, and nerves. Biber [42] quoted Kircmayr, Zacherl, and Seefelder reporting the same constatations. Those findings explain the symptomatology frequently encountered: mucous drainage and contractions of the proboscis during mimicking.

Dasgupta's patient's proboscis had the same external and inner layers and included a ring of hyaline cartilage [108].

The Proboscis Insertion (Fig. 6.4)

The insertion of the proboscis is most of the time medial to the inner canthus; we found it 41 times out of 71 this way but could be onto the medial third of the upper eyelid, and it was the case 17 times out of 71. Most rarely, it could be inserted onto the mid-third of the upper eyelid. We met this condition 7 times out of 7, associated with a coloboma of that same upper eyelid (cleft10).

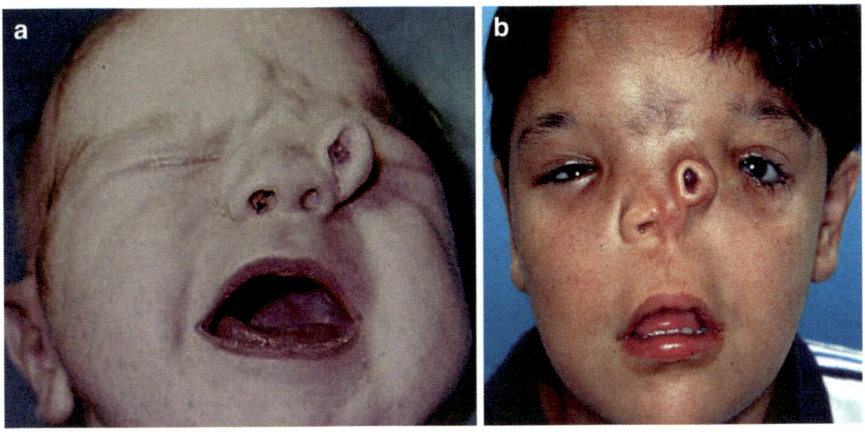

Fig. 6.5 Atypical types of proboscis. (**a**) Short proboscis partially attached along its shaft to the nasal area. (**b**) Proboscis inserted to the inner canthus with a very short shaft

Cases of proboscis attached to the lateral third of the upper eyelid have been reported. Still, they are quite different: they do not present a dimple at their distal extremity and are associated with cleft 9. We believe they are more appendages associated with cleft 9, as seen in other rare clefts (see chapter cleft 6, 7, and 8), which could be manifestations of the disorganization in mice equivalent mutation.

Specific associations are seen depending on the insertion site: inner canthus insertion is frequently associated with cleft 3, insertion to the medial third of the upper eyelid is frequently associated with eyebrow anomaly, and insertion to the mid-third of the upper lid is associated with cleft 10.

The Transition of Proboscis Toward the Supernumerary Nostril (Fig. 6.5)

Most of the time, the proboscis is fully pedunculated, but it could be partially attached by a more or less important part of its length to the nasal skin. Boo-Chai's [105] case displays a ¾ attached part, while the second JOST's case [49] proboscis is attached by its entire length. This fusion could be a transitional condition between the proboscis and the supernumerary nostril.

Uğurlu's case [90] is a perfect missing link between proboscis and supernumerary nostril.

6.6.2 *Supernumerary Nostril (Fig. 6.6)*

Of the 60 cases in the literature reported by Shen [98] and the three more reported since his publication, we could provide ourselves with the original papers for 21 and have 4 out of our clinical series. Thus, a whole of 67 cases have been brought to our knowledge.

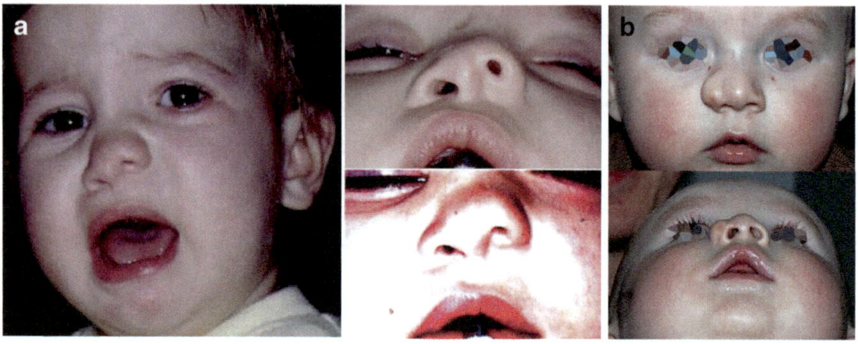

Fig. 6.6 Supernumerary nostril and transitional proboscis. (**a**) hemi-nasal hypoplasia. The affected nostril looks as a fusioned proboscis. (**b**) Right supernumerary nostril

The "no-data" lines in Table 6.1 are confusing about Shen's paper. His classification as medial and lateral does not always match our constatations from the pictures in the referenced paper when available.

With supernumerary nostrils, what is striking is their pleomorphism, which makes the treatment very difficult to systematize. This point will be discussed below.

In some cases, the supernumerary nostril presents itself as a minor form of proboscis or an "aborted proboscis, which is evident in Nakamura's case [63], conditions in which the proboscis is attached with the nose for a part of its length could be transitional forms of this malformation as seen in Coessen's [31] and Jost's [49] cases. Wilkinson's patient [94] could be, as well, considered as a transitional type of proboscis toward the supernumerary nostril but in which the aborted proboscis would be associated with hemi-arhinia.

The supernumerary nostril is never associated with a total hemi-arhinia. Moreover, our constatations are that in 15 of the 25 cases we got the data, there was a reduction in the size of the ipsilateral nasal components. In six patients, the nose was normal in size, but for the supernumerary nostril and four cases were inconclusive.

6.6.2.1 Bilateral Proboscis

Bilateral proboscis looks like a very specific condition; the reported cases are primarily rare, [80], but they are so similar that it could not be a fortuity. They are at every time associated with a total arhinia; the proboscises are inserted above the medial part of the upper lid, and there is a mid-brain anomaly: cyst or supernumerary cerebral lobe associated with a duplicated inter-frontal suture, which isolates a frontal Wormian bone.

6.6.2.2 Nasal Aplasia Associated with the Proboscis

The nasal development on the side of the proboscis is always, more or less, affected. We disagree with the authors who put "proboscis lateralis without nasal hypoplasia" in their classification.

There is, in all the cases in which we had access to their data (71 cases), an asymmetry between both nostrils.

- 21 out of 71 patients with proboscis had partial hemi-nasal hypoplasia.
- 46 out of 71 patients with proboscis had a total hemi-arhinia
- 4 out of 71 were missing data.

We will analyze the nasal anomalies below along with the phenotype "hemi-arhinia without proboscis".

6.6.3 Hemi-Arhinia Without Proboscis (Fig. 6.7)

The hypoplasia, in cleft 2, affects the whole tract: nostril aperture, nasal fossa, and choana are reduced in size, as well as the paranasal sinuses and the turbinates. In the total hemi-arhinia, all of them are missing; onto the skull base, the cribriform plate and ethmoidal roof are missing and sometimes let room for an encephalocele as in Chaisrisawadisuk [28], Boahene [3], and one of our cases.

The absence of an olfactory bulb has been demonstrated with MNRI several times.

The features in complete hemi-arhinia are that of a total absence of those anatomical structures: the septum is lying on the maxilla of the affected side, this maxilla, missing the antrum as a compact piece of bone, there is neither a nasal bone nor an ethmoidal bone.

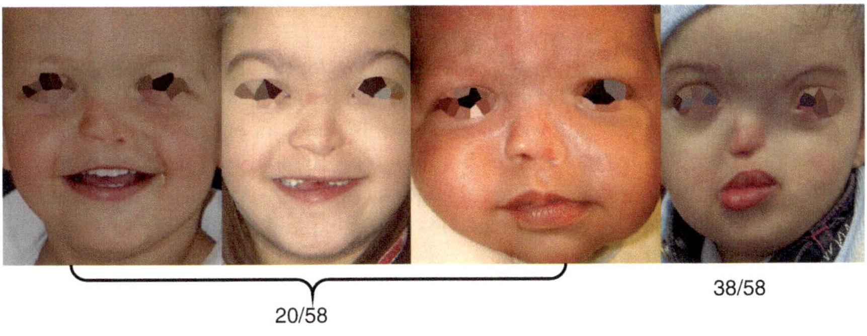

Fig. 6.7 Several degree of hemi-nasal hypoplasia without proboscis. From left to right: increasing severity of hemi-nasal hypoplasia. Numbers are those of cases in the series (58)

- 20 out of 58 patients without proboscis had partial hemi-nasal hypoplasia.
- 38 out of 58 patients without proboscis had a total hemi-arhinia.

Usually, hemi-arhinia has no consequence upon breathing and would not necessitate functional repair.

The anatomical characteristics of hemi-nasal hypoplasia or aplasia are identical whether or not associated with a proboscis.

6.6.4 *The Skeleton of Hemi-Arhinia with or Without Proboscis*

The modern technics of medical imaging have confirmed the noteworthy Selenkoff's constatations. They are helpful for surgical planning.

The presence or absence of a proboscis does not make a difference in the radiological presentation of the hemi-arhinia. The absence or reduction of the nasal aperture is the most striking aspect. The nasal bone is missing. The nasal fossa is reduced or absent. When absent, the nasal septum lies directly on the maxillary body. The antrum is reduced or missing, leaving a maxillary bone solely made of cortico-spongiose bone. The ethmoidal labyrinth is reduced or absent, the antrum being part of it. In complete aplasia, the lacrimo-nasal duct is missing; it is more or less affected in partial hemi-arhinia.

On the affected side, the cribriform plate is missing or reduced, and the width of the ethmoidal shelf is reduced.

6.6.5 *Total Arhinia*

The recent Shaw's [11] review in 2017 is a very comprehensive research. It was a substantial multicentric study that could find the data of 80 previously reported patients and added 21 new cases. Among this series, 40 patients have undergone genome sequencing. In 80% of the test, an SMCHD1 mutation was found. Simultaneously, the same research was done by Gordon, who investigated 14 patients and found an SMCHD1 mutation in all 14 patients.

The mutation yields a gain of function of this gene, an epigenetic regulator of ATPase function. Studies in Xenopus homologous Smchd1 gene demonstrated that its mutation yielded to misexpression of genes such as rx2a and six1, which regulate the size of the eye and nasal placode. This could explain the frequent association with ocular-associated malformation as seen in the Bosma association [8].

In total arhinia, both nasal tracts are missing, which frequently yields obstruction sleep apnea.

Ethmoid and paranasal sinuses are also missing, and the midfacial skeleton is underdeveloped Fig. 6.8.

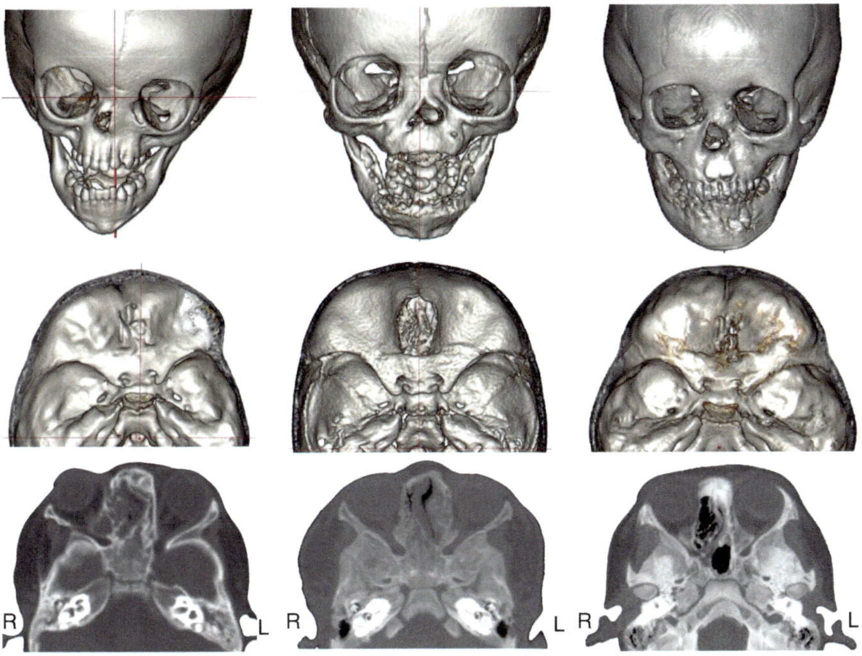

Fig. 6.8 The skeleton in hemi-arhinia. Left: complete left hemi-arhinia. Middle: partial left hemi-arhinia. Right: left proboscis with subtotal hemi-arhinia

6.7 The Cleft 12

Cleft 12 is the cranial counterpart of cleft 2; it manifests itself either by hypertelorism or encephalocele.

Advanced medical imaging is necessary to assess the skull base and interorbital area.

6.7.1 Hypertelorism

6.7.1.1 Clinical Aspects of Hypertelorism in Cleft 2–12

Sixty-five cases include hypertelorism: 25 light, 25 medium, and 15 severe.

Since the gravity was quoted from the authors' evaluation or the pictures cast in the papers and medical imaging is frequently missing, we could not distinguish true hypertelorism from canthal dystopia. Only 8 of the 151 patients underwent a surgical correction of hypertelorism.

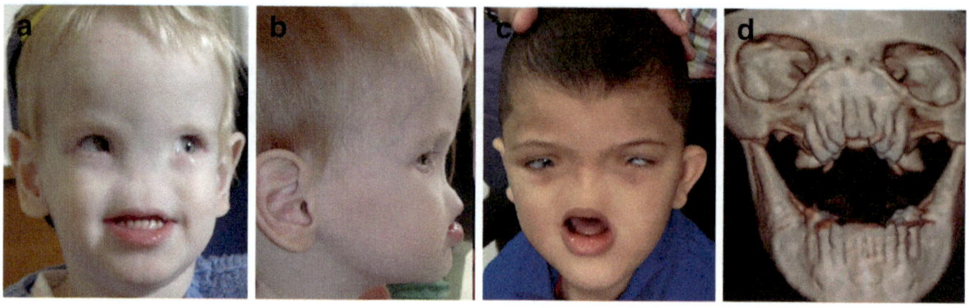

Fig. 6.9 Total arhinia. (**a**) Patient 1, frontal view. (**b**) Patient 2, lateral view. (**c**) Patient 2, frontal view. (**d**) Patient 2, CT scan

6.7.1.2 Analysis of the Interorbital Anomalies in Cleft 2–12 (Fig. 6.9)

To better understand the skull base and interorbital skeleton in cleft 2–12, we post-processed some available Dicom native data from CT scanners of patients.

Contrary to initial Tessier's assertions in 1977, he did not have access to that kind of data; on the side of cleft 2–12, the ethmoidal part of the skull base is narrowed. The olfactory groove is reduced, and the cribriform plate is missing (as described in Selenkoff's constatations [5]). More recent Tessier's conclusions in his 2009 publication about this point are more in line.

Thus, we would expect to meet hypotelorism in cases of cleft 2–12; instead, almost 50% of the patients display a more or less severe hypertelorism or at least a telecanthus.

From the careful analysis of five available native data of the CT scans of five patients, we made some exciting constatations: the skeletal bloc made of the frontal orbital process and the maxillary orbital process is rotated. This means that it goes to a more frontal orientation from an almost sagittal orientation. This move displaces laterally the inner canthal insertion. In older patients, we have seen a pneumatization of this piece of bone coming from the contralateral patent nasal fossa.

This skeletal deformation thus yields, at the least, a telecanthus and participates to some degree of hypertelorism. It, precisely fits with Tessier's description of the deformity in cleft 12:" *It is difficult to locate exactly on the frontal bone, whim is flattened while the frontal sinus is enlarged*" [1] (p 75, § 1, l. 8–10).

The ethmoidal labyrinth on the patent side is over-pneumatized, and the nasal tract is enlarged, which yields the global enlargement of the interorbital space.

6.7.2 Encephalocele (Fig. 6.10)

The encephalocele in cleft 12 could affect the cranial base yielding an ethmoidal encephalocele (Fig. 6.9); this is a very infrequent condition since we found it only in 3 out of the 151 cases.

Frontal encephalocele has been seen in 4 of the 151 patients.

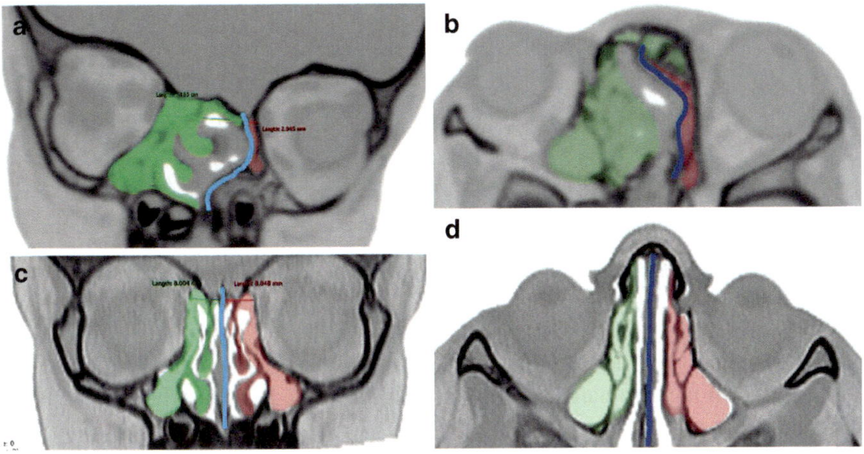

Fig. 6.10 Compared anatomy of the interorbital area: Comparison between a cleft 2–12 patient and an age matching normal patient's CT scan. (**a**, **b**) face and axial CT scan slices of a patient with total hemi-arhinia. (**c** and **d**) face and axial CT scan slices of a normal, age matching patient. Blue line marks the septum. Green areas are those of patent nasal and paranasal area. Red areas are those of affected side

6.8 Associated Malformations

6.8.1 Association with Other Clefts (Fig. 6.11)

6.8.1.1 Cleft Lip and Palate

As a general rule in this book (See classification of rare clefts), we consider the usual cleft lip as an association with rare clefts more than the downward continuation of clefts 1, 2, and 3.

We found 21 associations with unilateral cleft lip, not always on the same side as the cleft, and 2 cases associated with bilateral cleft lip.

6.8.1.2 Cleft 3

The association of a coloboma onto the lower eyelid, which could be interpreted as a partial cleft 3, is not infrequent; about this point, an observation is especially demonstrative: Tambwekar's case [87] in which a supernumerary nostril is associated with a true oculo-nasal cleft 3. We quoted even limited coloboma of the inferior eyelid at the inner canthus as cleft 3 and found 18 occurrences.

There are few cases of typical oculo-nasal cleft, 3. Still, most of the time, the coloboma is limited to the lower eyelid, medially to the lachrymal punctum, and the inner canthus is dystopic, being displaced downward. The lachrymal apparatus is disturbed.

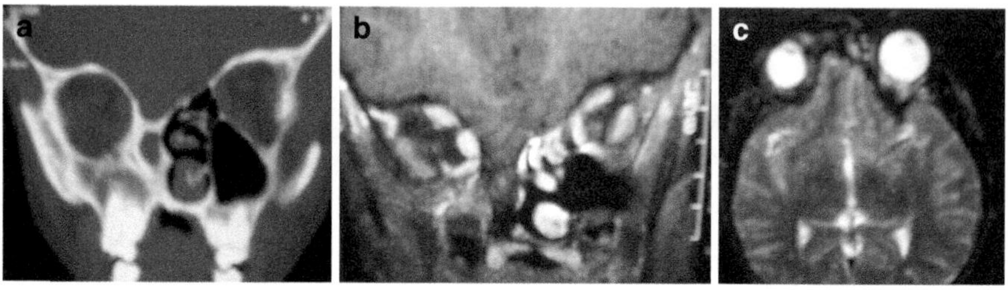

Fig. 6.11 Ethmoidal encephalocele in the setting of cleft 12. (**a**) CT scan, frontal view. (**b**) MRI, frontal view. (**c**) MRI, axial view

The association of cleft 3 with cleft 2 may be related to a common cause since, for instance, in Jagannathan's case [97], cleft 3 is on the left side while cleft 2 is on the right side.

Another reason for the association could be the role of the proboscis since it occurs more frequently when a proboscis is inserted into the inner canthus.

6.8.1.3 Other Rare Clefts

- Cleft 4 was associated three times.
- Cleft 10 was associated four times, 3 out of 4, with a proboscis inserted above the medial third of the upper eyelid.
- Cleft 11, three cases.
- Cleft 0, three cases.

6.8.1.4 Upper Lip Fistula

A fistula of the upper lip, slightly paramedian, has been noticed four times, twice in the literature and twice in our series. We hypothesize that it is a rudimentary nasal tract. In our cases, in which the CT scan data were available, we assessed that the fistula was heading to the atretic nasal tract.

6.8.2 Ophthalmologic Malformations

6.8.2.1 Lid Coloboma

In this series, the sum of clefts, which concerns the eyelids, cleft 3, 4, 10, and 11, is 27 (19%).

We have seen that the most significative, as well as the more frequent, was the cleft 3.

6.8.2.2 Canthal Dystopia

Canthal dystopia is a frequent association. Telecanthus is part of the enlargement of the intercanthal distance and could be related to several mechanisms. We see a patient with a telecanthus consecutive to a mucocele developed after the resection of a proboscis. Some other cases are related to dacryocystocele, but the frontalization of the orbital apophysis of the frontal bone and maxilla is the most frequent mechanism.

Downward canthal displacement is a constant association with the colobomas of the lower lid frequently associated with cleft 3.

6.8.2.3 Eyeball Malformations

Microphthalmia was present in 29 of 151 patients (20%). Other ocular malformations are encountered, iris coloboma most frequent in total arhinia and a part of Bosma's syndrome. Other unusual ocular malformations have been reported as the "cyclopean eyeball" of Meeker's patient [59].

6.8.2.4 Eyebrow Anomalies

Suppose there are few anomalies of the hairline in this series. In that case, a specific eyebrow anomaly has been seen in 10 patients, usually associated with a proboscis inserted over the medial third of the upper lid as in the Selenkoff's inaugural case. The head of the eyebrow is prolongated toward the missing nose area.

6.8.2.5 Lachrymal System Anomalies

The anomalies of the lachrymal system are frequent. Their consequences go from lagophthalmos to dacryocysts and dacryocystitis. In the proboscis setting, Sahu reported 20% of anomalies in his series.

The ophthalmologic malformations in the setting of proboscis were the topic of Sahu's comprehensive research [78], but his study missed other cleft 2–12 without proboscis.

6.8.3 The Cleft 2–12 in the Setting of Syndromes

Contrary to many rare clefts, cleft 2–12 occur infrequently in the setting of amniotic band syndrome (ABS). ABS was present in only one case; another could evocate disorganization in mice syndrome, Stanek's case [85].

Also, craniofacial microsomia was associated with cleft 1–12 only six times.

6.9 Differential Diagnosis (Fig. 6.12)

6.9.1 Differential Diagnosis from Other Rare Clefts

Amazingly, many publications of so-called Cleft 2 reported misdiagnosed rare clefts; about this point, Ozeks's [69] paper is peculiarly demonstrating since of the four patients, only the second is a cleft 12, others are 3, 1–13, and 1. In the overall review of his series of nasal clefts, Monasterio named his cases of hemi-arhinia 2 or 3 according to the displayed pictures in the publication.

The differential diagnosis with cleft 3 could be confusing when cleft 2 is associated with cleft 3, which is quite frequent. It is accessible in the presence of a proboscis but more difficult when the hemi-arhinia is partial without a proboscis.

Cleft 2–12 features are quite characteristic and are not a big deal to recognize. The only difficulty comes from confusion, in its definition, versus cleft 1–13. Both are along, almost the same path. The main difference lies in the quality of the defect: the cleft 1–13 deserves the name of cleft and could be called nasoschisis, while the cleft 2–12 corresponds with hypoplasia. The case that Tessier has selected to illustrate in Fig. 6.8 from his original paper displays a partial nasal hypoplasia that could be interpreted as a cleft when it is just a vertical retraction of a non-cleft soft triangle.

6.9.2 Maxillo-Nasal Dysplasia and Holoprosencephaly

Total arhinia, the sum of two lateral malformations, is sometimes confused with maxillo-nasal dysplasia, part of holoprosencephaly. The mechanisms of those two syndromes are very different since, in holoprosencephaly, the malformation is due to a midline defect that yields a deficiency of the whole components issued from the frontonasal process.

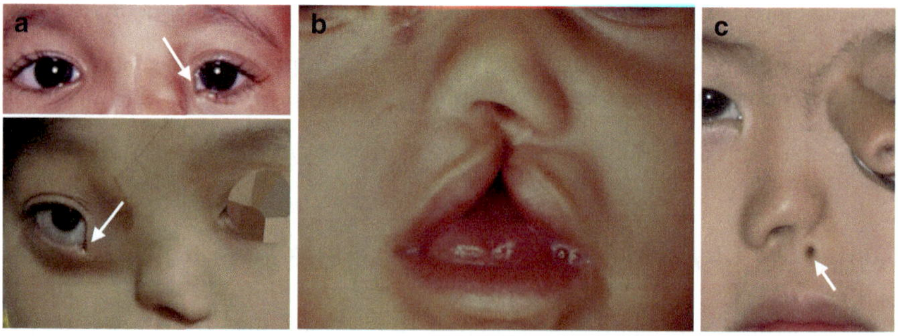

Fig. 6.12 Associations with cleft 2–12. (**a**) Minor medial coloboma of the lower lid usually associated with proboscis (the proboscis has been resected). (**b**) Unilateral cleft lip on the side opposite to the cleft 2. (**c**) Upper-lip fistula, heading toward hypoplastic nasal fossa

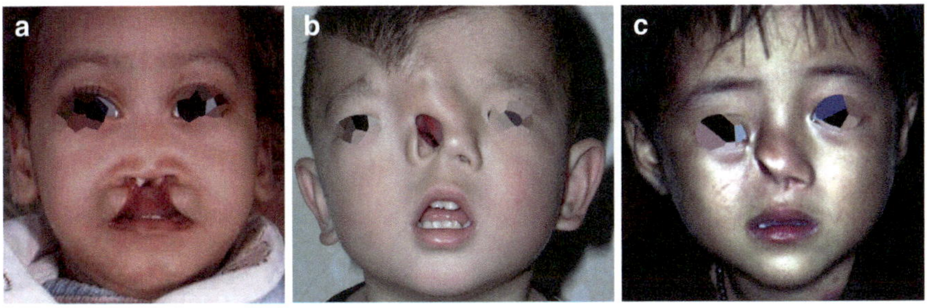

Fig. 6.13 Differential diagnosis. (**a**) Holoprosencephaly. (**b**) Cleft 1–13. (**c**) Cleft 3

If this malformation were considered a craniofacial cleft, it would have to be a cleft 0–14 since it is a midline defect. In the most severe form, there is a median cleft of the upper lip, the columella is missing, as well as the premaxilla and most of the septum, there is a hypotelorism, but the pathognomonic symptom is the more or less severe cerebral malformation in the spectrum of holoprosencephaly. If the medial components of the naso-maxillary complex are missing, the lateral ones, represented by the alae, are present (Fig. 6.13).

6.10 Treatment of Clefts 2–12

6.10.1 The Technics

The treatment of cleft 2–12 has to deal with several questions: what to do, when it is present, with the proboscis lateralis; what to do to repair the nasal hypoplasia; what to do with the hypertelorism.

6.10.1.1 Surgery with the Proboscis Lateralis (Fig. 6.14)

Most authors consider that the proboscis tissues would be the ideal material for reconstructing the missing hemi-nose. Moreover, it depends on the size and the pedicle of the proboscis. We have learned from its anatomy that there are vessels in the lipo-conjunctival layer; so, as it has been proved in many cases, the proboscis could survive with a subcutaneous pedicle.

In 19 patients, the proboscis has been resected. Once it has been used as a donor site for a composite graft for the nostril, another proboscis has been used as flaps, once as a migrating flap [53] and others as permanent flaps.

The proboscis could be managed in different ways.

The first technic is to open the proboscis, to change the cylinder toward a flat flap inserted in a vertical trench cut off the nasal dorsum.

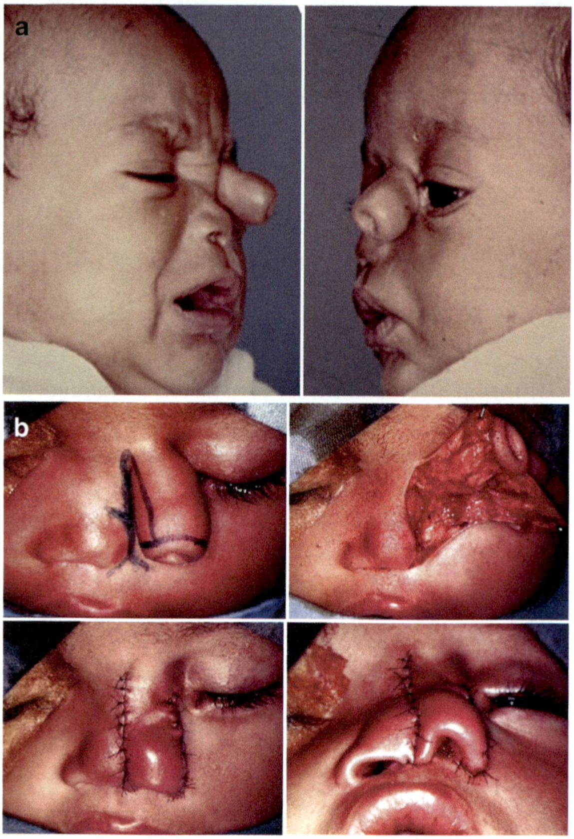

Fig. 6.14 Nasal reconstruction with proboscis. (**a**) Patient initial condition. (**b**) Intraoperative pictures

The second technic, which we call "proboscis adhesion," consists of the resection of the epidermal layer of the proboscis medial face and a band of skin along the nasal dorsum of the affected side and to suture the two raw surfaces altogether.

The third technic consists of the resection of most of the epidermal layer of the proboscis except the tip, which is kept to reconstruct the nostril circumference. The skin around the pedicle is incised in its whole thickness with respect to the subcutaneous pedicle.

To the location of the missing nostril, an arciform incision is made. A vertical tunnel is dissected, parallel to the dorsum nasi, to connect the upper and lower incisions. The row proboscis cylinder is passed through the tunnel, the proboscis tip reaches the lower incision to reconstruct the missing nostril, and the proboscis's volume reconstructs the nose's shape.

In cases of a supernumerary nostril, the supernumerary nostril must be respected. It is not a very big deal when the nostril of the affected side has a normal size, but when it is reduced, a part of the excess tissue of the supernumerary nostril can be used. There is no standard design; the local flap must be tailored to each situation.

6.10.1.2 Nasal Reconstruction

We cannot do better when talking about cleft 2–12 treatment than to side with Tessier's pieces of advice comprehensively detailed in the paper devoted to this topic.

Two coauthors of this chapter have published their experience in 2008 [109] about seven cases and the literature review.

Two points deserve a discussion: the technics for external nasal repair and the usefulness and the technics for reconstructing the nasal respiratory tract.

External Nasal Reconstruction

The cutaneous lining for the reconstruction of the nasal repair can be obtained from different areas in different ways.

As for acquired defects of the nose, one could use free grafts, a special notice for the case where a part of the proboscis was used for alar repair, but it was the only example of this technic and needed to be more conclusive.

As seen above, the proboscis has been used once as a migratory flap, but it is usually used as a permanent pedicled flap. To be fit for this purpose, the proboscis must be of a sufficient length and reach the tip of the nose, on the unaffected side (Fig. 6.14). From the pictures of results in reported cases from the literature, it looks as if the best results are obtained when the proboscis is put through a subcutaneous tunnel after epidermal resection of its shaft.

When there is no proboscis available, the best skin that matches the aesthetic requirement is the frontal skin.

The frontal flap can be harvested in two ways (Fig. 6.15) as a vertical or oblique flap with its pedicle in the glabellar area. It was the design used by Millard in his

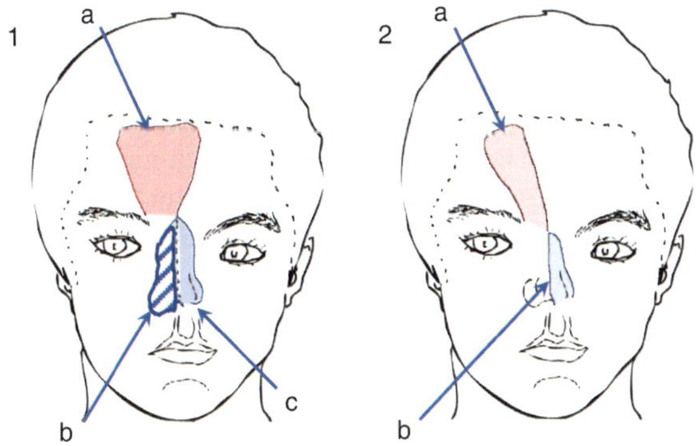

Fig. 6.15 Nasal reconstruction with frontal flap. *1*: vertical frontal flap for whole nasal unit reconstruction. (**a**) Frontal flap. (**b**) Nasal internal lining with a vertical pedicle. (**c**) Nasal internal lining with a horizontal pedicle. *2*: oblique frontal flap for hemi-nasal reconstruction. (**a**) Oblique frontal flap for hemi-nasal reconstruction. (**b**) Nasal internal lining with a horizontal pedicle

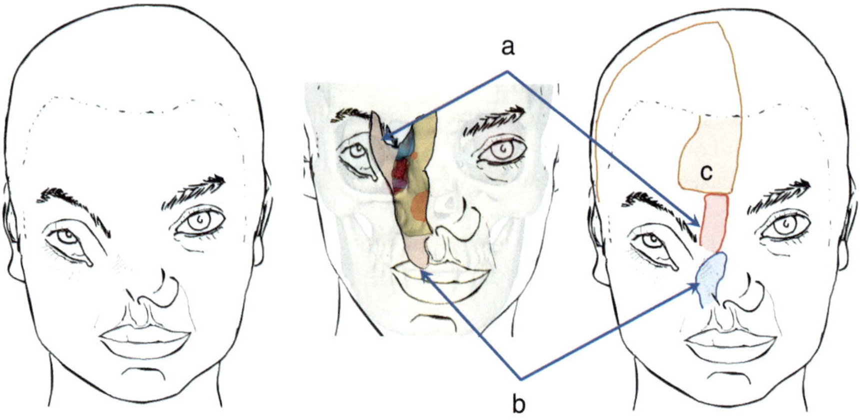

Fig. 6.16 Tessier's procedure for hemi-arhinia. The raising of flaps (**a**, **b**) intended for inner lining give access to the medial canthal area. The canthal dystopia as well as dacryocystorhinostomy, when feasible, are performed at the same time. The external nasal reconstruction, in this case, is performed with a Converse's scalping flap (**c**) In red: the dilated lachrymal sac. In purple: the right medial canthal ligament. In orange: the drilled part of maxilla. In green: a mucocoele

paper "hemirhinoplasty" [110] which was devoted to acquire nasal mutilations but is worth to be read and whose advice should be followed for cleft 2–12.

Tessier was a Gillies's scalping flap enthusiast, the other type of frontal flap. It is the type of design he supported in the arhinia paper [2]; in some occurrences, he has combined a vertical frontal flap with a scalping flap (Fig. 6.16).

Other technics, such as remotely migrating flaps, Washio's flaps, and free flaps, have no room for this purpose.

Nasal Framework Building

Obtaining a pleasing projection and length for the reconstructed nose requires an underlying framework. Bone grafts are the usual technic for the dorsum, they can be a straight graft secured to the frontal bone with mini-plating or an L-shape graft, but with the L-shape graft, it is more difficult to obtain a slim columella.

The bone is harvested from the iliac crest, skull, or costal graft. Some authors advertise a chondro-costal graft, expecting a growth.

The tip of the nose could benefit from a conchal cartilage graft or bi-tissular conchal graft to improve the lining of the vestibule.

Reconstruction of the Nasal Respiratory Tract

For the internal lining, free epidermal grafts or local flaps may be used when an attempt is made at constructing an internal nasal respiratory tract.

For hemi-arhinia, reconstructing a complete nasal tract is not used since the patency in the unaffected side is sufficient to ensure normal breathing. But to ensure a correct nostril shape, we have to rebuild a nasal vestibule, which will be marsupialized toward the patent nasal tract, through the septum. Most authors, like ourselves, use a local flap with an inferior pedicle at the nasal threshold location; when it is impossible for a nasolabial flap to fit.

The reconstruction of a fully functional nasal respiratory tract is required only in cases in which the patient presents itself with obstructive apnea syndrome. It occurs only in total arhinia. When severe obstructive apnea syndrome exists in young patients, building a skeletal crossing is not easy. The bone resection, usually by drilling with a burr, has to go through a narrow space of the hypoplastic maxillary. There is little room between the skull base and the palatal shelves; this narrow space is overcrowded with tooth buds in young children. Blind drilling could be very dangerous, entering the skull base or oral cavity or hurting tooth buds.

Brusati [111] advocated the elegant intervention, which created the skeletal cavity thanks to a Lefort II down-fracture of the maxillary, which is safe for the tooth buds only after a certain age. Both patients, in his publication, were, respectively, 6 and 12 years old and did not suffer from obstructive apnea. Local flaps ensured the lining of the nasal tract.

Tessier's proposition to overcome the risks linked to the skull base and tooth buds pleaded for a facial bipartition, which would, at the same time, yield to a maximal enlargement of the bone passage and avoid hurting the tooth buds.

A Simple and Effective Technic for Minor Forms of Cleft 2

In the minor forms of cleft 2, the hyporhinia could be limited: an ala could be present, as well as a hypoplastic nostril. Even in those minor forms, the nasal fossa is atretic.

In those conditions, our proposal for treatment is a two-time nasal repair. The first step is an early stage: (Fig. 6.17) relocation of the alae and a release of the threshold stenosis thanks to a cutaneous flap with subcutaneous pedicle as demonstrated in schematic drawing and patient pictures.

The second time (Fig. 6.18) for repairing those types of partial cleft is an open rhinoplasty with a reconstruction of the missing dome with a cartilage graft.

Our approach to open rhinoplasty is an incision running inside the nostril along the plica nasi at the caudal border of the alar cartilage. At the bottom of the columella, it crosses following the labio-columellar fold. The subcutaneous dissection plane leaves the perichondrium intact, and attached to the cartilage. Since the skin is very thin, this dissection is facilitated by a strong saline injection. After having freed the skin off the lateral face of the medial crus of the alar cartilage and crossed the cephalic rim of this medial crus, the skin comes with cellular tissue, which usually fills the space between both medial crus and contains the columellar pedicle (veins and arterial supplies).

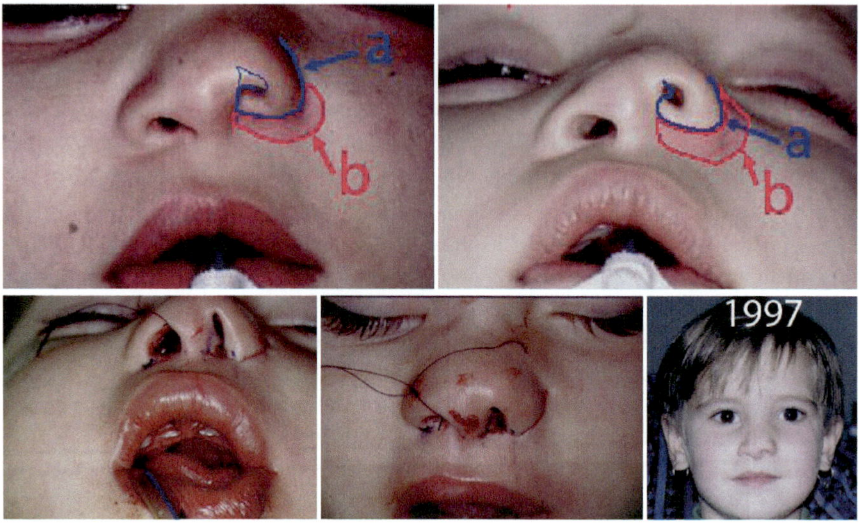

Fig. 6.17 (**a**) Lateral rhinotomy that totally frees the ala. (**b**) Cutaneous flap with a subcutaneous pedicle, translated to enlarge the nasal threshold. The ala is reinserted onto the lateral edge of the flap incision done symmetrical with the nasolabial fold of the unaffected side. The pyriform aperture has been drilled off for enlargement

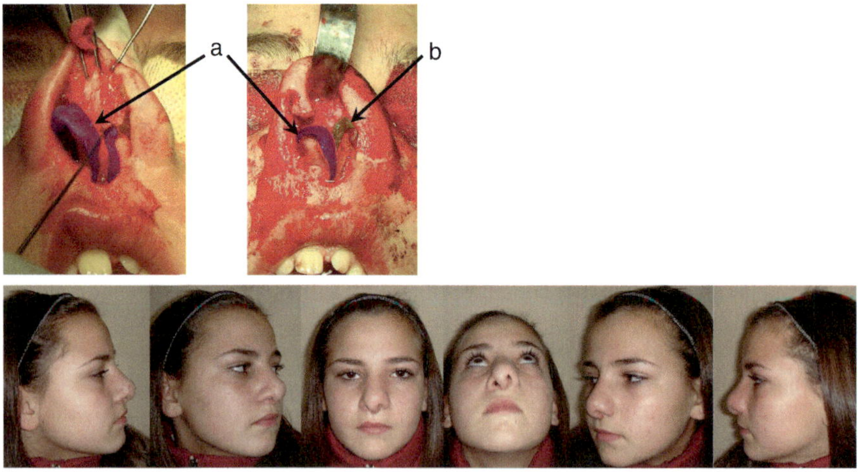

Fig. 6.18 Open rhinoplasty as a second stage, same patient than in Fig. 6.16. (**a**) Alar cartilages are highlighted in blue. (**b**) The cartilage graft is highlighted in yellow

Since there is a gap in those patients, we find a stump or nothing left of the medial crus on the affected side. It is helpful to reach what is left of the lateral crus to find the triangular cartilage and do "a retro" dissection of the lateral crus to bring out the lack of substance, the missing cartilage, in the dome area, which corresponds to the cleft.

The skin is caudally dissected from the perichondrium of the triangular cartilages on both sides, then from the periosteum and pyramidal muscles.

We used, at that time to separate the two alar cartilages from each other, which gives great access to the septum. From that time, the septum is dissected in sub perichondral plan so one can harvest what is needed to reconstruct the missing part of the alar cartilage.

The repair of the cartilaginous frame could be very precise.

Then the skin of the nose could be draped over the reconstructed frame; the point is to restore the empty triangle, which is the most difficult to achieve good symmetry.

Under such conditions where the airway is regular through the unaffected side, we don't attempt to reconstruct a nasal fossa in the affected side since it is of no use. We do a marsupialization of the nasal vestibule of the cleft side to the normal nasal fossa, which means creating a septal perforation.

6.10.1.3 Inter-Orbital Surgery

Surgery for Hypertelorism

Except in cases of association with other rare clefts, the hypertelorism, even if present (69 out of 148), is rarely severe (30 light, 27 mild and 12 severe). No more than 7 patients underwent hypertelorism surgery; most were box osteotomy, and one of our patients had a unilateral box osteotomy. Another had a craniofacial bipartition and a nasal tract reconstruction, creating a skeletal passage lined with a skin flap.

Canthoplasty

The medial canthus is frequently displaced downward and outward. This displacement is often associated with a lower lid coloboma which could be a part of a cleft 3. Thus, as advocated by Tessier, medial canthoplasty is an important part of the treatment of those patients. It could easily be performed with nasal reconstruction and, when feasible, with a dacryocystorhinostomy.

When there is an association of cleft 3 with cleft 2–12, the ascending medial process of the maxilla is missing and will require a bone graft to permit the canthopexy.

Dacryocystorhinostomy

According to Sahu's statistics [78], anomalies of the lachrymal system occur in 20% of the cases. Tessier's advice for treating lachrymal impairment, when required, is to wait until the natural process of dilatation has enlarged the dacryocyst to have a sufficient amount of lachrymal tissue. But, simultaneously, access to the nasal fossa is difficult.

The favorable conditions for the realization of a dacryocystorhinostomy are not frequently matched; if so: the intubation with the Lester Jone tube is helpful, and the tube must be left in place for a long time, at least 2 months.

When the dacryocystorhinostomy is not feasible, and there are some issues related to the dacryocyst, the excision of the lacrimal sac must be performed.

6.10.2 The Surgical Indications

Surgical timing in infants with a disfiguring condition has been the subject of many discussions. It is generally admitted that to allow a normal social integration and consider the psychological formation of self-imaging, surgical rehabilitation would have to be done before the age of 6 years, before entering primary school.

But two conditions could interfere with this timing and must be addressed: the management of proboscis lateralis and the possible obstructive sleep apnea condition.

6.10.2.1 In Case of Proboscis Lateralis

A proboscis lateralis must be addressed earlier since it is most distressing. The decision is whether to keep it, if it could be used, or to resect it if it is inappropriate for hemi-nasal reconstruction. If it has a sufficient length and a reliable pedicle, it is considered by most authors as the best material to reconstruct the missing part of the nose. If it is too short of reaching a correct position and it is to be resected, one must consider the possibility of using a part for a composite graft.

Care must be given to remove any epithelial remnant when the proboscis is resected. We have observed a case in which a considerable cyst developed after an incomplete resection during early childhood.

6.10.2.2 In Case of Obstructive Sleep Apnea

Obstructive sleep apnea syndrome would occur uniquely in the case of total arhinia and could require early nasal permeation. When it is performed as a life-saving procedure, only the internal lining is required, and the reconstruction of the external nasal pyramid can be set aside for a later procedure.

In our experience and cases of total arhinia found in the literature, the patients went across early childhood without significant problems. Thus, the question is: is it worth performing complex, tissue-consuming surgery to try to reconstruct a nasal airway that will be frequently hampered by secondary stenosis?

We would tend to strictly reserve functional surgery for life-threatening conditions when no other way to fix obstructive apnea syndrome could be found. We prefer to leave the patient who does not have an issue with breathing, alone.

6.11 Authors Cases

6.11.1 *Case One (Figs. 6.19, 6.20, and 6.21)*

A boy was referred for treatment after a failed attempt elsewhere to create a nasal airway; the pit is, in fact, the scarring from this precedent procedure. The patient has a CFM with left microtia and facial palsy.

Our first surgery combines the creation of a skeletal nasal aperture by drilling, lining the new cavity with a local flap and repairing the missing alae with a frontal flap on a subcutaneous pedicle. The second stage was the treatment of hypertelorism by bipartition and iteration of nasal reconstruction. The previous frontal flap was moved as internal lining, and a new glabellar flap was harvested thanks to the orbital narrowing. This flap, too short, must be mobilized later to fit. The final nasal surgery was an iliac bone graft to the dorsum. In the meantime, an ear reconstruction has been performed.

6.11.2 *Case Two (Figs. 6.22 and 6.23)*

A woman referred for the sequels of hemi-arhinia with proboscis. She has been operated on elsewhere three times. First, the resection of her proboscis. Second, a frontal flap, and third, a revision of the nasal repair. Pictures of the previous condition are from her archives.

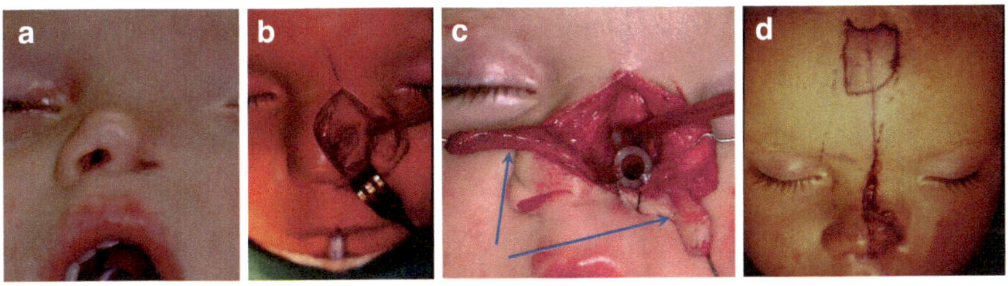

Fig. 6.19 Author's case 1. (**a**) Initial condition, the pit is the scarring from a first surgical attempt. (**b**) The left pyriform aperture is totally missing. (**c**) A new aperture has been drilled off. Blue arrows point toward the flaps designed for internal lining. (**d**) The alar is reconstructed by a frontal flap with a subcutaneous pedicle

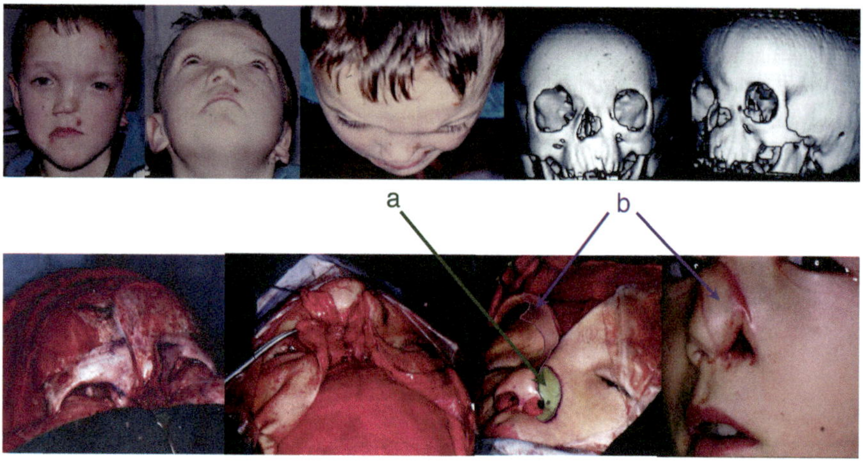

Fig. 6.20 Author's case 1. Second surgery: craniofacial bipartition. (**a**) Frontal flap for the external lining. (**b**) Migrating flap for the internal lining

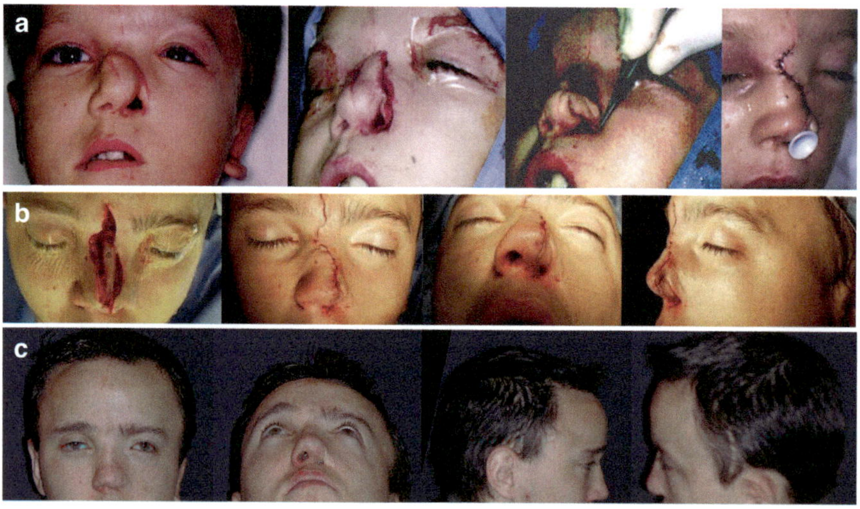

Fig. 6.21 Author's case 1. (**a**) Migration of the second frontal flap. (**b**) Iliac bone graft to the dorsum. (**c**) Final result

We made an iliac bone graft for nasal repair, a bone graft for orbital repair, a resection of the dacryocyst and a canthopexy.

6.11.3 Case Three (Fig. 6.24)

A boy with total arhinia without any sleep apnea: external reconstruction without attempt at airway reconstruction.

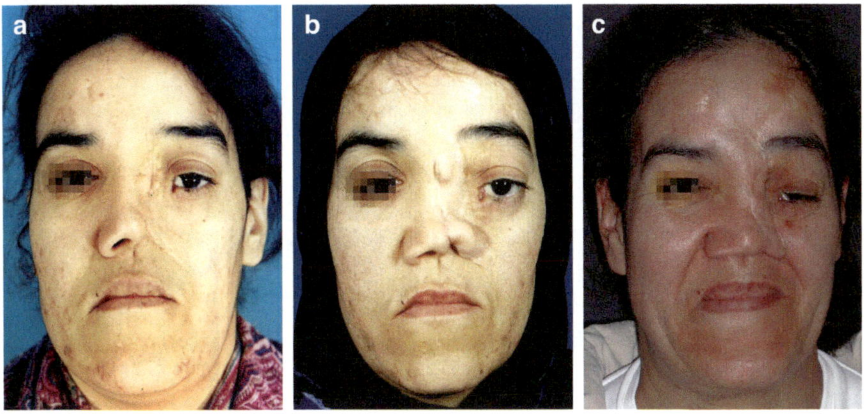

Fig. 6.22 Author's case 2: Secondary case. (**a**) Initial condition, picture from patient's archives, the proboscis has been resected previously. (**b**) Result after a first procedure done elsewhere. (**c**) Condition at our first examination after a second procedure in another institution

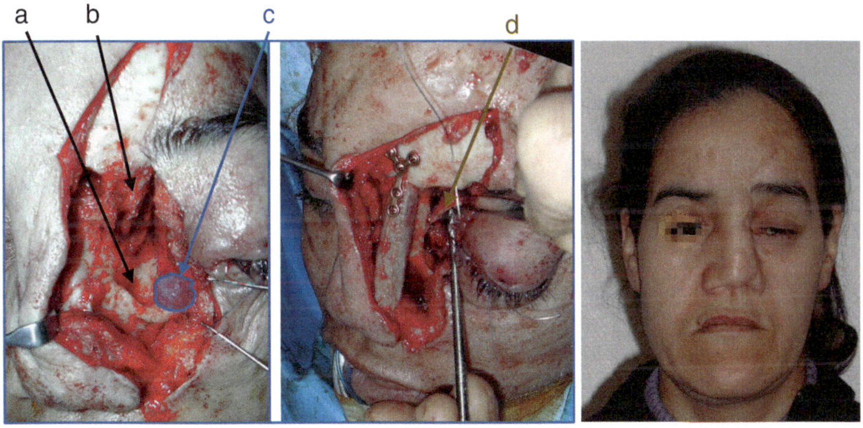

Fig. 6.23 Surgery and final result. (**a**) Absence of lachrymo-nasal duct and bone deformation by the dacryocyst. (**b**) Communication with the frontal sinus at the former proboscis insertion. (**c**) The dacryocysts to be resected. (**d**) Graft to reconstruct the upper-medial orbital corner and canthopexy

6.11.4 Case Four (Fig. 6.25)

A girl with total arhinia. In this case, an attempt at creating an airway is made by using the inferiorly based nasal flap as the internal lining. The external nose is reconstructed with a vertical frontal flap. A poor late result due to a growth defect required a second frontal flap after a skin expansion.

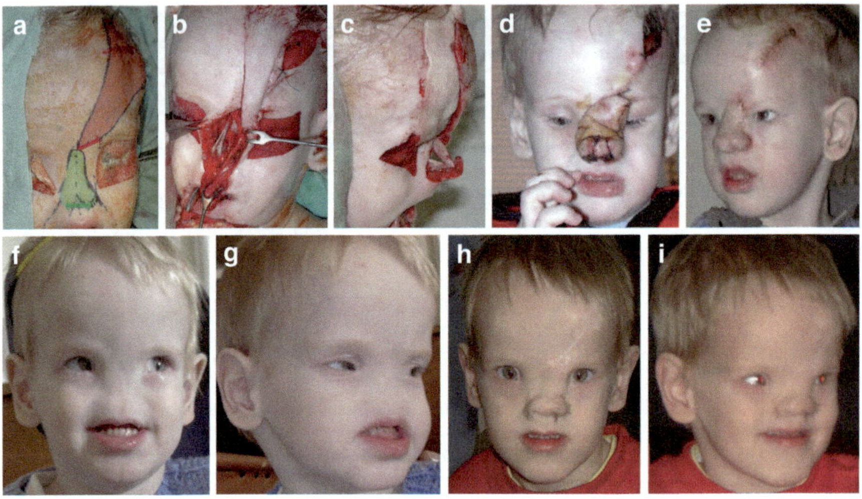

Fig. 6.24 External nasal reconstruction: frontal flap with costal bone graft. (**a**) Outlining of flaps: red frontal flap, green nasal flap. Double arrows mark the pedicles. (**b**, **c**) Costal grafts. (**d**) Intermediate condition before severing the frontal flap pedicle. (**e**) Early result after severing the pedicle. (**f**, **g**) Initial presentation. (**h**, **i**) Result after 1 year

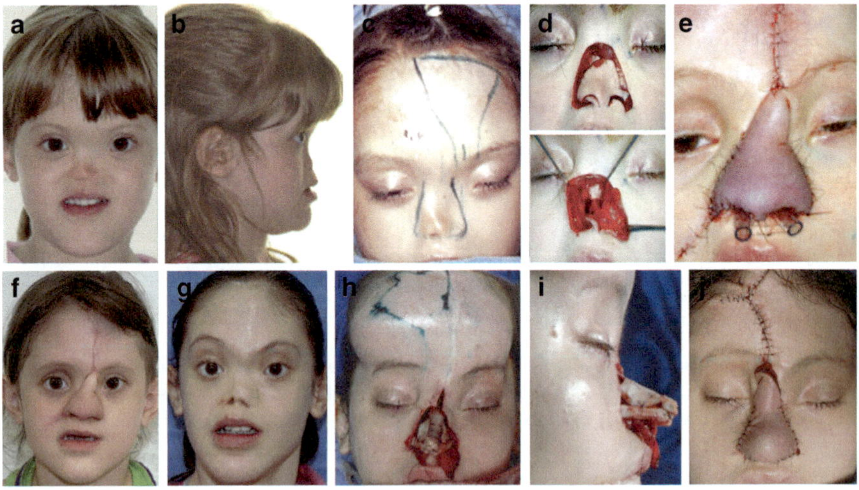

Fig. 6.25 Full nasal reconstruction. (**a**, **b**) Total arhinia. (**c–e**) Reconstruction, inferior flap for airway lining, frontal flap for external reconstruction. (**f**) Early result. (**g**) Poor late result due to a lack of growth. (**h–j**) Second reconstruction with an expanded frontal flap over a cartilage and bone frame

References

1. Tessier P. Anatomical classification of facial, cranio-facial and latero-facial clefts. J Maxillofac Surg. 1976;4:69–92. https://linkinghub.elsevier.com/retrieve/pii/S0301050376800136.
2. Tessier P, Ciminello FS, Wolfe SA. The arrhinias. Scand J Plast Reconstr Surg Hand Surg. 2009;43(4):177–96. https://doi.org/10.1080/02844310802517259.
3. DKO B, Bartley GB, Clay RP, Thompson DM. Heminasal proboscis with associated microphthalmos and encephalocele. J Craniofac Surg. 2005;16(2):300–6. http://journals.lww.com/00001665-200503000-00018.
4. Förster A. Die Missbildungen des Menschen, systematisch dargestellt, text and atlas, vol. Text & Atlas; 1861. p. 168.
5. Selenkoff A. Ein Fall von Arhinencephalia unilateralis bei einem erwachsenen Manne. Arch Für Pathol Anat Physiol Für Klin Med. 1884;95(1):95–101. https://doi.org/10.1007/BF01931120.
6. Geoffroy Saint Hilaire I. Histoire générale et particuliére des anomalies de l'organisation chez l'homme et les animaux, vol. Atlas. Paris: Bailliére; 1837. https://ia800106.us.archive.org/17/items/BIUSante_35541/BIUSante_35541.pdf.
7. Grünberg K. Chapter IV: Die Gesichtsspalten und die zu ihnen in genetischer Beziehung stehenden anderweitigen Mißbildungen des Gesichts. In: Swalbe E, editor. Die morphologie der missbildüngen des menschen und der tiere. Jena: verlag von Gustav Fischer; 1909. p. 113–204. https://archive.org/details/b21506899_0002.
8. Bosma JF, Henkin RI, Christiansen RL, Herdt JR. Hypoplasia of the nose and eyes, hyposmia, hypogeusia, and hypogonadotrophic hypogonadism in two males. J Craniofac Genet Dev Biol. 1981;1(2):153–84.
9. Thiele H, Musil A, Nagel F, Majewski F. Familial arhinia, choanal atresia, and microphthalmia. Am J Med Genet. 1996;63(1):310–3. https://doi.org/10.1002/(SICI)1096-8628(19960503)63:1<310::AID-AJMG51>3.0.CO;2-N.
10. Gordon CT, Xue S, Yigit G, Filali H, Chen K, Rosin N, et al. De novo mutations in SMCHD1 cause Bosma arhinia microphthalmia syndrome and abrogate nasal development. Nat Genet. 2017;49(2):249–55. http://www.nature.com/articles/ng.3765.
11. Shaw ND, Brand H, Kupchinsky ZA, Bengani H, Plummer L, Jones TI, et al. SMCHD1 mutations associated with a rare muscular dystrophy can also cause isolated arhinia and Bosma arhinia microphthalmia syndrome. Nat Genet. 2017;49(2):238–48. https://www.nature.com/articles/ng.3743.
12. Rahimov F, Ribeiro LA, de Miranda E, Richieri-Costa A, Murray JC. GLI2 mutations in four Brazilian patients: how wide is the phenotypic spectrum? Am J Med Genet A. 2006;140A(23):2571–6. https://onlinelibrary.wiley.com/doi/10.1002/ajmg.a.31370.
13. KEA A-E. Proboscis Lateralis: a report of two cases. Int J Pediatr Otorhinolaryngol. 2004;68(4):503–5. https://linkinghub.elsevier.com/retrieve/pii/S0165587603004865.
14. Abulezz T. Congenital heminasal aplasia: clinical picture, radiological findings, and follow-up after early surgical intervention. J Craniofac Surg. 2019;30(3):e199–202. http://journals.lww.com/00001665-201905000-00090.
15. Acarturk S, Kivanc K, Atilla E, Sekucoglu T. Proboscis lateralis: evaluation of the anomaly and a review of two cases. Plast Reconstr Surg. 2006;117(7):140e–6e. http://journals.lww.com/00006534-200606000-00050.
16. Agarwal S, Latta S. Proboscis lateralis. Indian J Otolaryngol Head Neck Surg Off Publ Assoc Otolaryngol India. 2010;62(1):79–80.
17. Ajike SO, Mohammed R, Johnson AO, Chaha K, Samaila MO. Lateral proboscis (elephant tusk) with orofacial clefts: a report of a rare case. Case Rep Pediatr. 2018;2018:1–4. https://www.hindawi.com/journals/cripe/2018/6820972/.
18. Akkuzu G, Akkuzu B, Aydin E, Derbent M, Ozluoglu L. Congenital partial arhinia: a case report. J Med Case Rep. 2007;1(1):97. https://jmedicalcasereports.biomedcentral.com/articles/10.1186/1752-1947-1-97.

19. Al-Helo S, Taghi AS, Mahboba S. Unusual case of accessory nose associated with unilateral complete congenital choanal atresia. Saudi Med J. 2008;29(9):1342–3.
20. MHA B. Half nose. J Laryngol Otol. 1984;98(9):915–6. https://www.cambridge.org/core/product/identifier/S002221510014770X/type/journal_article.
21. Belet N. Proboscis lateralis: a case report. Clin Dysmorphol. 2002;11(3):219–20. http://journals.lww.com/00019605-200207000-00015.
22. Belet N, Belet Ü, Tekat A, Küçüködük Ş. Proboscis lateralis: radiological evaluation. Pediatr Radiol. 2002;32(2):99–101. http://link.springer.com/10.1007/s00247-001-0602-6.
23. Bhandari PS. Simultaneous and symmetrical reconstruction of heminose and restoration of nasal airway in congenital absence of heminose. Br J Plast Surg. 2004;57(6):575–8.
24. Binns JH. Congenital tubular nostril (proboscis lateralis). Br J Plast Surg. 1969;22(3–4):265–8. https://linkinghub.elsevier.com/retrieve/pii/S0007122669801177.
25. Bothra N, Naik M, Ali MJ. Multiple lacrimal drainage anomalies in proboscis lateralis. Orbit. 2021;40(3):255–7. https://www.tandfonline.com/doi/full/10.1080/01676830.2020.1767157.
26. Ali MJ, Singh S, Naik MN. Image-guided lacrimal drainage surgery in congenital arhinia-microphthalmia syndrome. Orbit. 2017;36(3):137–43. https://doi.org/10.1080/01676830.2017.1280059.
27. Bryant JR, Stein JR, Boyajian MK, Manrique M, Mantilla-Rivas E, Aivaz M, et al. Heminasal reconstruction utilizing Presurgical planning, template-based cartilage reconstruction and tissue expansion. J Craniofacial Surg. 2020;31(6):1724–6.
28. Chaisrisawadisuk S, Khampalikit I, Moore MH, Anderson PJ, Chaisrisawadisuk S. Proboscis Lateralis with basal encephalocele: a report of clinical management and reconstructive approach. Cleft Palate Craniofac J. 2022:105566562210963. https://doi.org/10.1177/10556656221096323.
29. Chauhan DS, Guruprasad Y. Proboscis lateralis. J Maxillofac Oral Surg. 2010;9(2):162–5.
30. Chen MT, Yeong EK. Supernumerary nostrils. Br J Plast Surg. 1992;45(7):557–8. https://linkinghub.elsevier.com/retrieve/pii/000712269290156R.
31. Coessens B, De Mey A, Lejour M. Correction of supernumerary nostrils. Int J Pediatr Otorhinolaryngol. 1992;23(3):275–80. https://linkinghub.elsevier.com/retrieve/pii/016558769290110B.
32. D'assumpção EA. Proboscis lateralis: case report. Plast Reconstr Surg. 1975;55(4):494–7. https://journals.lww.com/plasreconsurg/Citation/1975/04000/PROBOSCIS_LATERALIS__Case_Report.21.aspx.
33. David LR, Sanger C, Fisher D, Argenta LC. Proboscis lateralis: a rare craniofacial anomaly, reconstruction, and long-term evaluation. J Craniofac Surg. 2008;19(4):1107–13. https://journals.lww.com/00001665-200807000-00043.
34. Das D, Das G, Gayen S, Konar A. Median facial cleft in amniotic band syndrome. Middle East Afr J Ophthalmol. 2011;18(2):192. http://www.meajo.org/text.asp?2011/18/2/192/80713.
35. Erich JB. Nasal duplication. Report of case of patient with two noses. Plast Reconstr Surg. 1962;29(2):159–66.
36. Bell Tawse H. Supernumerary nostril and cavity. Proc R Soc Med. 1920;13(Laryngol_Sect):28–30. https://doi.org/10.1177/003591572001300713.
37. Eroğlu L, Uysal OA. Proboscis lateralis: report of two cases. Br J Plast Surg. 2003;56(7):704–8. https://linkinghub.elsevier.com/retrieve/pii/S0007122603003564.
38. Fawzy HAAR, Ghareeb F, Farghaly AS, Al Barah A, El Sheikh Y. Patterns and management of congenital nasal clefts. Menoufia Med J. 2015;28(1):99. http://www.mmj.eg.net/text.asp?2015/28/1/99/155960.
39. Fisher M, Zelken J, Redett RJ. Heminasal agenesis: a reconstructive challenge. J Craniofac Surg. 2014;25(3):e239–41. https://journals.lww.com/00001665-201405000-00135.
40. Fischer H, Eppstein R, von Gregory H, Gubisch W. Nasal reconstruction in Heminasal deficiency (proboscis Lateralis): two case reports, with airway reconstruction in one case. Facial Plast Surg. 2014;30(03):365–70. https://doi.org/10.1055/s-0034-1376880.

41. Franklin Bishop BW. Lateral nasal proboscis. Br J Plast Surg. 1964;17:18–21. https://doi.org/10.1016/S0007-1226(64)80004-7.
42. Biber JJ. Proboscis lateralis: a rare malformation of the nose its genesis and treatment. J Laryngol Otol. 1949;63(12):734–41. https://www.cambridge.org/core/product/identifier/S0022215100047125/type/journal_article.
43. Galiè M, Clauser LC, Tieghi R, Kawamoto HK, Wolfe SA, Bianchi AE. The arrhinias: Proboscis lateralis literature review and surgical update. J Cranio-Maxillofac Surg. 2019;47(9):1410–3. https://linkinghub.elsevier.com/retrieve/pii/S101051821831148X
44. Ghieh F, Karami R, Sittah GA. Proboscis lateralis with heminasal hypoplasia. J Craniofac Surg. 2019;30(3):e254–5. http://journals.lww.com/00001665-201905000-00112.
45. Guerrero JM, Cogen MS, Kelly DR, Wiatrak BJ. Proboscis lateralis. Arch Ophthalmol. 2001;119(7):1071–4.
46. Hassani ME, Karimi H, Hassani H, Hassani A, Jalili-Manesh M. Heminasal proboscis, a rare craniofacial cleft. J Craniofac Surg. 2014;25(1):e7–9. http://journals.lww.com/00001665-201401000-00069
47. Horoz U, Kuroki T, Shimoyama M, Yoshimoto S. Approach to half-nose and proboscis lateralis. J Craniofac Surg. 2018;29(8):2234–6. http://journals.lww.com/00001665-201811000-00052.
48. Jian XC, Su HB, Chen XO. Triple nostrils associated with cleft lip and palate. Br J Plast Surg. 1995;48(1):53. https://linkinghub.elsevier.com/retrieve/pii/0007122695900330
49. Jost G, Mookherjee R, Dionyssopoulos A. Proboscis lateralis: treatment of two atypical cases. Aesthet Plast Surg. 1995;19(2):165–8. http://link.springer.com/10.1007/BF00450253.
50. Khoo BC. The proboscis lateralis–a 14-year follow-up. Plast Reconstr Surg. 1985;75(4):569–77.
51. Kirkpatrick TJ. Lateral nasal proboscis. J Laryngol Otol. 1970;84(1):83–9. https://www.cambridge.org/core/product/identifier/S0022215100071668/type/journal_article.
52. Kukreja HK. Half nose. J Laryngol Otol. 1973;87(6):599–602. https://www.cambridge.org/core/product/identifier/S0022215100077367/type/journal_article.
53. Lelli GJ, Maher EA, Milite JP, Dyleski R. Proboscis lateralis. Ophthal Plast Reconstr Surg. 2008;24(6):499–501. https://journals.lww.com/00002341-200811000-00024.
54. Magadum SB, Khairnar P, Hirugade S, Kassa V. Proboscis lateralis of nose-a case report. Indian J Surg. 2012;74(2):181–3.
55. Mahindra S, Daljit R, Jamwal N, Mathew M. Lateral nasal proboscis. J Laryngol Otol. 1973;87(2):177–81. https://www.cambridge.org/core/product/identifier/S0022215100076763/type/journal_article.
56. Martin S, Hogan E, Sorenson EP, Cohen-Gadol AA, Tubbs RS, Loukas M. Proboscis lateralis. Childs Nerv Syst. 2013;29(6):885–91. http://link.springer.com/10.1007/s00381-012-1989-0.
57. Mathur NN, Garg R. Proboscis lateralis. Indian J Otolaryngol Head Neck Surg Off Publ Assoc Otolaryngol India. 1999;51(1):74–5.
58. Mclaren L. A case of cleft lip abd palate with polypoid nasal tubercule. Br J Plast Surg. 1955;8:55–9. https://linkinghub.elsevier.com/retrieve/pii/S0007122655800112.
59. Meeker LH. Cyclopean eye and lateral proboscis with normal half face. Arch Ophtalmol. 1947;38(2):159. http://archopht.jamanetwork.com/article.aspx?doi=10.1001/archopht.1947.00900010164003
60. Mladina R, Manojlovic S, Markov-Glavaš D. An unusual case of heminasal aplasia: Proboscis lateralis or cystic Teratoma? J Craniofac Surg. 2003;14(1):5.
61. Motohashi N, Kuroda T, Cohen MM. Half nose with ipsilateral eye and ear anomalies and facial asymmetry: report of a case with cephalometric analysis and orthodontic treatment. Cleft Palate Craniofac J. 1999;36(4):353–60. https://doi.org/10.1597/1545-1569_1999_036_0353_hnwiea_2.3.co_2.
62. Nagase T, Kobayashi S, Ohmori K. Achieving natural shading of the nostril in the reconstruction of a half nose. Br J Plast Surg. 1998;51(2):131–4. https://linkinghub.elsevier.com/retrieve/pii/S0007122697901521.

63. Nakamura K, Onizuka T. A case of supernumerary nostril. Plast Reconstr Surg. 1987;80(3):436–41. http://journals.lww.com/00006534-198709000-00018.
64. Sah BP. Supernumerary nostril associated with dermoid cyst: a rare case report and review of literature. Am J Med Case Rep. 2014;2(3):52–4. http://pubs.sciepub.com/ajmcr/2/3/3/index.html.
65. Aslanabadi S, Djalilian H, Zarrintan S, Sokhandan M, Hashem-Zadeh H, Lotfi AR. Supernumerary nostril together with esophageal atresia, imperforate anus and patent ductus arteriosus: a case report and review of the literature. Pediatr Surg Int. 2009;25(5):433–6. http://link.springer.com/10.1007/s00383-009-2351-9.
66. Numanoglu V, Ermis B, Dursun A, Battal F, Ornek Z, Dogan SM, et al. Supernumerary nostrils together with oesophageal atresia and patent ductus arteriosus. Clin Dysmorphol. 2007;16(4):269–70. https://journals.lww.com/00019605-200710000-00009.
67. Onizuka T, Tai Y. Supernumerary Nostril. Plast Reconstr Surg. 1972;50(4):403–5. http://journals.lww.com/00006534-197210000-00025.
68. Kingsly P, Dhanraj P, Gupta AK, Babu S. Heminasal aplasia: a report of two cases. Indian J Otolaryngol Head Neck Surg Off Publ Assoc Otolaryngol India. 2007;59(1):58–9.
69. Ozek C, Gundogan H, Bilkay U, Cankayali R, Guner U, Gurler T, et al. Rare craniofacial anomaly: Tessier no. 2 cleft. J Craniofac Surg. 2001;12(4):355–61. http://journals.lww.com/00001665-200107000-00008.
70. Poed LB, Hochhauser L, Bryke C, Streeten BW, Sloan J. Proboscis lateralis with associated orbital cyst: detailed MR and CT imaging and correlative embryopathy. AJNR Am J Neuroradiol. 1992;13(5):1471–6.
71. Powar RS, Tubaki VR. Supernumerary nostril with complete unilateral cleft lip: a case report and review. Cleft Palate Craniofac J. 2007;44(6):657–9. http://journals.sagepub.com/doi/10.1597/06-115.1.
72. Rao PB. Proboscis lateralis. J Laryngol Otol. 1963;77(12):1028–31. http://www.journals.cambridge.org/abstract_S0022215100061715.
73. Raposo C, Lim R, Jarrahy R. Rare craniofacial clefts. In craniofacial disorders, Plastic surgery keys. https://doi.org/10.1055/b-0038-162658. https://plasticsurgerykey.com/craniofacial-disorders-8/.
74. Rawat SS, Gupta HKD. Congenital double columella. Br J Plast Surg. 1975;28(3):153–4. https://linkinghub.elsevier.com/retrieve/pii/0007122675901186.
75. Reddy KA, Rao AK. Triple nostrils: a case report and review. Br J Plast Surg. 1987;40(6):651–2. https://linkinghub.elsevier.com/retrieve/pii/0007122687901640.
76. Rontal M, Duritz G. Probocis lateralis: case report and embryologic analysis. Laryngoscope. 1977;87(6):996–1006.
77. Rosen Z, Gitlin G. Bilateral nasal proboscis. AMA Arch Otolaryngol. 1959;70:10–24. http://archotol.jamanetwork.com/.
78. Sahu ES, Shroff PH, Sahu A, Bhargava A, Sharma B. Ophthalmic manifestations of proboscis lateralis. BMJ Open Ophthalmol. 2021;6(1):e000558. https://bmjophth.bmj.com/lookup/doi/10.1136/bmjophth-2020-000558.
79. Kaur B, Bansal S, Saikia UN, Gupta P. Congenital lateral nasal proboscis with orbital mass. Int J Clin Rhinol. 2014;7(3):139–41. https://doi.org/10.5005/jp-journals-10013-1216.
80. Sarsmaz K, Lafci O, Cayonu Kahraman N, Ergun E, Celen S, Caglar AT. A rare case of bilateral proboscis lateralis: prenatal US and MRI findings. J Clin Ultrasound. 2021;49(6):632–5. https://doi.org/10.1002/jcu.22982.
81. Govila A. Proboscis lateralis type IV–a report from the Indian subcontinent. Acta Chir Plast. 1991;33(1):34–9.
82. Shaye DA, Hakizimana A, Ndamyiyumva E, Umuganwa P, Tuyishimire G, Ncogoza I, et al. Proboscis lateralis: a unique window into nasal embryology. Facial Plast Surg Aesthetic Med. 2020;22(4):307–8. https://doi.org/10.1089/fpsam.2020.0107.
83. Singh I, Gathwala G, Kalra GS, Malhotra V. Proboscis lateralis of nose. Indian J Pediatr. 2001;68(5):467–8. http://link.springer.com/10.1007/BF02723031.

84. Skevas A, Tsoulias T, Papadopoulos N, Assimakopoulos D. Proboscis lateralis, a rare malformation. Rhinology. 1990;28(4):285–9.
85. Stanek J, de Courten-Myers G, Spaulding AG, Strub W, Hopkin RJ. Case of complex craniofacial anomalies, bilateral nasal proboscides, palatal pituitary, upper limbs reduction, and amnion rupture sequence: disorganization phenotype? Pediatr Dev Pathol. 2001;4(2):192–202. https://doi.org/10.1007/s100240010131.
86. Takcı S, Korkmaz A, Simşek-Kiper PO, Utine GE, Boduroğlu K, Yurdakök M. Congenital partial arhinia: a rare malformation of the nose coexisting with holoprosencephaly. Turk J Pediatr. 2012;54(4):440–3.
87. Tambwekar SR, Aiyer PM, Vij VK. Supernumerary nostril in association with incomplete naso-ocular cleft. Plast Amp Reconstr Surg. 1997;100(3):682–4. http://journals.lww.com/00006534-199709000-00022.
88. Thorne MC, Ruiz RE, Carvalho J, Lesperance MM. Proboscis lateralis: case report and review. Arch Otolaryngol Neck Surg. 2007;133(10):1051. https://doi.org/10.1001/archotol.133.10.1051.
89. Udagawa A, Hamajima A, Okamura T, Lee S, Yoshimoto S, Ichinose M. Hemi aplasia of the nose with complete cleft lip and palate of the contralateral side. J Plast Reconstr Aesthet Surg. 2009;62(10):e349–52. https://linkinghub.elsevier.com/retrieve/pii/S1748681508005202
90. Uğurlu K, Karşidag S, Ozçelik D, Sadikoğlu B, Baş L. Repair of proboscis lateralis. Scand J Plast Reconstr Surg Hand Surg. 2005;39(3):184–7.
91. Vaid S, Shah D, Rawat S, Shukla R. Proboscis lateralis with ipsilateral sinonasal and olfactory pathway aplasia. J Pediatr Surg. 2010;45(2):453–6. https://linkinghub.elsevier.com/retrieve/pii/S0022346809008276.
92. Verma P, Pal M, Goel A, Singh I, Bansal V. Proboscis lateralis: case report and overview. Indian J Otolaryngol Head Neck Surg Off Publ Assoc Otolaryngol India. 2011;63(Suppl 1):36–7.
93. Tadashi U, Iida H, Hiroyuki O. Supernumerary nostrils associated with cleft lip and palate. Br J Plast Surg. 1996;49(7):499. https://linkinghub.elsevier.com/retrieve/pii/S0007122696900429.
94. Wilkinson G. Rare congenital deformity of the nose in an infant. Proc R Soc Med. 1910;3(Laryngol_Sect):83–5. https://doi.org/10.1177/003591571000300659.
95. Williams A, Pizzuto M, Brodsky L, Perry R. Supernumerary nostril: a rare congenital deformity. Int J Pediatr Otorhinolaryngol. 1998;44(2):161–7. https://linkinghub.elsevier.com/retrieve/pii/S0165587698000445.
96. Xu Y, Fan F, Wang H. Supernumerary nostril: an extremely rare case. Int J Pediatr Otorhinolaryngol Extra. 2012;7:89–91.
97. Jagannathan M, Dixit V, Nayak BB, Joshi A. Supernumerary nostril with a contralateral naso-ocular cleft. Eur J Plast Surg. 2003;26(1):44–6. https://doi.org/10.1007/s00238-003-0464-2.
98. Shen C, Shetye PR, Flores RL. Nasal duplication: a review of literature and case report. Cleft Palate Craniofac J. 2021;58(5):628–36. https://doi.org/10.1177/1055665620962671.
99. Yildirim SV. Proboscis lateralis: a case report. Int J Pediatr Otorhinolaryngol. 2001;61(2):179–82.
100. Mehta L, Petrikovsky B, Tydings L, Lundberg J. Lateral nasal proboscis: antenatal diagnosis and counseling. Obstetr & Gynecol. 1999;94(5):3.
101. Yoo SW, Jeong HM, Lee SH, Lee JH. A case of congenital heminasal hypoplasia with an intranasal cyst: an extremely rare occurrence. Int J Pediatr Otorhinolaryngol. 2013;77(4):585–7. https://linkinghub.elsevier.com/retrieve/pii/S0165587612007276.
102. Zbar RIS, Rai SM, Ghimire P. Repair of congenital nasal anomalies involving redundancy of structures. The Cleft Palate-Craniofacial Journal [Internet]. 2003 Mar [cited 2022 Dec 17];40(2):214–7. http://journals.sagepub.com/doi/10.1597/1545-1569_2003_040_0214_rocnai_2.0.co_2.
103. Shanmuganathan P, Chong DK. Accessory nostril associated with Choanal atresia. J Craniofac Surg. 2021;32(8):2845–7.

104. Oshima J, Sasaki K, Aihara Y, Myojo R, Sasaki M, Shibuya Y, et al. Accessory columellas: a case series on surgical method and short-term postoperative course. J Plast Reconstr Aesthetic Surg JPRAS. 2022;S1748-6815(22):00495–8.
105. Boo-Chai K. The oblique facial cleft. Br J Plast Surg. 1970;23:352–9. https://linkinghub.elsevier.com/retrieve/pii/S0007122670800741.
106. Sakamoto Y, Miyamoto J, Nakajima H, Kishi K. New classification scheme of proboscis lateralis based on a review of 50 cases. Cleft Palate Craniofac J. 2012;49(2):201–7. https://doi.org/10.1597/10-127.1.
107. Förster A. Die Missbildungen des Menschen: systematisch dargestellt. Jena: Druck und Verlag von Friedrich Mauke; 1861. p. 344. https://archive.org/details/b21309036.
108. Dasgupta G, Kacker SK, Bhan AK. Proboscis. J Laryngol Otol. 1971;85(4):401–6. https://www.cambridge.org/core/product/identifier/S002221510007359X/type/journal_article.
109. da Silva FR, Alonso N, de Freitas AT, Busato L, Dall'Oglio Tolazzi AR, de Oliveira e Cruz GA, et al. The surgical repair of half-nose. J Plast Reconstr Aesthet Surg. 2010;63(1):15–21. https://linkinghub.elsevier.com/retrieve/pii/S1748681508009868.
110. Millard DR. Hemirhinoplasty. Plast Reconstr Surg. 1967;40(5):440–5. http://journals.lww.com/00006534-196711000-00003.
111. Brusati R, Colletti G. The role of maxillary osteotomy in the treatment of Arhinia. J Oral Maxillofac Surg. 2012;70(5):e361–8. https://linkinghub.elsevier.com/retrieve/pii/S0278239112000985.

Chapter 7
Cleft 3/11

Nivaldo Alonso, Renato da Silva Freitas, Cristiano Tonello, and Philippe Pellerin

Pearls

- Tessier cleft number 3 (TC3) is one of the most difficult and challenging malformations to correct by involving all the facial anatomical structures.
- TC3 was found more associated with discontinuity of the eyebrow and no frontal bone deformities, a minor and major form of Tessier 10 cleft than with Tessier cleft 11.
- TC3 cleft was also found to be associated with many different facial cleft and amniotic bands syndrome.
- Age and type of surgical treatment depend on the severity of the eye exposition and the nasal cleft.

N. Alonso (✉)
Plastic Surgery, Universidade de São Paulo, São Paulo, Brazil

Hospital de Reabilitação Anomalias Craniofaciais Universidade de São Paulo, Bauru, Brazil

R. da Silva Freitas
Plastic Surgery Unit, Hospital de Clínicas, Universidade Federal do Paraná, Curitiba, Brazil

Craniofacial Surgery, Assistance Center for Cleft Lip and Palate (CAIF), Hospital do Trabalhador, Curitiba, Brazil

C. Tonello
Curso de Medicina Bauru Faculdade de Odontologia Bauru Universidade de São Paulo, Bauru, Brazil

Hospital de Reabilitação Anomalias Craniofaciais Universidade de São Paulo, Bauru, Brazil

P. Pellerin
Centre Hospitalier Régional Universitaire de Lille, Lille, France

N. Alonso et al. (eds.), *Facial Reconstruction of Unusual Facial Clefts*,
https://doi.org/10.1007/978-3-031-40926-4_7

7.1 History

These unusual facial clefts have been known and described since a long time ago, and many old references can be found in the literature. R. Morian, in 1886, over a century ago, proposed a classification for these facial clefts in Berlin during the German Medical Society Meeting [1]. Tessier Cleft 3 (TC3) is still commonly called an oculo-nasal cleft Morian type 1, and it is very interesting how accurate Morian's first description, like Tessier's in 1976, is without any particular type of images we have today. However, the most widely accepted and easily understood classification was proposed by Tessier, and this malformation is known worldwide as Tessier Cleft 3 [2]. There are similarities between the two classifications. Morian used the terminology including all the facial structures involved, and Tessier gave numbers to his clinical findings based on the orbit and boundaries between facial structures and cranial structures (Fig. 7.1).

Tessier proposed an extensive approach aiming to reconstruct the lip, nose, piriform aperture, and medial canthus in the same stage but also stated that these cleft demand planning, staged, sequential approach to producing the ideal result at the complete facial growth. Before Tessier's proposal for complete staged surgical treatment, very few descriptions of protocols of procedures [3, 4]. Some old references show an isolated reconstruction of facial structure as demonstrated by Delpech J could be seen in some individual surgical treatments [5] (Fig. 7.2).

Monasterio and Taylor published one of the largest series among 495 patients 68 had TC3 cleft and provided some staged ideas in sequence for surgical treatment [6]. Our previous experience in 2010 was to treat 21 patients and present our protocol for this rare facial malformation [7].

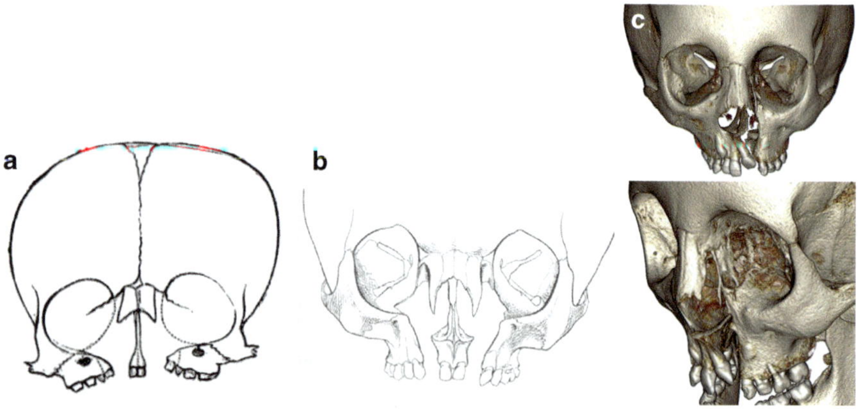

Fig. 7.1 Correlation between old facial cleft classification and new CT scan. (**a**) Morian I—Oculo-nasal cleft, (**b**) Tessier Cleft 3, (**c**) 3D CT Scan Tessier Cleft 3

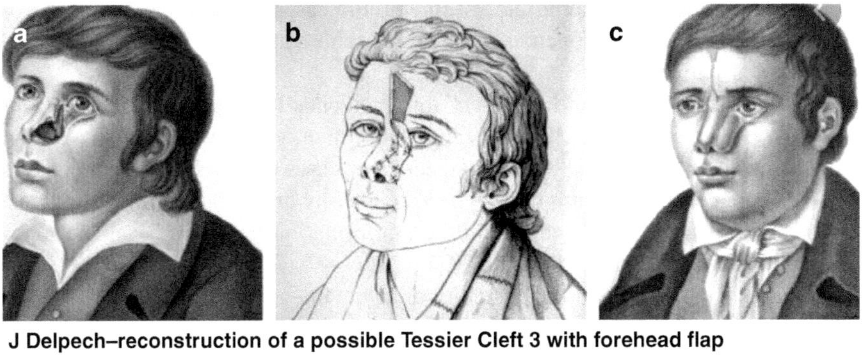

Fig. 7.2 Historical description of surgical treatment of TC3. (**a**) left TC3, (**b**) forehead flap, (**c**) final reconstruction

7.2 Anatomical Findings

The Tessier number 3, oculo-nasal cleft, represents one of the most challenging malformations to correct for the craniofacial surgeon. TC3 is a rare malformation, with few cases published in the literature [8–15]. Also, a small number of techniques to correct was already published [2, 13, 16–19]. This malformation is a paranasal-medial orbito-maxillary cleft running across the lacrimal segment of the lower eyelid and over the lacrimal groove. The frontal process of the maxilla may be absent, as well as the medial wall of the maxillary sinus. It passes around the nasal ala in the nasolabial groove to finally cross the lip and the alveolus like a "harelip" [2]. Kawamoto said that the lip deformities are located in the same region as the common clefts of the lip [20].

It may be expressed as only a coloboma in the lower eyelid and a simple notch in the alar base, or in its more severe manifestation, as a complete soft tissue and bony cleft of the face and cranium with microphthalmia and anophthalmia. Its localization coincides with the embryonic junction of the maxillary and frontonasal processes, and therefore, this cleft makes embryologic sense [16]. The Cleft 11 may represent the northbound prolongation of the cleft into the medial third of the upper eyelid and eyebrow and upward onto the forehead, As stated by Tessier, this deformity was not found in all cases but in complex cases associated with severe facial deformation, six cases in our series. Our series shows us more association with Tessier Cleft 10 and 9. Amniotic band syndrome has also been implicated in the process of facial clefting and could be seen in our series; more information about etiology is in the previous chapters.

The involvement of the eye itself is variable. When microphthalmos is present, the problem of restoring facial symmetry is more complex. An important point is a real condition in which the eye is normal but unprotected because of the eyelid deformity. Early provision of soft tissue protection is of paramount importance. The treatment of TC3 begins soon after birth by using ophthalmic ointment to protect the cornea and globe, avoiding ulcers; in extreme cases, the cornea could be protected by purse-string conjunctival suture done with conjunctive, as was described in one of our patients [21].

This facial malformation has a very low incidence [20, 22, 23]. In one of our publications, we presented 21 patients, and since then, very few patients have been included in the literature [7]. Our actual series of cases comprises 77 patients, and we distribute the patients into three types grouped by anatomical clinical findings. This division was done to understand the malformation better and evaluate long-term follow-up treatment and results. Many patients have an association of clinical signs that give us an idea of the difficulty of achieving good final results (Table 7.1 and Figs. 7.2, 7.3, 7.4, 7.5, and 7.6).

Type **Ia—TC3** associated with Cleft 10, with eyebrow discontinuity (no adjacent frontal bone involvement), medial palpebral ligament displacement, coloboma lower eyelid, lateral paranasal cleft including soft tissue and bone, and cleft lip and palate.

Type **Ib—TC**3 isolate like **Ia without** eyebrows discontinuity.

Type **II—TC**3 is associated with other facial clefts and facial malformation.

Type **III—TC3** medial palpebral ligament displacement, coloboma lower eyelid, lateral paranasal cleft including soft tissue and bone without cleft lip and palate.

If we associate types of Ia, Ib, and III, we found around 50% of our patients. The other 50% were severe cases associated with facial malformations, including craniosynostosis, encephaloceles, and amniotic bands.

Radiological findings of the different types have similar features like ascending ramus of the maxilla, and the lacrimal system is always compromised, the cleft runs between the punctum and caruncle, and the lacrimal sac and duct are mostly absent.

Table 7.1 Patients with TC3 anatomical findings

Type Ia TC3 associated to Cleft 10, with eyebrown discontinuity, medial palpebral ligament displacement, coloboma lower eyelid, lateral paranasal cleft including soft tissue and bone and cleft lip and palate
Type Ib TC3 isolate like **Ia without** eyebrown discontinuity
Type II TC3 associated with others facial clefts and facial malformation
Type III TC3 medial palpebral ligament displacement, coloboma lower eyelid, lateral paranasal cleft including soft tissue and bone **without** cleft lip and palate

Cleft 3 - Number of Patients	
Type Ia	**10**
Type Ib	**18**
Type II	**39**
Type III	**10**
Total	**77**

Others Facial Malformation associated	
Tessier # 10	**12** patients
Tessier# 2	01
Tessier# 8	02
Tessier# 9	08
Tessier# 11	06
Median cleft	01
Pai S	01
Treacher Collins	01
OAV S	01
Plagiocephalie	03
Choanal atresia	03
Amniotic bands	**11**
Anophtalmia/microphtalmia	**10**

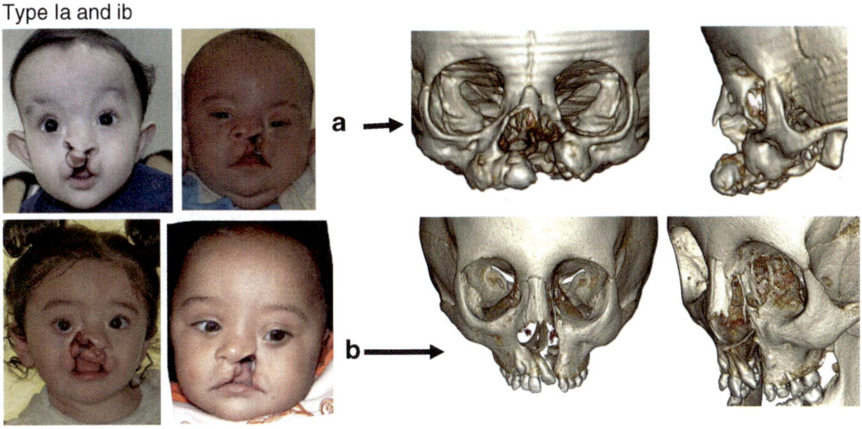

Fig. 7.3 Clinical findings in our series. (**a**) **Type Ia TC**3 associated to Cleft 10, with eyebrown discontinuity, medial palpebral ligament displacement, coloboma lower eyelid, lateral paranasal cleft including soft tissue and bone and cleft lip and palate. (**b**) **Type Ib TC**3 isolate like **Ia without** eyebrown discontinuity

The medial part of the maxilla until the frontal process is always absent, even in those without cleft lips. The alveolar cleft is always in between the lateral incisor and the canine. Some vertical dystopias of the orbit could be present because of the anteromedial commitment of the maxilla. When present, the cleft lip and palate are always complete; the opposite in Tessier Cleft 4, where most of the cleft palate was incomplete even if the cleft lip was present.

Several theories have been discussed about rare facial clefts [24, 25]. The mesodermal penetration theory, proposed by Pohlman, Veau, and Starkstates, to explain the etiology of facial clefts presumes that the failure occurs along potential lines of fusion as the result of a lack of mesodermal penetration [26]. Coady et al. state that craniofacial clefts have long been reported in association with limb and body wall constriction bands, with an incidence between 8.4 and 63% of cases [27]. The great majority of clefts in the ring constriction group were in quite specific axes. We found 11 cases (14.2%) of amniotic band syndrome in our series.

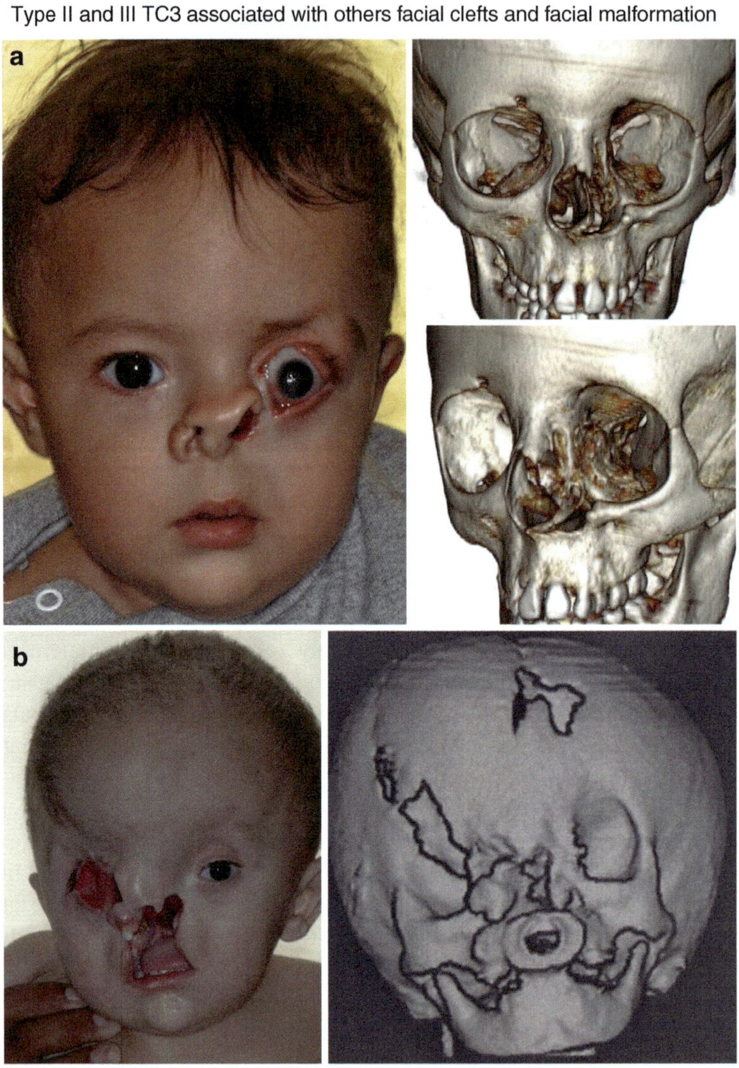

Fig. 7.4 Clinical findings in our series. (**a**) TC3 on the left side associated to right TC2, absence of fronto-maxillary process, coloboma in the left lower and upper eyelid. (**b**) TC3 bilateral associated with multiples clefts, TC9, TC10, TC8 right side, and complete cleft lip and palateb

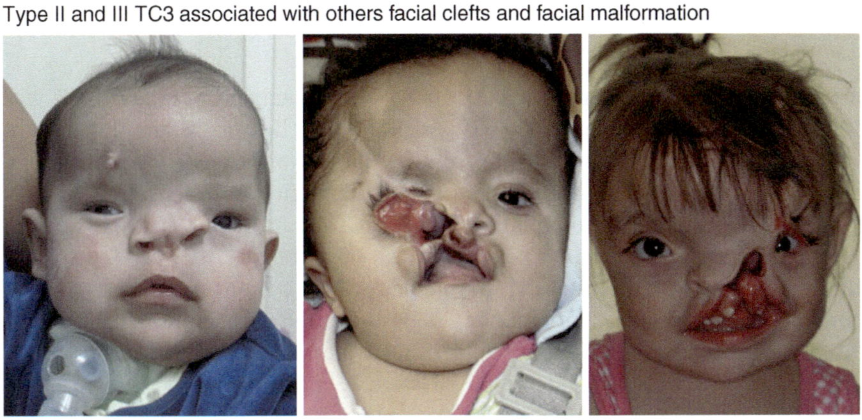

Fig. 7.5 Clinical findings in our series. (**a**) Left TC3 associated with hyperteleorbitism and skin appendage, (**b**) right TC3 associated to TC9 and TC10 anophthalmia, amniotic bands and coloboma upper and lower eyelid, (**c**) left TC3 associated to TC9 and TC10

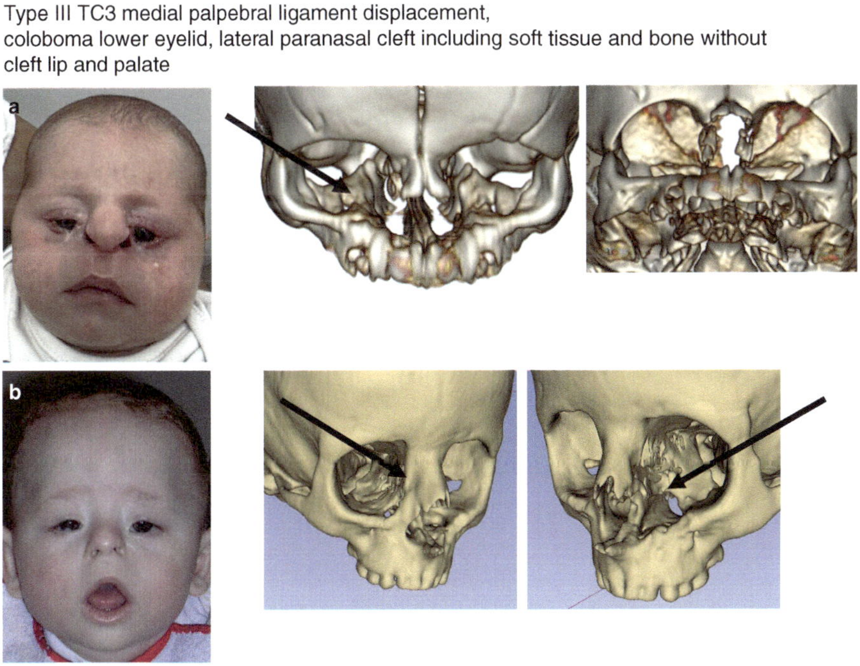

Fig. 7.6 Clinical findings in our series. (**a**) Bilateral TC3 without CLP, huge maxillary hypoplasia, no lacrimal system. (**b**) TC3 asymmetric bilateral, right side hypoplastic, and wide bone loss on the left side

7.3 Our Clinical Cases

In our series, 57 female gender patients were predominant, bilateral TC3 was almost 50%, and 10 patients had TC3 without cleft lip and palate cleft. These patients without cleft lip and palate are difficult to explain only by the theory of embryologic lines fusion and amniotic bands constriction (Table 7.1). In contrast to Tessier's observation relating TC3 with Cleft 11, in our series, it was not as often as expected (only six patients). Many different clefts were found, and Cleft 10, eyebrow discontinuity, and number 9 were more prevalent. Another clinical observation was that number 9 was associated with amniotic bands syndrome (ABS) in many patients. The lacrimal system was absent in all our cases, and microphthalmia and anophthalmia were related to more complex cases. Choanal atresia was diagnosed in 03 patients associated with ABS [28] (Figs. 7.7, 7.8).

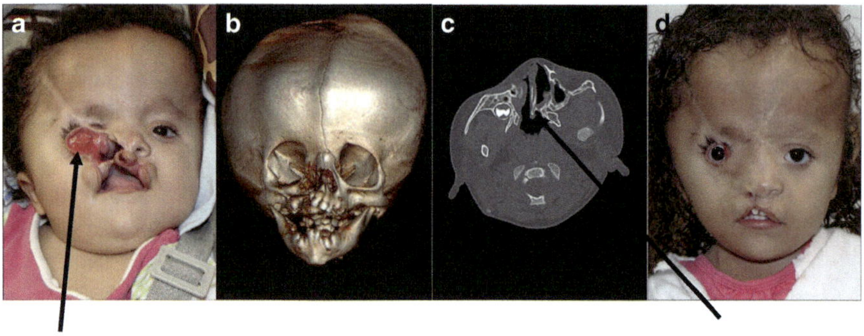

Fig. 7.7 (**a, b**) Clinical cases choanal atresia and ABS. TC3 cleft with number 10 with ABS and Choanal atresia and anophtalmia. (**a**) Arrow anophthalmia, (**b**) Ct scan with bone deformities, (**c**) left choanal atresia, (**d**) postoperative after first operation

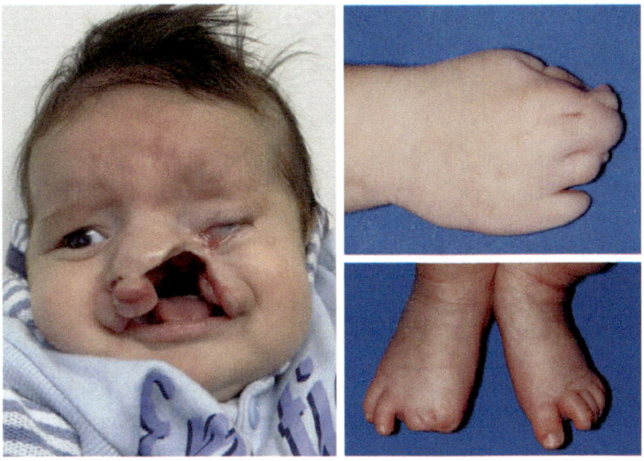

Fig. 7.8 Clinical cases ABS. TC3 associated to ABS

7.4 Surgical Treatment

The principles for treating these unusual clefts are based on clinical diagnosis and staged planning according to functional needs. The surgical objectives for TC3 are to close the lower eyelid coloboma, reconstruct the frontal process of the maxilla, create a septum between the nose and the maxillary sinus, repair the transverse diameter of the orbit and elongate the nasal area, lining, and all the nasal structures. All the stages can be done in a single initial procedure when possible. Depending on the eye exposition, emergency surgery or any adjuvant procedure should be done to protect the eyeball [21].

Important landmarks for surgery Fig. 7.9.

- In unilateral cases, the first point on the noncleft side is the insertion of the medial palpebral ligament. Then transposition of this point to the same level on the cleft side will be the parameter for reinsertion of the cleft medial ligament.
- Lip marking, the first point is the alar insertion cleft side and noncleft side and measurement of the distance between alar insertion and medial palpebral canthus. Depending on this, the decision is made to recruit local flaps from glabella, upper eyelid, and jugal area.
- The nasal lining is, in TC3 cases, used from the nasal mucosa coming from the cranial nasal lining or from the muco-septal flap to reconstruct the nasal lining or close nasal maxillary communication.
- Our technique for lip repair is always a type of Millard modification [29] or for bilateral lip adhesion first and could be Spina's technique or Mulliken's [30, 31].
- Lateral lip element should be used for elongating the nose just above the cranial part of alar cartilage, and the lateral incision is always parallel to the white roll or vermillion. On the lateral lip element, a skin incision, parallel to vermillion, will be necessary to create two lateral flaps, one for lip repair and the other to elongate the nose. Then, inferior rotation of the upper lip is achieved. The initial skin incision must be at the same distance as the cutaneous-mucosa transition in

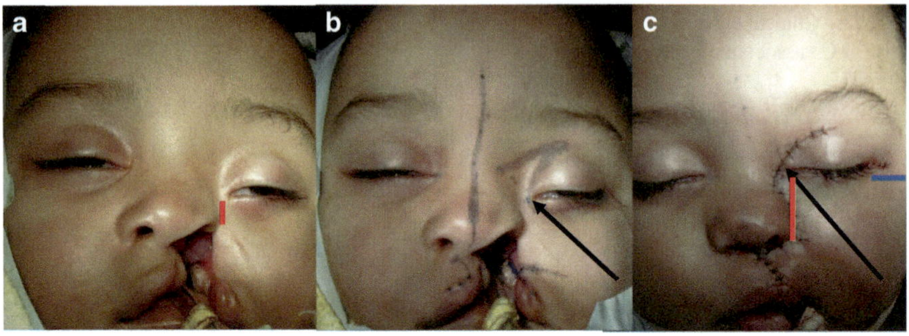

Fig. 7.9 (**a**) Surgical markings for type I TC3. (**b, c**) Surgical markings glabellar flap for lower eyelid and nose. Surgical markings when the lower eyelid has normal size only displaced. Elongation of para lateral nasal dimension with interposition of jugal flap red line in (**a**) and (**c**). Lateral cantholisys for lower eyelid mobilization line blue

the medial segment of the philtrum. The extension of this flap may be the minimum to adapt to nasal ala. In bilateral cases, we have indicated the Spina technique, lip adhesion, uni or bilateral, depending on protrusion of pre-maxilla and tension, performed between 3 and 6 months. Creating an oral muscular sphincter, mild pressure will be positioned under the pre-maxilla. Definitive lip repair is undergone around 3–4 years of age or before, depending on the severity of the deformity. This technique permits refinement of the lip contour and well positioning of the scar; camouflaging the scar permits better cosmetic results.

Specifically, to TC3, a radical orbital dissection was indicated. The connection of the orbital septum with the periosteum opposes the displacement of the eyelid. Reinsertion of the lower eyelid to the medial palpebral ligament through a transnasal canthopexy and a lateral cantholysis must be performed. The striking shortness of the vertical distance between the eyelid and lip seems to present a difficult obstacle to normalization. The transposition of jugal flaps increases the distance between the canthus and the lip. Closure of the eyelid coloboma, restoration and modeling of the orbit and maxilla by bone grafting, formation of an inter-nasal septum, and closure of the labio-maxillary cleft are also necessary.

Also, minor eyelid clefts may be treated, bringing the lower eyelid medial and upward displacement usually as a separate operation. In the cases of severe clefts, a one-stage reconstruction of the cheek and lower palpebral cleft should be attempted. In less complicated forms, the reconstruction of a deformed medial palpebral angle and lower eyelid may be performed later at the age of 4–5 years unless the eyelid coloboma is accompanied by considerable eversion, thus necessitating earlier reconstruction because of eye protection. Orbital floor reconstruction should be evaluated as soon as the paranasal cleft is closed and could be done at the age of 4–5 years old in the time for any other associated procedure.

We have used a Z-plasty by using one of the arms of the Z to raise the medial canthus, while the other corrects the vertical dimension of the nose. In more severe cases, a glabellar flap is necessary when lower eyelid deficiency is significant, which will be inferiorly rotated to the nasal ala. In bilateral complex cases, a bilateral glabellar flap can create enough tissue to reconstruct the nose's size bilaterally (Figs. 7.10, 7.11).

The soft tissue and skin deficiency demands reconstruction, ideally with a tissue of texture, consistency, and color. An expander permits the excision of grossly scarred cleft tissues and resurfaces with tissues whose color match, contour, and vascularity are significantly improved. The pre-expansion of the forehead provides

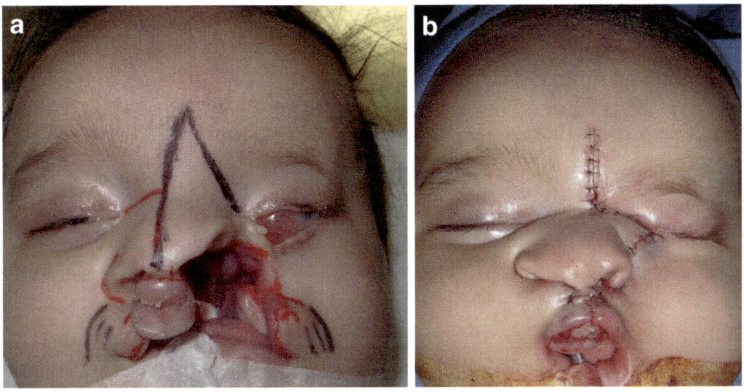

Fig. 7.10 Surgical markings glabellar flap for lower eyelid. (**a**) Marking for glabellar flap, (**b**) flap used to elongate the nose bilateral cleft lip corrected with Mulliken's technique

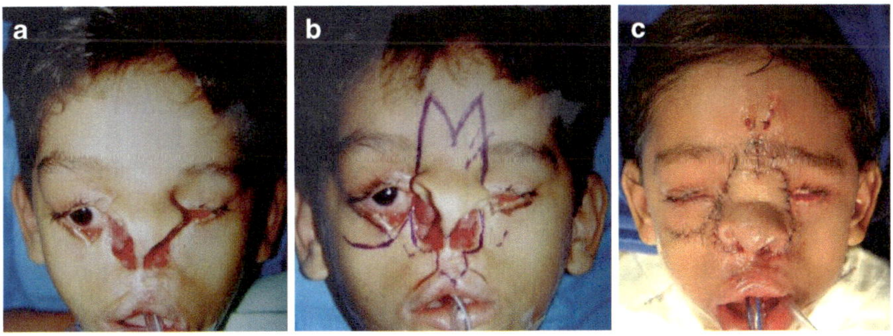

Fig. 7.11 Surgical markings bilateral glabellar flap. (**a**) Bilateral TC3 with coloboma of the lower eyelid, (**b**) Bilateral glabellar flap with nasal mucosal flap for linning Canthopexy and lower eyelid reconstruction, (**c**) final immediate result

sufficient extra color-matched skin for major nasal reconstruction with primary closure of the donor site. When the cleft is associated with hypertelorism, the subperiosteal expansion of the temporo-zygomatic soft tissues before orbital translocation releases those distorting laterally pulling soft tissues and permits stable tension-free orbital skeletal and periorbital soft tissue correction. The tissue expansion was used in the secondary correction of facial clefts in eight patients. We never used it primarily. Theoretically, tissue expansion may give the advantages of excision of grossly scarred cleft tissue, improvement of the soft-tissue vascularity before bone grafting, coverage of the cleft region with tension-free tissue, allowing for the release of tissue tractional forces restricting hypertelorism and orbital dystopia correction, and use of forehead flap with primary closure of the donor site. The incision lines in Tessier Cleft 3 clefts are on the supratarsal fold, paranasal, or philtrum for most of the time, which permits the scar camouflage.

The lacrimal system is always compromised. The nasolacrimal duct is most of the time absent and the sac is abnormal or hypoplastic and causes repeated local infections. The lower canaliculus is malformed and beyond repair; total extirpation of the sac and the duct remain is, therefore, the treatment of choice. When the nasolacrimal duct is involved, treatment includes total excision, since repeated infection tends to develop in the hypoplastic lacrimal system.

Important points to plan the staged procedures in TC3; eye exposition, size of the lower eyelid, size of the para-lateral nasal cleft, and unilateral or bilateral cleft. Based on these points, the surgical plan could be done. The presence of anophthalmia significantly increases the difficulty of correcting the deformity. For secondary cases, repositioning the alar base incision on the cranial portion of nasal lower lateral cartilage and advancing in different plans the nasal mucosa and the skin could be used to better place the nasal alar base [32].

In type II TC3, some different deformities should need another approach like encephalocele and craniosynostosis. Other challenges are anophthalmia and microphthalmia, and they need orbit expansion early and orbit reconstruction for eye prosthesis in the future. Some of our cases have amniotic bands syndrome in limbs, hands, and feet, which also need surgical care parallel to facial deformities.

Usually, the nasal ala in patients with TC3 cleft is dislocated superiorly, and the distance between the medial canthus and ala is so short. Therefore, it is necessary to perform any flap to bring the ala inferiorly to the upper lip. The flap with the medial pedicle—on the dorsum—was used sometimes. However, the scar will be located on the glabella area, and differently in older patients, the scar is visible but necessary when the distance between the inner canthus and lateral alar base is too short. Another option is to make an incision on the alar groove, until a good position in this segment. Then a gap is created that is necessary to bring a flap from a lateral side. This incision will be longer as necessary. In this case, the prolongation of the incision on the nasal ala for 3 mm at least permits it to rotate downward.

The involvement of the lower eyelid includes the absence of lacrimal duct and canaliculus, detachment of medial canthus, and dislocated lateral and inferiorly.

The purpose is to fix the lower eyelid to the medial canthus and recreate a new lacrimal way. Everything to protect the cornea and eyeball. A flap from the upper lid to the lower in the medial canthus can be used. The upper eyelid is always a nice donor to the lower eyelid, so in the medial area as in the lateral. To TC3, the myocutaneous flap from the upper eyelid could be mobilized through this incision a refixation of the medial canthus may be done. The lacrimal way may be compromised in several areas. Punctum, sac, or duct may be altered by facial clefts, specifically facial number 2, 3, and 4 clefts. TC3 cleft passes across the lacrimal punctum, and obstruction may be present. In our series, sac and duct in number 3 cleft were absent or atrophic in almost all patients, differently from number 4 cleft, where they are sometimes present but atrophic or dilated. In unusual cases, extreme measurements should be taken to preserve the eyeball, and conjunctive could be used to protect the vision as was described in one of our cases [18]. The reconstruction of the cul-de-sac may utilize an everted conjunctiva or a lateral advancement flap with all components of the lower eyelid. Dacryo-cyst-rhinostomy or conjunctivo-rhinostomy will be indicated depending on the anatomy found. It is important to mention here that we observed a relevant incidence in our service of choanal atresia, 13 patients representing 13.26% of our series of unusual facial clefts, from those 3 patients had TC3 and 10 patients with TC4 [28] and early diagnostic could avoid tracheotomy [28].

We have treated this facial malformation and conducted a retrospective analysis of our series consisting of 77 cases of TC3. In our previous paper, published with another cleft center, it was presented to 21 patients [7]. Most patients come to the center in their first year of life. The typical presentation of TC3 is with short nose deformity including alar base, displacement of medial canthus, and cleft lip and palate. Another typical deformity, the coloboma of the lower eyelid, was also identified in all patients. Hydrocephaly was observed in the most severe cases, as encephalocele. Mental retardation and short-life prognosis were the rules in these severe deformities. Plagiocephaly (three patients) was the type of cranium deformation found that could be classified as number 10 or 9 clefts in most of them.

Long-term follow-up was presented in many patients and many different refining was necessary mainly in the eyelid area and nasal alar base.

7.5 Case Description

The patient came to our service at 3 months of age. He was born after 38 weeks of gestation with no setbacks. Parents are nonconsanguineous. No history of use of drugs or other complications during this period. Unilateral cleft lip left involvement of ala, paranasal, and medial canthus, and disproportion between the upper eyelid and lower eyelid. She presented a wide unilateral cleft with a skin appendage in the upper lip cleft. He was managed with eye gel and corneal hydration with saline

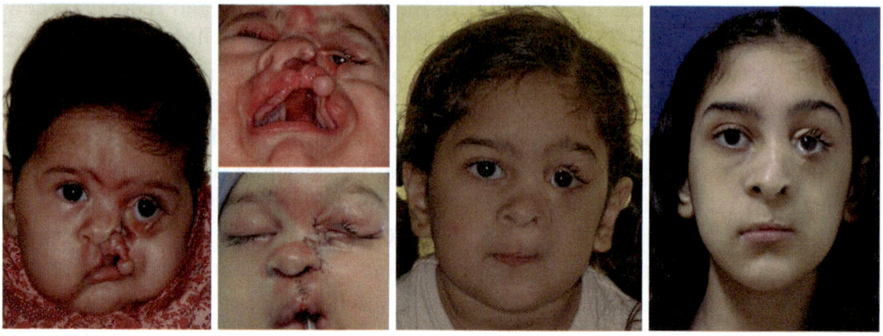

Fig. 7.12 Clinical cases long-term follow-up—eyelid and nasal reconstruction

solution and was submitted to total reconstruction at 6 months of life. Lower eyelid coloboma reconstruction was performed using a flap, from the medial segment, and upper eyelid and canthopexy were performed with contralateral palpebral ligament fixation. In the first evaluation, the patient had on the left-side upper lip clefts with involvement of the nasal floor, vertical dimension of the left orbit was increased. Wide subperiosteal undermine; no bone graft was done in this initial surgery. At the time of palatoplasty, radiologic evaluation was done, and there was no need for a bone graft in the orbit. After a long-term follow-up, we decided not to graft this patient, as can be seen in the long-term follow-up 12 years later. The upper eyelid presents very long eyelashes, and the disproportion was adjusted with time (Fig. 7.12).

This second patient was sent to us as having regular cleft lip and palate, but was evident the short distance between the left nasal alar base and the eyelids and the displacement of the medial canthus. Nasal elongation was done with the interposition of a lateral face flap with lower eyelid incision and lateral cantholysis. It is essential to wide and extended lateral undermining over the infraorbital nerve, and in orbit, the floor is also involved subperiosteally. In this case, the nasal lining was mobilized from the upper part of the nasal mucosa under the nasal bone. For lip repair, we used a Millard-modified technique in our service at that time [29] (Fig. 7.13).

In bilateral cases like our next patient, we do need a large forehead flap to reconstruct the lower eyelid and, at the same time, provide tissue to elongate the left side. Lip repair could be done in stages, as is performed by one of the coauthors of this work. Lip repair was performed during facial cleft repair in this patient using Mulliken's technique. After 6 months, palatoplasty was performed (Fig. 7.14).

In this last case, in a patient with TC3 without cleft lip and palate, the CT images show us the medial orbit and maxillary reconstruction with bone graft and medial ligament repositioning (Fig. 7.14).

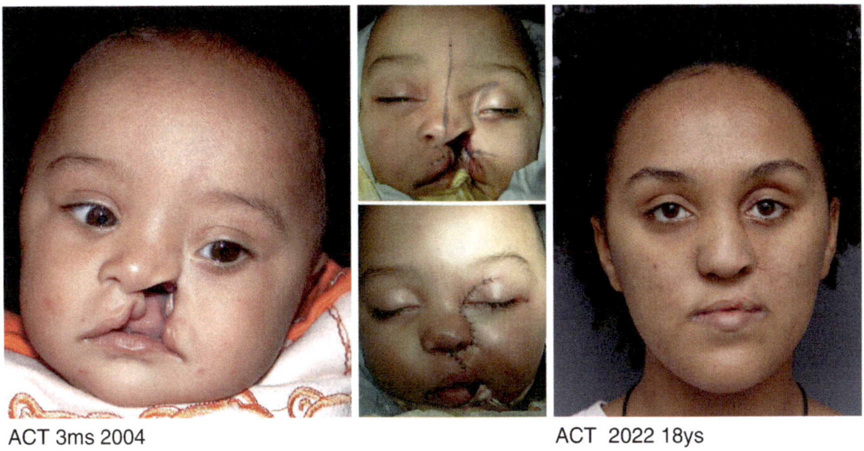

Fig. 7.13 (**a**) Clinical cases long-term follow-up—eyelid repositioning

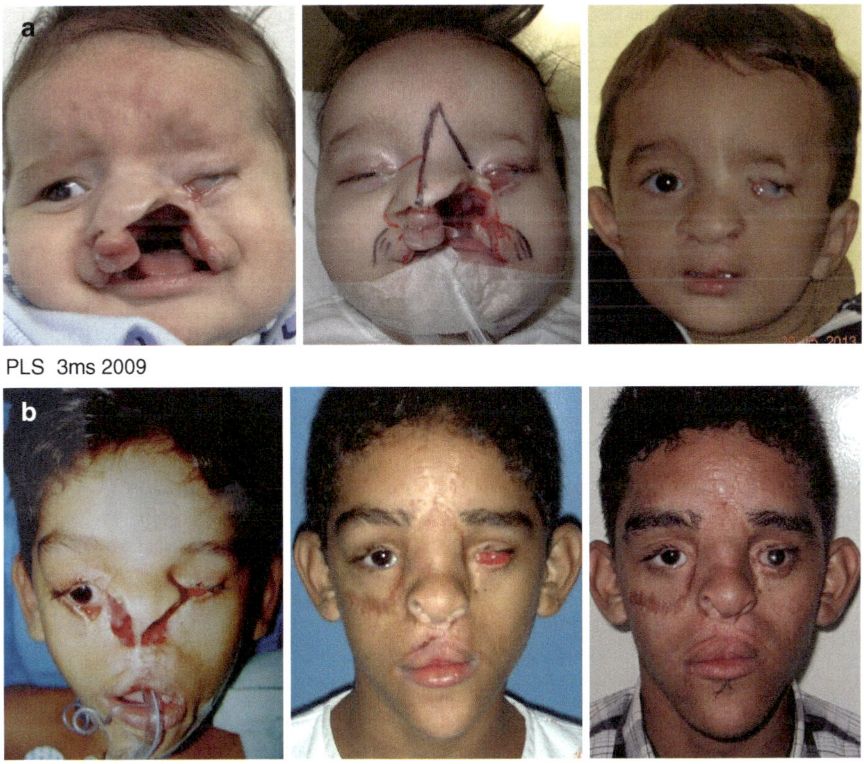

Fig. 7.14 (**a**) Clinical cases long-term follow-up—glabellar flap unilateral. (**b**) Clinical cases long-term follow-up—glabellar flap bilateral. (**c**) Clinical cases—orbital reconstruction with bone graft

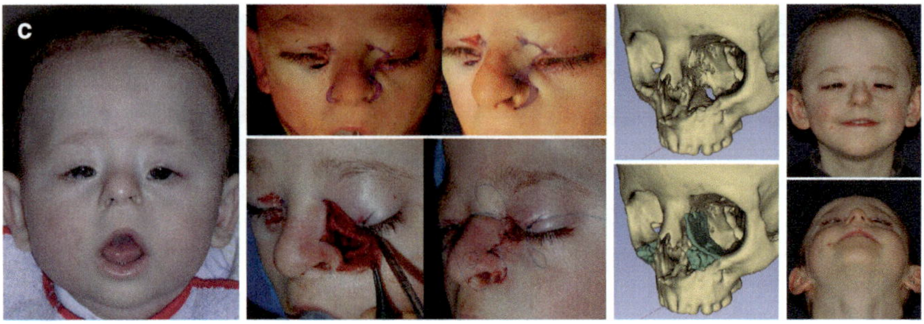

Fig. 7.14 (continued)

References

1. Morian, R. Uber die schrage Gesichtsspalte. sitzung der berliner medicinischen gesellschaft 1886.
2. Tessier P. Anatomical classification of facial, cranio-facial, and latero- facial clefts. J Maxillofac Surg. 1976;4:69–92.
3. Jalaguier A, colobome facial bilateral. Double fente congénitale bucco-orbitaire. Autoplasties successives. Guérison. In: Jalaguier AD, editor. titres et travaux scientifiques. Paris: Asselin et Houzeau; 1912. p. 29–31. https://archive.org/details/BIUSante_110133x096x07/page/n65/mode/2up.
4. Butcher H. Reports in operative surgery. Dublin Quarterly J Med Sci. 1860;XXIX:258.
5. Delpech JM. Observations et réflexions sur l'opération de la rhinoplastique, observation premiére. In: Chirurgie Clinique de Montpellier ou Observations et Réflexions tirées des travaux de chirurgie clinique de cette école. Paris: Chez Gabon, libraire, rue de l'école de Médecine; 1828. p. 221–35.
6. Monasterio FO, Taylor JA. Major craniofacial clefts: case series and treatment philosophy. Plast Reconstr Surg. 2008;122(2):534–43. http://journals.lww.com/00006534-200808000-00027.
7. da Silva FR, Alonso N, Busato L, Ueda WK, Hota T, Medeiros SH, et al. Oral-nasal-ocular cleft: the greatest challenge among the rare clefts. J Craniofac Surg. 2010;21(2):390–5.
8. Xu Y, Mu Y, Chen R, Zheng Z, Zhang W. Two rare cases of simultaneous Tessier number 3 cleft, contralateral cleft lip, and signs of amniotic band syndrome. J Cranio-Maxillofac Surg. 2016;44(6):672–5. https://linkinghub.elsevier.com/retrieve/pii/S1010518215003790.
9. Mishima K, Sugahara T, Mori Y, Sakuda M. Three cases of the oblique facial cleft. J Cranio-Maxillofac Surg. 1996;24(6):372–7. https://linkinghub.elsevier.com/retrieve/pii/S1010518296800394.
10. Allam KA, Lim AA, Elsherbiny A, Kawamoto HK. The Tessier number 3 cleft: A report of 10 cases and review of the literature. J Plast Reconstr Aesthet Surg. 2014;67(8):1055–62. https://linkinghub.elsevier.com/retrieve/pii/S174868151400182X.
11. Gawrych E, Janiszewska-Olszowska J, Chojnacka H. Tessier type 3 oblique facial cleft with a contralateral complete cleft lip and palate. Int J Oral Maxillofac Surg. 2010;39(11):1133–6. https://linkinghub.elsevier.com/retrieve/pii/S0901502710002377.
12. Wenbin Z, Hanjiang W, Xiaoli C, Zhonglin L. Tessier 3 cleft with clinical Anophthalmia: two case reports and a review of the literature. Cleft Palate Craniofac J. 2007;44(1):102–5. https://doi.org/10.1597/05-155.
13. Golinko MS, Pemberton JD, Phillips J, Johnson A, Hartzell LD. The Arkansas Tessier number 3 cleft experience: soft tissue and skeletal findings with primary surgical management: four-step approach. J Craniofac Surg. 2018;29(7):1834–41. https://journals.lww.com/00001665-201810000-00039.

14. Alonso N, Tonello C. Rare facial clefts. In: Hamdan U, Rogers-Vizena C, Vyas R, Sommerlad B, Low D, editors. Interdisciplinary cleft care global perspectives. San Diego CA: Plural; 2023. p. 689–701. http://www.pluralpublishing.com.
15. Alonso N, da Silva Freitas R. Craniofacial clefts and others related deformities. In: Plastic surgery indications and practice. p. 455–71.
16. van der Meulen JCH. Oblique facial clefts: pathology, etiology, and reconstruction. Plast Reconstr Surg. 1985;76(2):212–24. http://journals.lww.com/00006534-198508000-00007.
17. Kim EN, Moss WD, Yamashiro DK, Tuncer FB, Siddiqi FA. Management of Tessier type 3 cleft with a novel reverses palatal expander. J Craniofac Surg. 2021;32(8):e814–6. https://doi.org/10.1097/SCS.0000000000007866.
18. Hyeon OJ, Park YW. Anatomical repair of a bilateral Tessier No. 3 cleft by midfacial advancement. Maxillofac Plast Reconstr Surg. 2018;40(1):9. https://doi.org/10.1186/s40902-018-0147-3.
19. Chen PKT, Chang FCS, Chan FC, Chen YR, Noordhoff MS. Repair of tessier no. 3 and no. 4 craniofacial clefts with facial unit and muscle repositioning by midface rotation advancement without z-plasties. Plast Reconstr Surg. 2012;129(6):1337–44. http://journals.lww.com/00006534-201206000-00020.
20. Kawamoto HK. The kaleidoscopic world of rare craniofacial clefts: order out of chaos (Tessier classification). Clin Plast Surg. 1976;3(4):529–72.
21. Tonello C, Paula RG, Paula IP, Nunes RB, Kokitsu-Nakata NM, Alonso N. Eyeball preservation with purse-string conjunctival closure for melting corneal ulcer in rare facial cleft. Cleft Palate Craniofacial J. 2020:1055665620980632.
22. Smith HB, Verity DH, JRO C. The incidence, embryology, and oculofacial abnormalities associated with eyelid colobomas. Eye. 2015;29(4):492–8. http://www.nature.com/articles/eye2014335.
23. Moore MH. Rare craniofacial clefts. J Craniofac Surg. 1996;7(6):408–11. http://journals.lww.com/00001665-199611000-00003.
24. van der Meulen JC, Mazzola R, Vermey-Keers C, Strieker M, Raphael B. A morphogenetic classification of craniofacial malformations. Plast Reconstr Surg. 1983;71(4):560–72. http://journals.lww.com/00006534-198304000-00022.
25. Losee JE, Kirschner RE, Whitaker LA, Bartlett SP. Congenital nasal anomalies: a classification scheme. Plast Reconstr Surg. 2004;113(2):676–89. http://journals.lww.com/00006534-200402000-00034.
26. Dee CT, Szymoniuk CR, Mills PED, Takahashi T. Defective neural crest migration revealed by a zebrafish model of Alx1-related frontonasal dysplasia. Hum Mol Genet. 2013;22(2):239–51.
27. MSE C, Moore MH, Wallis K. Amniotic band syndrome: the association between rare facial clefts and limb ring constrictions. Plast Reconstr Surg. 1998;101(3):640–9. http://journals.lww.com/00006534-199803000-00010.
28. Tonello C, Martins DA, Baptista MA, Mondelli F, Kokitsu Nakata NM, Feitosa LB, et al. Tessier 3 and 4 clefts and choanal atresia: an unusual association? Cleft Palate Craniofacial J. 2022;59(10):1228–32. https://doi.org/10.1177/10556656211042172.
29. DYS T, Alonso N, Rocha DL. Evaluation of primary cleft nose repair: severity of the cleft versus final position of the nose. J Craniofac Surg. 2010;21(5):1519–24. https://journals.lww.com/00001665-201009000-00046.
30. Spina V, Lodovici O. Conservative technique for the treatment of unilateral cleft lip: reconstruction of the midline tubercle of the vermilion. Br J Plast Surg. 1960;13:110–7. https://linkinghub.elsevier.com/retrieve/pii/S0007122660800276.
31. Mulliken JB, Wu JK, Padwa BL. Repair of bilateral cleft lip: review, revisions, and reflections. J Craniofac Surg. 2003;14(5):609–20.
32. Van Slyke AC, Burge J, Bos R, Parker G, Chong DK. The anatomical subunit approach to managing tessier numbers 3 and 4 craniofacial clefts. Plast Reconstr Surg-Glob Open. 2022;10(9):e4553. https://doi.org/10.1097/GOX.0000000000004553.

Chapter 8
Cleft 4

Nivaldo Alonso, Renato da Silva Freitas, Cristiano Tonello, and Philippe Pellerin

Pearls

- Tessier 4 (TC4) facial cleft is a rare and complex craniofacial malformation classified as lateral facial cleft.
- The cleft lip in TC4 is lateral to the regular cleft lip and palate.
- TC4 has similarities to other lateral facial Clefts 3, 5, 6, and 7 and can be found in association.
- Most TC4 have incomplete cleft palate, which could suggest TC3 is related to embryological lines but temporally late fusion or specific vascular problems.
- Age and type of procedure depend on the severity of the eye exposition.

N. Alonso (✉)
Plastic Surgery, Universidade de São Paulo, São Paulo, Brazil

Craniofacial Surgery, Hospital de Reabilitação Anomalias Craniofaciais Bauru USPUniversidade de São Paulo, Bauru, Brazil

R. da Silva Freitas
Plastic Surgery Service of Hospital das Clinicas, Universidade Federal do Paraná, Curitiba, Brazil

Craniofacial Surgery, Assistance Center for Cleft Lip and Palate (CAIF), Hospital do Trabalhador, Curitiba, Brazil

C. Tonello
Curso de Medicina Bauru Faculdade de Odontologia Bauru Universidade de São Paulo, Bauru, Brazil

Hospital de Reabilitação Anomalias Craniofaciais Universidade de São Paulo, Bauru, Brazil

P. Pellerin
Centre Hospitalier Régional Universitaire de Lille, Lille, France

N. Alonso et al. (eds.), *Facial Reconstruction of Unusual Facial Clefts*,
https://doi.org/10.1007/978-3-031-40926-4_8

8.1 History

As was described in the previous chapter on TC3, Morian 1887 and Tessier 1976 have some very interesting actual drawings about this very unusual facial cleft, TC4, named by Morian as oro-ocular Morian II or oblique orbito-maxillary cleft or Tessier Cleft 4 (TC4) [1, 2] (Fig. 8.1).

Jalaguier 1909 presented one of the first techniques to repair this facial cleft (Fig. 8.2). Different flaps were used to close a bilateral cleft to protect the eye and facial reconstruction [3] (Fig. 8.2). Tessier (1977) published his book and standardized techniques to repair TC4. Multiple zetaplasties were suggested to be associated

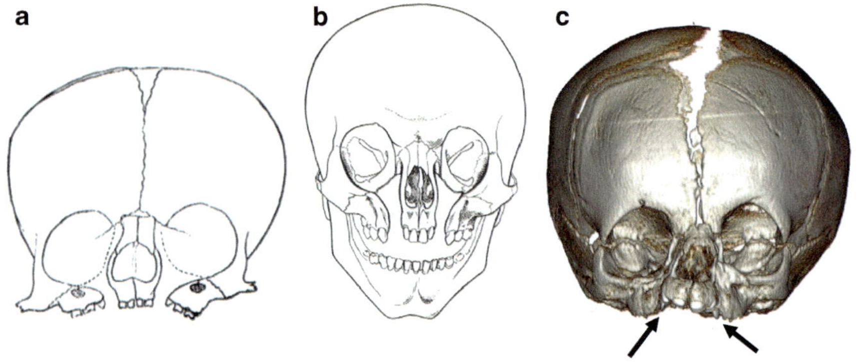

Fig. 8.1 Correlation between old classification and 3D CTscan. (**a**) Morian II medial oro-ocular, (**b**) Tessier Cleft 4, (**c**) Bilateral Tessier Cleft 4 CT Scan

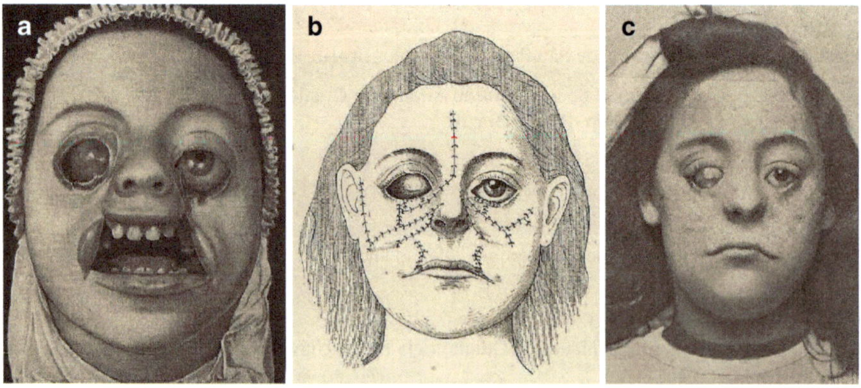

Fig. 8.2 Historical surgical procedures by Jalaquier 1909. (**a**) BilateralTC4 with eye exposition and lower eyelid colobomas. (**b**) Forehead Flap, local flap described previously. (**c**) Described Post operative

with canthopexies and nasal reconstruction [4] (Fig. 8.3). After this publication, many surgeons suggested modifications for this kind of unusual facial malformation [5]. Resnick and Kawamoto reported eight cases treated with interdigitating local flaps to close the soft-tissue defect associated with calvarium bone grafting to restore orbital continuity and correct the maxilla cleft. The authors emphasized that this procedure could provide early protection to the eye, a better position of the medial canthal ligament, reconstitution of the bony orbit, and immediate improvement in facial appearance [6]. Van der Meulen proposed modifying Tessier's technique, associating a lateral canthotomy and a Z-plasty with a facial flap similar to Esser's Flap to do medial advancement of the lower eyelid [7] (Fig. 8.4).

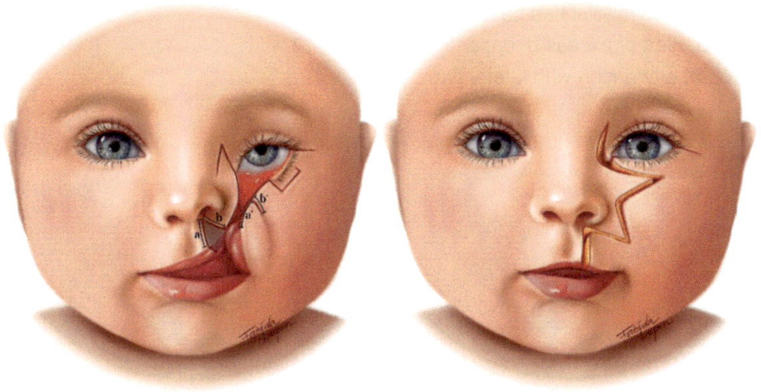

Fig. 8.3 Tessier's first surgical description

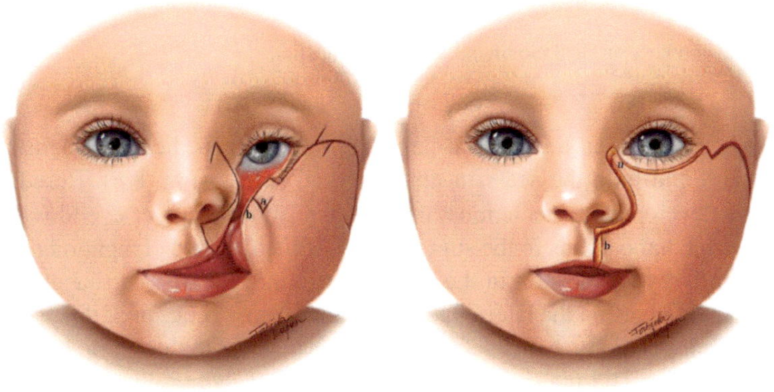

Fig. 8.4 van der Meulen's modification for TC4

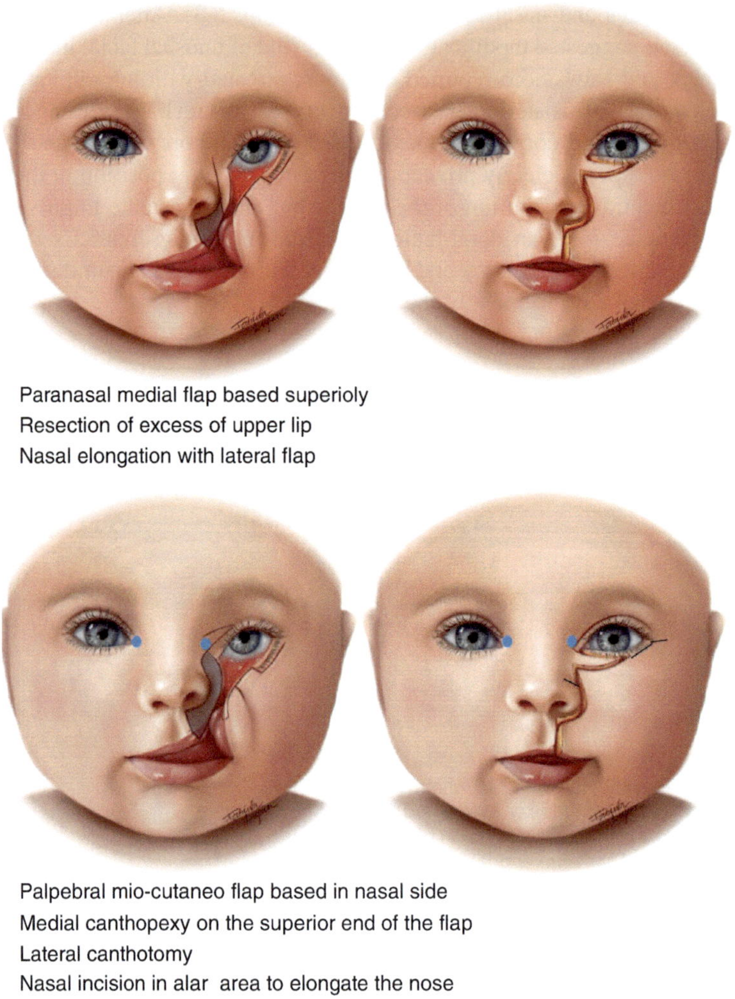

Fig. 8.5 Kawamoto's surgical modification/our modification

Longaker et al. used a paranasal flap with a superior pedicle to reconstruct the lower eyelid and hide the scars in the paranasal sulcus (Fig. 8.5). Based on this article, we developed our technique, using a flap from the upper eyelid with transposition of medial canthus in the superior part of the flap and elongation of the alar base vertically by an incision in the cranial portion of the alar cartilage (Fig. 8.5). Two dissection plans on the lateral facial flap allow more rotation of this lateral flap, and the muscles could be better visualized and reattached to the lateral border of the piriform aperture. The incision in the middle third of the nose to bring the lateral flap provides a better alar base position. The nose's lining and elongation are done simultaneously using nasal mucosa and skin from the glabellar area. The point of rotation of the upper eyelid flap is the correct position of the medial palpebral ligament [8–10].

Many of these papers have presented short experiences with its treatment, frequently using one of these techniques mentioned above with the introduction of small modifications [11–16]. Multiple local flaps have been used to close soft-tissue defects, elevate the medial canthus, and protect the globe. Functional aspects have always been focused on as the primary goal of surgical reconstruction. Some of these modifications, however, can lead to suboptimal results with conspicuous facial scars, poor color matching of the cheek and nasal flaps, and unnatural facial expression from the unrepaired facial musculature. Scar position in aesthetic units of the face is vital to achieving more adequate results. Long-term follow-up is essential to the observer if the scars stay in the same place after facial growth. We have quite a significant number of secondary lower eyelid reconstructions in older patients with TC4 reconstructed early. Some tricks were used to keep the paranasal scars imperceptible, like deep suture with nonabsorbable suture in the piriform aperture (trans osseous suture), two plane dissection in the lateral facial flap muscular and subcutaneous plane, and no tension on suture of the rotation facial flap with an extension of the lower eyelid incision associated to lateral cantholisis.

8.2 Anatomical Findings

TC4 is described as an oblique facial cleft and, like the others, has a very low incidence [17, 18]. Its clinical presentation ranges from a simple unilateral cleft to wide bilateral defects with significant bone fissures. The fissure usually extends from the medial canthal ligament, crosses the inferior orbital rim and orbital floor, medially to the infraorbital foramen, runs through the maxillary sinus, and ends over the alveolar bony, between the lateral incisor and canine [2]. Consequently, the orbital contents, including the eyeball, may prolapse into the maxillary sinus through the inferior orbital rim and floor defect. In the soft tissues, the coloboma passes outside the inferior lacrimal punctum. The nasolacrimal duct and sac can be found normal, but the inferior lacrimal canaliculus and the distal portion of the nasolacrimal are always compromised or absent.

The nose is not directly affected by the cleft but is shorter on the side of the cleft, with a smaller distance between the alar cartilage and the inner palpebral canthus. When the upper lip is affected, the cleft is between the philtral crest and labial commissure. The absence of piriform aperture involvement is one of the differences with TC3 in most patients. Eyeball malformation, with microphthalmia or anophthalmia, may be present, associated with exposure keratopathy, secondary to eyelid coloboma. Tessier Cleft 10, described as a cranial extension of TC4, was observed in only in few patients in this series (three patients). This suggests an uncommon association and possibly lack of correlation between both clefts. Amniotic bands in the limbs, however, were evidenced in many patients (10 patients) and could be an essential etiologic factor for these facial clefts [19–22].

Table 8.1 Patients with TC4 anatomical findings

Type Ia medial canthus displacement, coloboma lower and upper eyelid, paranasal cleft between piriform aperture and infraorbital nerve,cleft lip and palate
Type Ib medial canthus displacement, coloboma lower and upper eyelid, paranasal cleft between piriform aperture and infraorbital nerve, cleft lip and palate **with anophthalmia or microphthalmia**
Type II associated with others facial malformations and clefts
Type III only medial canthus displacement, coloboma lower and upper eyelid, paranasal cleft between piriform aperture and infraorbital nerve **without cleft lip and palate**

Others Facial Malformation associated		
Tessier 3	01	
Tessier 5	05	
Tessier 6		**12**
Tessier 7		**16**
Tessier 8	03	
Tessier 9	03	
Tessier 10	03	
OAV	02	
Choanal atresia		**12**
Amniotic bands		**10**
Anophthalmia/microphthalmia		**15**

Cleft 4	Number of patients
Type Ia	42
Type Ib	15
Type II	26
Type III	03
Total	86

Only 92 patients were published in the literature until our previous paper, 2008, when we added 21 patients [13]. A review of English literature demonstrates more than 85 patients, totaling 173 patients with TC4. Our actual series of patients is 86 from São Paulo, Curitiba, and Lille. We collected all data and images possible from all patients, and based on this, we distributed the patients, using Tessier's publications and according to clinical findings in three anatomical types. One of the reasons for this division was that patients with other malformations associated had different numbers and types of procedures done. The presence or absence of microphthalmia or anophthalmia significantly changes the number of procedures and final cosmetic results—clinical classification of TC4 in 86 patients (Table 8.1).

- Type Ia: medial canthus displacement, coloboma lower and upper eyelid, the paranasal cleft between piriform aperture and infraorbital nerve, cleft lip, and palate.
- Type Ib: medial canthus displacement, coloboma lower and upper eyelid, the paranasal cleft between piriform aperture and infraorbital nerve, cleft lip, and palate with anophthalmia or microphthalmia.
- Type II: any TC4 associated with others' facial malformations and clefts.
- Type III: only medial canthus displacement, coloboma lower and upper eyelid, the paranasal cleft between piriform aperture and infraorbital nerve without cleft lip and palate.

In this series of patients, we could observe initial differences from TC3, fewer patients without complete cleft lip and palate in TC4 than TC3, and the type of cleft palate most of the time incomplete in TC4 than TC3. Higher incidence of choanal atresia in TC4 than in TC3. There is more TC4 without other facial malformation than TC3 and more incidence of amniotic band syndrome (Figs. 8.6, 8.7, and 8.8).

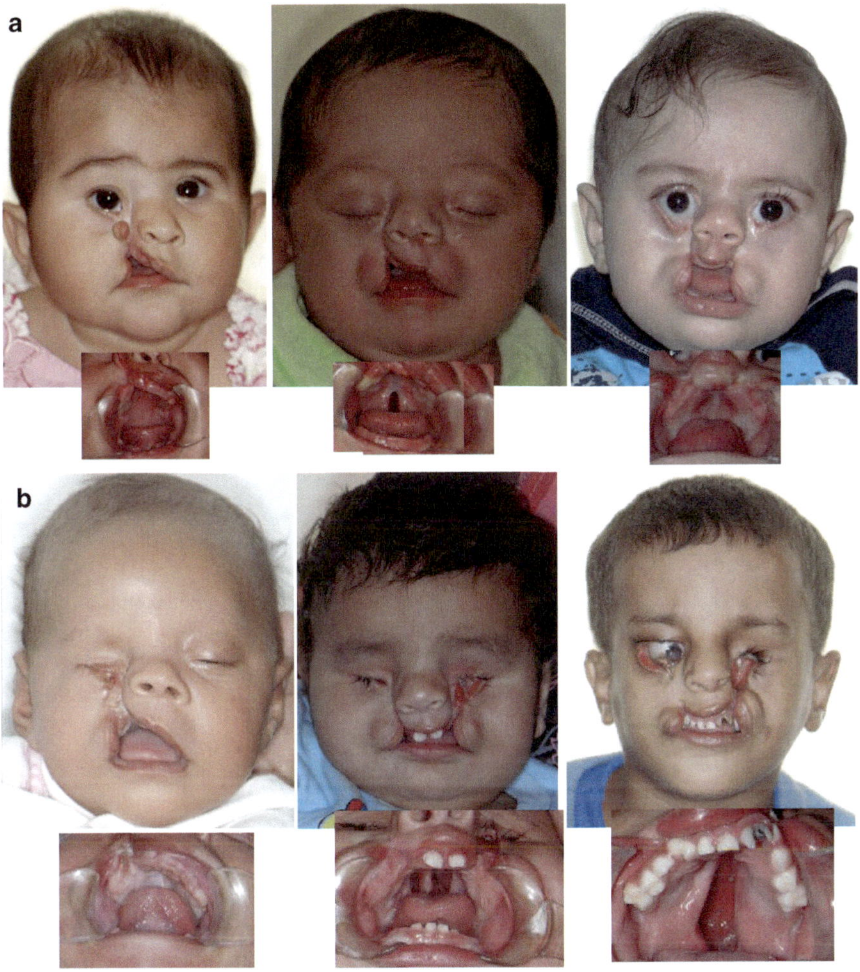

Fig. 8.6 Anatomical findings TC4. (**a**) **Type Ia** medial canthus displacement, coloboma lower and upper eyelid, paranasal cleft between piriform aperture and infraorbital nerve, cleft lip and palate. Unilateral, Bilateral and incomplete bilateral. (**b**) **Type Ib** medial canthus displacement, coloboma lower and upper eyelid, paranasal cleft between piriform aperture and infraorbital nerve, cleft lip and palate **with anophthalmia or microphthalmia. Unilateral, Bilateral and Asymmetric Bilateral**

Type II associated with others facial malformations and clefts

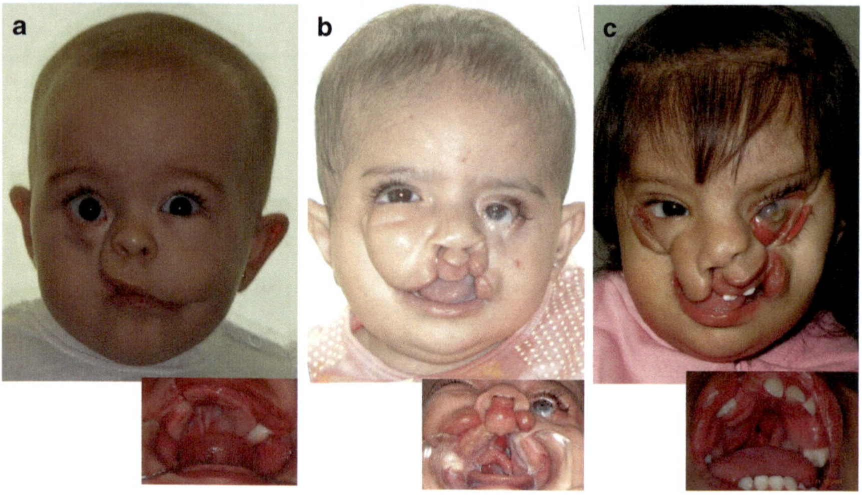

Fig. 8.7 Anatomical findings TC4. (**a**) TC4, Tessier cleft 6, maxillary duplication, Tessier cleft 7, macrostomia, no cleft palate. (**b**) TC4, Tessier cleft 6, macrostomia, bilateral cleft lip and palate. (**c**) TC4, Tessier cleft 5, Tessier cleft 6, Tessier cleft 8, macrostomia, amniotic bands syndrome, microphtalmie

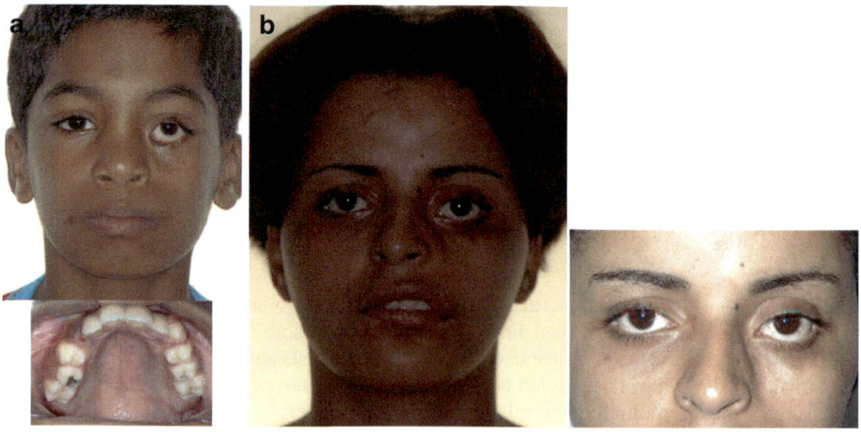

Fig. 8.8 Anatomical findings TC4. **Type III** only medial canthus displacement, coloboma lower and upper eyelid, paranasal cleft between piriform aperture and infraorbital nerve **without cleft lip and palate**

Radiological images, when correlated with the clinical features, suggest no close relationship exists between the soft and bone tissue defect. The frontal process of the maxilla is always involved as the maxilla itself, but the piriform aperture can be compromised eventually. The cleft lip is lateral to the well know "harelip," but the bone cleft passes between the canine and lateral incisor, closer to the canine than the regular cleft lip and palate (Figs. 8.9 and 8.10).

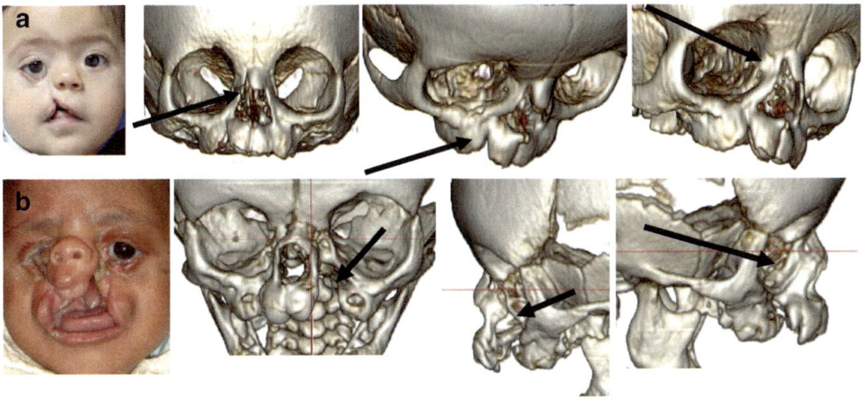

Fig. 8.9 Radiological findings TC4 uni/bil. (**a**) Right unilateral TC4 hypoplastic ascending ramus maxilla. Alveolar bone cleft between canine and lateral incisor. (**b**) Bilateral TC4 no lacrimal bone and wide left maxillary cleft

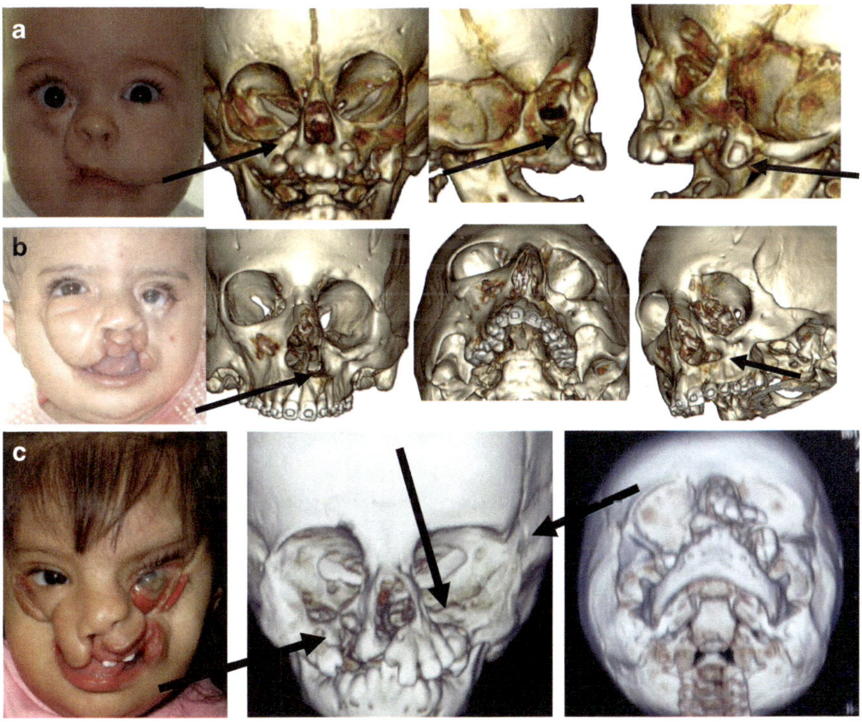

Fig. 8.10 Radiological findings TC4 associated clefts. (**a**) Maxillary duplication left, maxillary cleft medial to nerve, Tessier cleft 4+6. (**b**) Right deformity of zigoma, piriform aperture hypoplastic, Tessier 4+6. (**c**) Hypoplastic maxilla bilateral, enlargement orbital bilateral, Tessier 4+5+8+9

8.3 Our Cases

We analyzed 86 patients from three different centers 52 female and 34 male, 40 unilateral and 46 bilateral. One-third of the patients have another cleft associated with TC3, whereas almost 50% had other facial malformations. Additional observations were 12 choanal atresias in this series of patients and critical clinical findings for early diagnosis and treatment. As mentioned, Tessier Cleft 10 was noted in only three patients, but Tessier Cleft 5, 6, and 7 were present in 33 patients. We observed in 10 patients a bigger size of the upper eyelid on the side of TC4 and abnormal eyelashes that we do not consider any cleft. Only one patient had Tessier Cleft 3 associated. Differences between clefts 3 and 4 besides lateral facial cleft are apparent when we look at this associated facial malformation, reinforcing the idea of different embryological moments. Most of the patients with unilateral TC4 had incomplete or no cleft palate. We observed that one of the patients with a phenotype of TC4 had a radiological image suggesting TC3, with no bone in the piriform aperture on the left side in the radiological evaluation. Still, soft tissue was very typical of TC4 [10, 18] (Figs. 8.11, 8.12, 8.13).

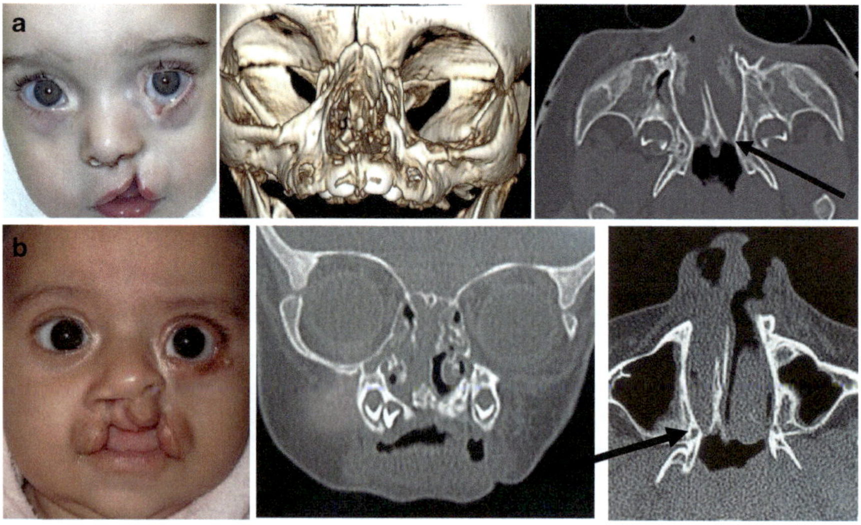

Fig. 8.11 Radiological findings TC4 Choanal atresia. (**a**) Bilateral total choanal atresia uni TC4. (**b**) Unilateral choanal atresia in opposite side of TC4

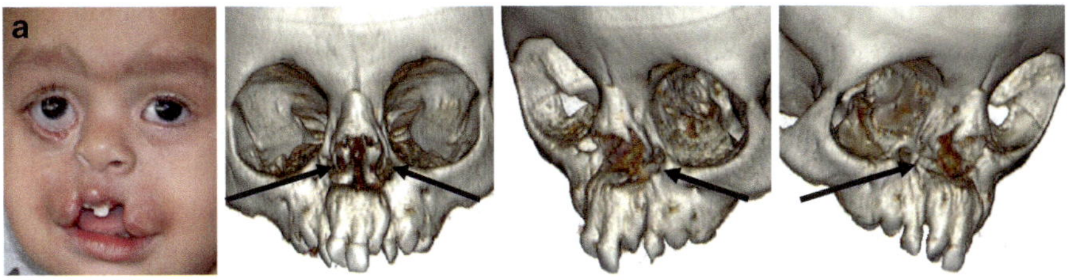

Fig. 8.12 Radiological findings TC4 Phenotype X bone deformity. (**a**) Clinical findings of TC4 but in CT no piriform aperture, CT more compatible to TC3

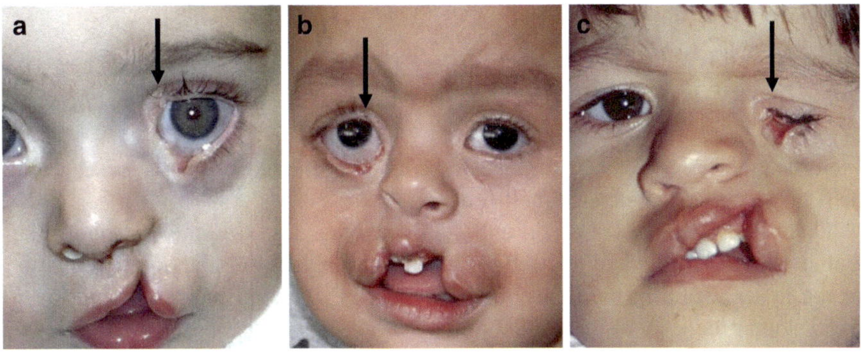

Fig. 8.13 Coloboma of the upper eyelid. (**a**) Upper eyelid coloboma with long eyelashes. (**b**) Coloboma with standard size of upper eyelid. (**c**) Microblepharia associated coloboma in both upper and lower eyelid

8.4 Surgical Treatment

The treatment of TC4 cleft has some principles. Initially, the priority is to protect the corneas. The soft tissue component is treated in the first months of life to restore facial appearance, evaluating each part (lip, nasal, and lower eyelid). The orbital bony defect may be addressed secondarily if necessary. Many patients do not have average facial growth potential; secondary procedures should be expected. Alveolar, maxillary, and orbital deformities should be evaluated and treated. Few articles published protocols for treating rare facial clefts, reflecting the rarity of this malformation. Still, some evident steps should be expected for long-term follow-ups, like soft tissue and scars corrections, orthognathic surgery, and rhinoplasties [12, 14, 16].

Treatment of rare facial clefts is complex to evaluate long-term results due to their low incidence. Its surgical repair is not a single-stage procedure but usually demands a planned, multistage approach. Primary surgical reconstruction aims to restore the oro-ocular distance and close hard and soft-tissue defects. Surgical reconstruction must consider restoring every compromised element—skin, soft tissues, and skeleton. Skin and soft tissue deficiency demand reconstruction, ideally using tissues with similar texture, consistency, and color.

Besides the rarity of this malformation, it is necessary to understand all its particularities. Patient born with TC4 cleft usually has corneal exposition and are prone to keratitis. This is the major problem in the first days of life, and immediate actions must be addressed to protect the eyeball. Eye ointment followed by surgery is necessary sometimes. The absence of orbital floor support makes the eyeball fall in the mouth and causes visual impairment like diplopia. When possible, mechanical occlusion using taping may help in the proposal. Some extreme measures could be necessary, like tarsorrhaphy or conjunctive purse-string suture [23]. Besides eye exposition, choanal atresia was found in 12 patients; the number should be considered very expressive and would need immediate treatment if it is bilateral. In some cases, patients could need a tracheotomy [24].

8.5 Surgical Markings

Important marking points are the size of the lower eyelid, the eyeball's presence, the cleft lip's size, and associated malformation.

Coloboma of the lower eyelid until half of the average size, mio cutaneous flap from the upper eyelid, and no need for lateral cantholysis after flap rotation fixation of the lower eyelid in the upper medial tendon. Paralateral incision going inside nasal skin at the level of the cranial portion of lower lateral cartilage and lip repair is done as a bilateral technique of Spina or for unilateral Millard's modification. An important observation is the medial lip marks because the cleft is lateral to the philtral crest. Excessive tissue in between could be resected, or part of it could be used in cases where the lower eyelid is too short, or the nasal cleft is too big, in anophthalmia or microblepharia (Figs. 8.14, 8.15, and 8.16).

Eyelid coloboma may have a variable grade of affection. Minor involvement involves the deformation of the lacrimal punctum and medial canthus dystopia. However, in significant cases, the deficiency of the lower eyelid is the most challenging subject in the repair of this kind of rare cleft. Flaps from the glabellar area, upper eyelid with medial pedicle, or paranasal area were already utilized to reconstruct the lower eyelid and treat the medial canthus dystopia. Even a skin graft was indicated to reposition the level of the palpebral margin. The choice of eyelid reconstruction must be based on the cleft anatomy, observing the deficiencies of soft tissue and the lower eyelid. The surgeons need to adequate the technique with the defect.

Bone grafting of the orbital floor is utilized. However, it should be used in a different stage of soft-tissue repair. The timing and type of maxilla bone graft have been individualized for each case. It has usually been made in a second-stage intervention. Bony reconstruction for skeletal defects on the face and orbit is generally only undertaken once the patient is 6 years of age and, more commonly, at age 7. The donor area may be calvarium, costal, or iliac crest. Sometimes, it is necessary to associate inlay and onlay bone grafts to reconstruct the whole facial framework adequately. Bone graft coverage with tension-free healthy tissues increases the

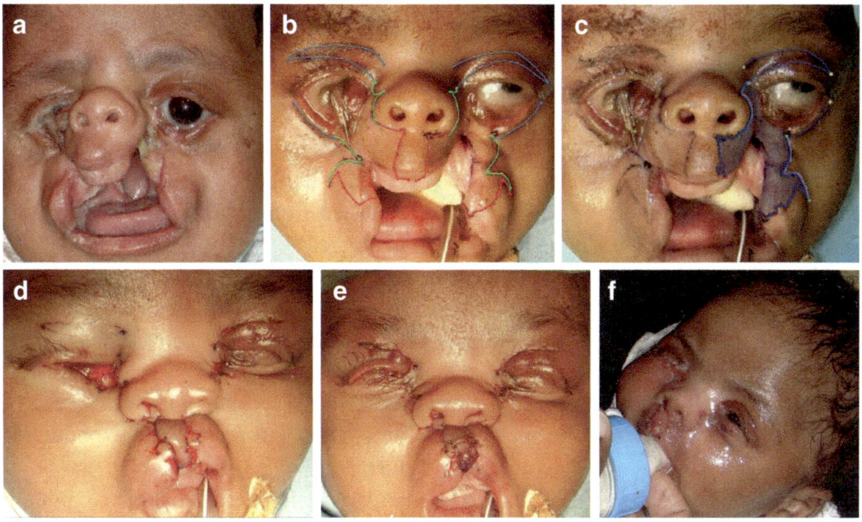

Fig. 8.14 Surgical marking for complete bilateral TC4. (**a**) Bilateral TC4. (**b**) Important points, upper/lower eyelid, bilayeral lip marks, lateral facial flap. (**c**) Tissue to be resected. (**d**) Flaps in position, right upper eyelid flap, marked to rotate. (**e**) Final position of the flap. (**f**) Day after the surgery

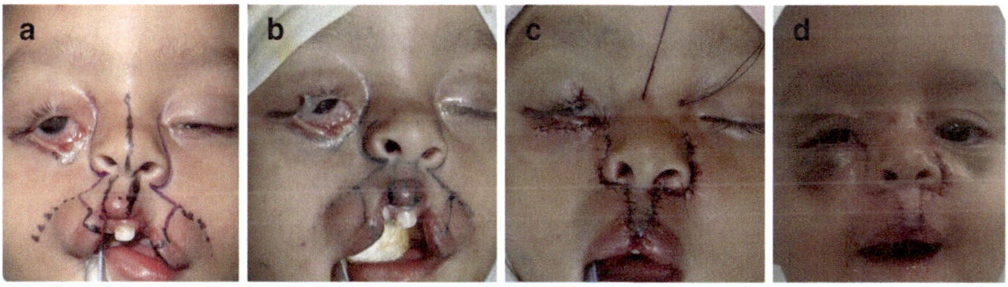

Fig. 8.15 Surgical marking for incomplete asymmetric TC4. (**a**) Paralateral nasal incision marks for lip repair Spina' technique. (**b**) Large upper eyelid. (**c**) Resection of coloboma upper eyelid, right medial canthopexy and limited left para nasal incision. (**d**) Final position of the scars

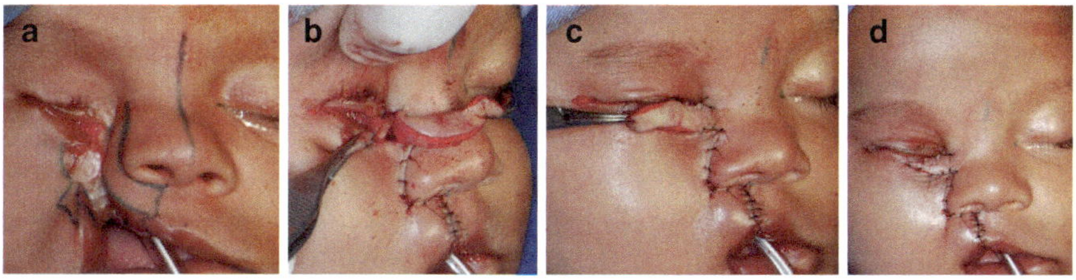

Fig. 8.16 Surgical marking anophthalmic cavity using the superior paranasal flap. (**a**) Marking paranasal flap in anophthalmic cavity. (**b**) Superior based paranasal flap rotation to fill out lower eyelid defect. (**c**) Flap in position. (**d**) Final aspect of lower eyelid

chance of graft integration, reducing the risk of its absorption and loss. Grafting of an orbital floor may correct the vertical orbital dystopia and enlargement, and of the anterior portion of the maxilla, correct the projection of the malar area. Alloplastic materials should not be used in children.

The advancement of tomographic study and prototyping is opening a new area of bone reconstruction. The volume of bone deficiency could be calculated previously and the bone shape and volume needed for reconstruction could be precisely reconstructed with autologous bone graft using this images.

Microphthalmia and anophthalmia are observed in TC4; the most common cause of this malformation is probably deficient closure of the fetal fissure of the invaginated optic vesicle [25]. An orbital expander may be indicated for cases of anophthalmia to enlarge the orbit and improve the maxillary growth and symmetry. The expander may be inserted in the first-stage procedure, associated with the closure of the soft-tissue defects. A permanent ocular prosthesis will replace the expander to improve the appearance and avoid social disturbs.

The retraction of the ala is a challenge, mainly when there is the desire to put the scar in the paranasal area. The undermining of nasal skin in the compromised side brings more tissue associated with the release of deep tissue adhesion to nasal bone and septum, which may correct the superior position of ala. In cases with more retraction, an incision between the ala and lateral sides of the nose is necessary.

For initial patients, we used Tessier's technique. Still, after a few years and for new patients, we have changed for paralateral nasal scars alternating from upper eyelid flap and nasal flap depending on the size of the lower eyelid defect. Tessier's initial technique brings excessive scars on the middle of the face. The original technique from Tessier is not utilized in our clinic anymore. Some patients who had this technique performed before were submitted to a secondary approach to bring the scars close to the nasal area. Secondary intervention may be necessary to correct medial and lateral canthal position, secondary ectropion, epiphora, lower eyelid skin deficiency, and further bony augmentation. Soft-tissue expansion, stretching uninvolved adjacent skin, allows the reconstruction of a large variety of defects by simply advancing or transposing the expanded normal tissue to the defect. Menard et al. published the most considerable experience using tissue expansion to reconstruct craniofacial clefts, including eight cases of TC4, three of them in the primary stage. They had only one case of expander extrusion [26]. However, our experience shows that tissue expansion is rarely necessary to reconstruct TC4.

Microsurgical flaps are another option for facial cleft reconstructions. Longaker and Siebert presented their experience with microsurgical reconstruction, including two patients with TC4. They used mainly para-scapular flaps, bringing a good volume of tissues to the face [27]. One patient was successfully submitted to a secondary forearm microsurgical flap in our series. Unlike tissue expansion, microsurgical reconstruction should be used only in secondary defects, with limited local tissue reconstructive options. Lipofilling is an alternative to improve the quality of the result, bringing volume and better texture to the face.

Our considerable experience treating this rare craniofacial disorder allowed us to develop some technical modifications, whose advantages could be evidenced in our practice. The original Tessier technique obtained reasonable results, but the scars needed to respect the face's natural folds and anatomical units. Later, looking for better cosmetic results, we started using the Kawamoto procedure, using a vertical nasal flap with a superior basis and a linear scar in the paranasal area. But, we could have achieved a better color match of the skin flap in some patients. More recently, however, we have realized that linear scar in the paranasal area could also be applied in Tessier's technique if the incisions were made more medially than originally described. The lower eyelid reconstruction and medial canthus reposition could also be performed by designing the upper eyelid flap in a lower position, close to the upper lid fold, or using the Kawamoto flap, depending on the site of soft tissue excess. Furthermore, regarding labial defects, the same principles and markings used for unilateral cleft lip from our modification of Millard's and Spina's technique for bilateral cleft lip could also be applied in TC4 [28–30]. These technical modifications have substantially improved our results, camouflaging scars into natural folds and anatomical limits without prejudicing functional outcomes.

8.6 Our Cases

Patient with TC4 on the left side submitted to correction early in life and had a secondary eyelid correction with inferior pedicle nasal flap and later one another refinement to move facial scars medially; after 17 years, we can observe good scars well-placed (Fig. 8.17).

Some patients operated with different approaches from 7 to 20 years of follow-up (Figs. 8.18 and 8.19).

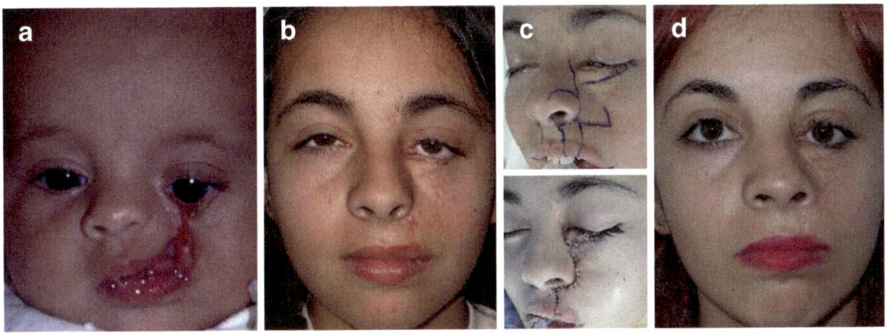

Fig. 8.17 Long-term follow-up of Tessier's technique with refinements. (**a**) Left unilateral TC4. (**b**) After first secondary eyelid correction. (**c**) Refinements to medially position scars. (**d**) Final result 17 years late

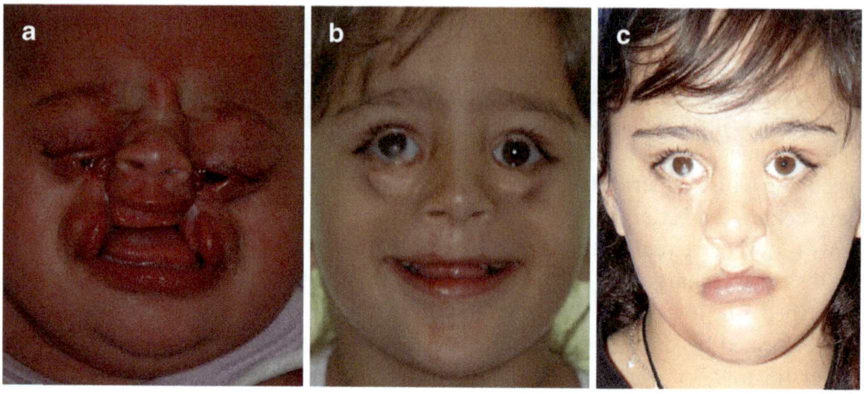

Fig. 8.18 Long-term follow-up secondary advancement rotation flap. (**a**) Bilateral TC4. (**b**) Mismatched colour. (**c**) Secondary refinements new advancement rotation flap

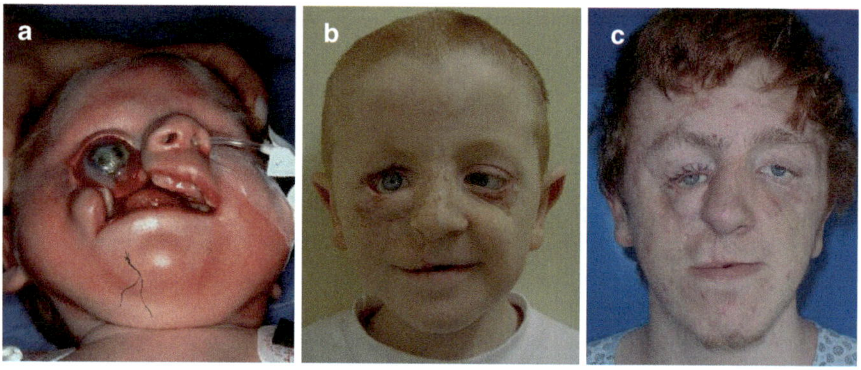

Fig. 8.19 Long-term follow-up after many surgeries. (**a**) severe right TC4, (**b**) After many surgeries, including forehead flap, orbital bone graft and eye prosthesis, (**c**) 20 years late after some refinements. Long-term follow-up unilateral TC4 normal nasal growth. (**d**) left TC4, (**e**) 9 years late no orbital bone graft, nasal elongation on the cleft side. Long-term follow-up bilateral asymmetric TC4 with choanal atresia. (**f**) Bilateral TC4 with choanal atresia, (**g**) 10 years late. Long-term follow up improvement of eye protection. (**h**) Right TC4 with eye exposure, (**i**) 8 years late after early surgery

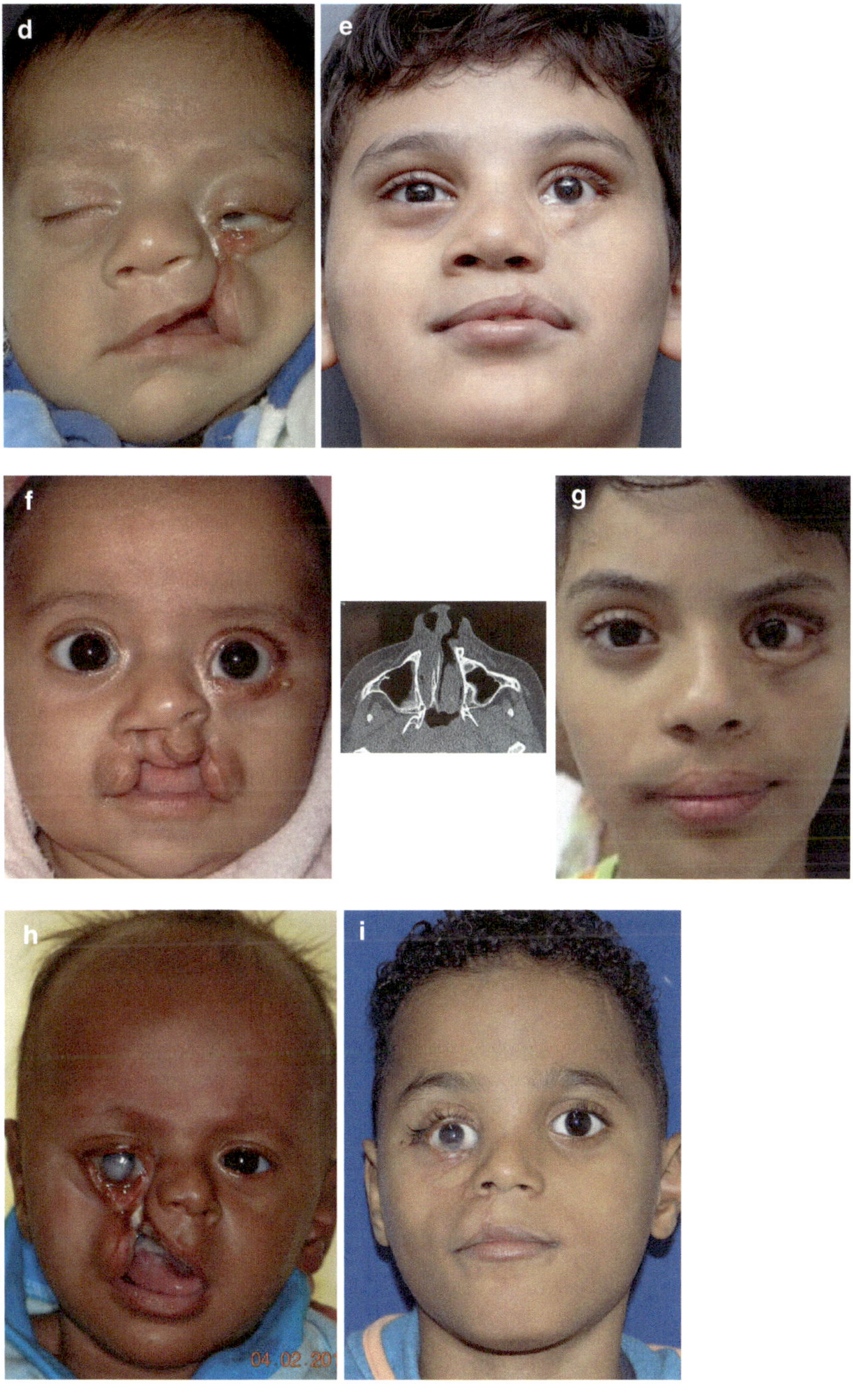

Fig. 8.19 (continued)

References

1. Morian R. Über die schräge Gesichtsspalte (about oblique facial clefts). Arch Klin Chir. 1887;35:245–88.
2. Tessier P. Anatomical classification of facial, craniofacial, and latero-facial clefts. J Maxillofac Surg. 1976;4:69–92. https://linkinghub.elsevier.com/retrieve/pii/S0301050376800136
3. Jalaguier A, colobome facial bilateral. Double fente congénitale bucco-orbitaire. Autoplasties successives. Guérison. In: Jalaguier AD, editor. Titres et travaux scientifiques. Paris: Asselin et Houzeau; 1912. p. 29–31. https://archive.org/details/BIUSante_110133x096x07/page/n65/mode/2up.
4. Tessier P. Classification Anatomique Des Fentes Faciales Cranio-Faciales Et Latéro-Latérales, Leur Rëpartition Autour De L'orbite. In: Rougier J, Société française d'ophtalmologie, editors. Chirurgie plastique orbito-palpébrale. Paris; New York: Masson; 1977.
5. van der Meulen JCH, Vaandrager JM. Facial clefts. World J Surg. 1989;13(4):373–83. https://doi.org/10.1007/BF01660750.
6. Resnick JI, Kawamoto HK. Rare craniofacial clefts: tessier no. 4 clefts. Plast Reconstr Surg. 1990;85(6):843–9. http://journals.lww.com/00006534-199006000-00001.
7. van der Meulen JCH. Oblique facial clefts: pathology, etiology, and reconstruction. Plast Reconstr Surg. 1985;76(2):212–24. http://journals.lww.com/00006534-198508000-00007.
8. Longaker MT, Lipshutz GS, Kawamoto HK. Reconstruction of Tessier no. 4 clefts revisited. Plast Reconstr Surg. 1997;99(6):1501–7.
9. Alonso N, da Silva Freitas R, e Cruz GA, Goldenberg D, AR DOT. tessier no. 4 facial cleft: evolution of surgical treatment in a large series of patients. Plast Reconstr Surg. 2008;22(5):1505–13. http://journals.lww.com/00006534-200811000-00024.
10. Alonso N, da Silva Freitas R. Craniofacial clefts and others related deformities. In: Plastic Surgery Indications and Practice. p. 455–71.
11. Van Slyke AC, Burge J, Bos R, Parker G, Chong DK. The anatomical subunit approach to managing Tessier numbers 3 and 4 craniofacial clefts. Plast Reconstr Surg-Glob Open. 2022;10(9):e4553.
12. AbdollahiFakhim S, Shahidi N, Bayazian G. A bilateral tessier number 4 and 5 facial cleft and surgical strategy: a case report. Iran J Otorhinolaryngol. 2013;25(73):259–62.
13. Aköz T, Erdoğan B, Görgü M, Kutlay R, Dağ F. Bilaterally involved tessier no. 4 cleft: case report. Cleft Palate Craniofac J. 1996;33(3):252–4. https://doi.org/10.1597/1545-1569_1996_033_0252_bitncc_2.3.co_2.
14. Balaji S. Single stage correction of bilateral Tessier 4 cleft. Indian J Dent Res. 2017;28(1):105. http://www.ijdr.in/text.asp?2017/28/1/105/203616.
15. Chen PKT, Chang FCS, Chan FC, Chen YR, Noordhoff MS. Repair of tessier no. 3 and no. 4 craniofacial clefts with facial unit and muscle repositioning by midface rotation advancement without z-plasties. Plast Reconstr Surg. 2012;129(6):1337–44. http://journals.lww.com/00006534-201206000-00020.
16. Mishra R, Purwar R. Formatting the surgical management of Tessier cleft types 3 and 4. Indian J Plast Surg. 2009;42(3):174. http://www.ijps.org/text.asp?2009/42/3/174/57192.
17. Smith HB, Verity DH, JRO C. The incidence, embryology, and oculofacial abnormalities associated with eyelid colobomas. Eye. 2015;29(4):492–8. http://www.nature.com/articles/eye2014335.
18. Alonso N, Tonello C. Rare facial clefts. In: Hamdan U, Rogers-Vizena C, Vyas R, Sommerlad B, Low D, editors. Interdisciplinary cleft care global perspectives. San Diego CA: Plural Publishing; 2023. p. 689–701. http://www.pluralpublishing.com.
19. Adeosun OO, James O, Akinmoladun VI, Owobu T. Amniotic band syndrome associated with orofacial clefts: a report of two cases: amniotic band syndrome. Oral Surg. 2012;5(4):185–9. https://doi.org/10.1111/j.1752-248X.2012.01163.x.
20. Assouan C, Ambroise B, de Boutray M, Labbé D, Bénateau H, Veyssiere A. Tessier number 4 bilateral craniofacial cleft associated with amniotic band syndrome: 22 years of follow-up. J

Stomatol Oral Maxillofac Surg. 2018;119(3):208–11. https://linkinghub.elsevier.com/retrieve/pii/S2468785517302410.

21. Bagatin M, Sarkissian R, Larrabeejr W. Craniofacial manifestations of the amniotic band syndrome. Otolaryngol Head Neck Surg. 1997;116(4):525–8. https://doi.org/10.1016/S0194-5998(97)70303-6.
22. MSE C, Moore MH, Wallis K. Amniotic band syndrome: the association between rare facial clefts and limb ring constrictions. Plast Reconstr Surg. 1998;101(3):640–9. http://journals.lww.com/00006534-199803000-00010.
23. Tonello C, Paula RG, Paula IP, Nunes RB, Kokitsu-Nakata NM, Alonso N. Eyeball preservation with purse-string conjunctival closure for melting corneal ulcer in rare facial cleft. Cleft Palate Craniofac J. 2021;58(9):1195–200. https://doi.org/10.1177/1055665620980632.
24. Tonello C, Martins DA, Baptista MA, Mondelli F, Kokitsu Nakata NM, Feitosa LB, et al. Tessier 3 and 4 clefts and Choanal atresia: an unusual association? Cleft Palate-Craniofacial J. 2022;59(10):1228–32. https://doi.org/10.1177/10556656211042172.
25. Warburg M, Jensen H, Prause JU, Bolund S, Skovby F, Miranda MJ. Anophthalmia-microphthalmia-oblique clefting syndrome: confirmation of the Fryns anophthalmia syndrome. Am J Med Genet. 1997;73(1):36–40.
26. Menard RM, Moore MH, David DJ. Tissue expansion in the reconstruction of Tessier craniofacial clefts: a series of 17 patients. Plast Reconstr Surg. 1999;103(3):779–86.
27. Longaker MT, Siebert JW. Microsurgical Correction of Facial Contour in Congenital Craniofacial Malformations: The Marriage of Hard and Soft Tissue. Plast Reconstr Surg. 1996;98(6):942–50. http://journals.lww.com/00006534-199611000-00003.
28. Spina V. The advantages of two stages in the repair of bilateral cleft lip. The Cleft Palate J. 1966;3(1):56–60.
29. Spina V, Kamakura L, Lapa F. Surgical_Management_of_Bilateral_Cleft_Lip. Surg Management Bilateral Cleft Lip. 1978;1(5):497–505.
30. da Silva FR, Bertoco Alves P, Shimizu GKM, Schuchovski JF, Lopes MAC, Maluf I, et al. Beyond fifty years of Millard's rotation-advancement technique in cleft lip closure: are there many "Millards"? Plast Surg Int. 2012;2012:731029.

Chapter 9
Cleft 5

Renato da Silva Freitas, Nivaldo Alonso, Cristiano Tonello, and Philippe Pellerin

Pearls

- Tessier Cleft 5 (TC5) facial cleft is an extremely rare congenital malformation. Less than 40 cases have been described in the English literature.
- TC5 has a frequent association with Clefts 8 and 4.
- The critical differential is diagnostic with cleft number 6; a computed tomography (CT) scan should be necessary often.
- TC5 is similar to Cleft 6 and 7, macrostomia, and palatal deformity.
- Surgical treatment is more predictable than any other facial cleft.

R. da Silva Freitas (✉)
Plastic Surgery Unit, Hospital de Clínicas, Universidade Federal do Paraná, Curitiba, Brazil

Craniofacial Surgery, Assistance Center for Cleft Lip and Palate (CAIF), Hospital do Trabalhador, Curitiba, Brazil

N. Alonso
Plastic Surgery, Universidade de São Paulo, São Paulo, Brazil

Craniofacial Surgery, Hospital de Reabilitação Anomalias Craniofaciais Bauru USP Universidade de São Paulo, Bauru, Brazil

C. Tonello
Curso de Medicina Bauru Faculdade de Odontologia Bauru Universidade de São Paulo, Bauru, Brazil

Hospital de Reabilitação Anomalias Craniofaciais Universidade de São Paulo, Bauru, Brazil

P. Pellerin
Centre Hospitalier Régional Universitaire de Lille, Lille, France

N. Alonso et al. (eds.), *Facial Reconstruction of Unusual Facial Clefts*, https://doi.org/10.1007/978-3-031-40926-4_9

9.1 Historical Considerations

TC5 is highly uncommon. Our paper published in 2009 found 26 cases reported in the English literature, and we added six new patients with TC5 [1, 2]. The incidence of this group of malformations is less than 0.25% among all facial clefts [3–5]. All known cases are sporadic, without genetic or syndromic association [6].

Many terms have already been proposed to call this malformation. The American Association of Cleft Palate Rehabilitation classified it as an orofacial canthal cleft; Morian (1887) as a type III lateral oro-ocular coloboma [7]; Karfik (1966) as an "accurate oblique cleft"; Boo-Chai (1970) as a type II oro-ocular cleft; and van der Meulen (1983) as lateral maxillary dysplasia [8]. Tessier 1976 published his classification worldwide and was accepted as Tessier Cleft (TC5) [9]. Tessier postulated that Cleft 9 would be a northbound version of this TC5 (Fig. 9.1). Our revision did not find a close relationship between these two clefts, even if we found three patients with this association. If there is an association between these, we believe it is sporadic. However, some of our cases were associated with TC4 and TC8.

TC5 is a lateral orbitomaxillary cleft. The cleft begins in the upper lip, near the oral commissure, extending upward through the jugal area, until the lower eyelid in the middle third as a coloboma. These clefts may be bilateral. The skeletal involvement begins on the premolar site, running lateral to the infraorbital nerve, until the orbital floor. The distance between the oral commissure and eyelid is shortened, giving the appearance of the "Joker." The cleft stops in the lateral portion of the orbit floor, generally not extending into the inferior orbital fissure. All oblique clefts may be associated with eyeball anomalies, such as microphthalmia or anophthalmia. The medial canthal ligament is almost always in the normal position, and the lateral is generally dystopic (Fig. 9.2). Tomographic scans may demonstrate an alveolar cleft ascending through to the anterior maxilla, with the involvement of the orbital floor. The medial portion of the orbital rim was hypoplastic bilaterally [4, 9] (Figs. 9.3, 9.4, 9.5). One fascinating point is that the aspects of the cleft palate in these patients have some differences from TC4, TC3, and TC6. We found an abnormality in 07 (seven) patients with TC5, short palate with lateral adhesion to the jugal mucosa with hypoplastic muscles and hypertrophic uvula. Looking closely, it is

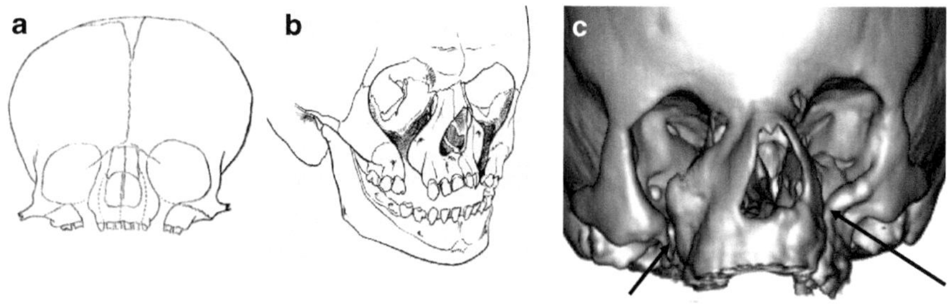

Fig. 9.1 Similar TC5 classification. (**a**) Morian III. (**b**) Tessier cleft 5, (**c**) 3D CT scan, Tessier cleft 5 right side, Tessier 4 left side

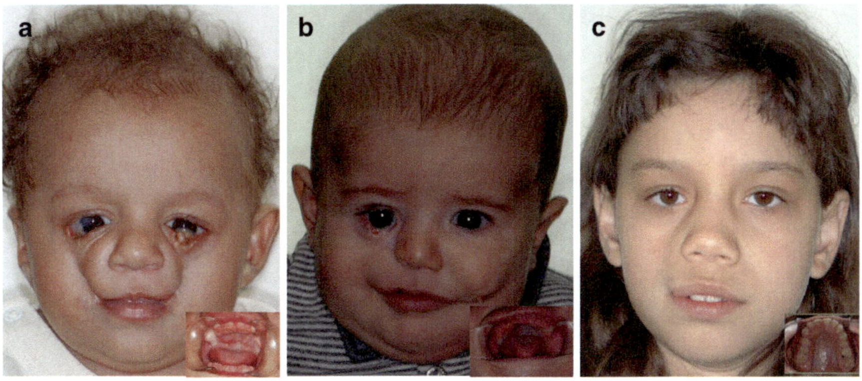

Fig. 9.2 Clinical findings. (**a**) Bilateral TC5, (**b**) right TC5 left TC6, (**c**) right unilateral TC5

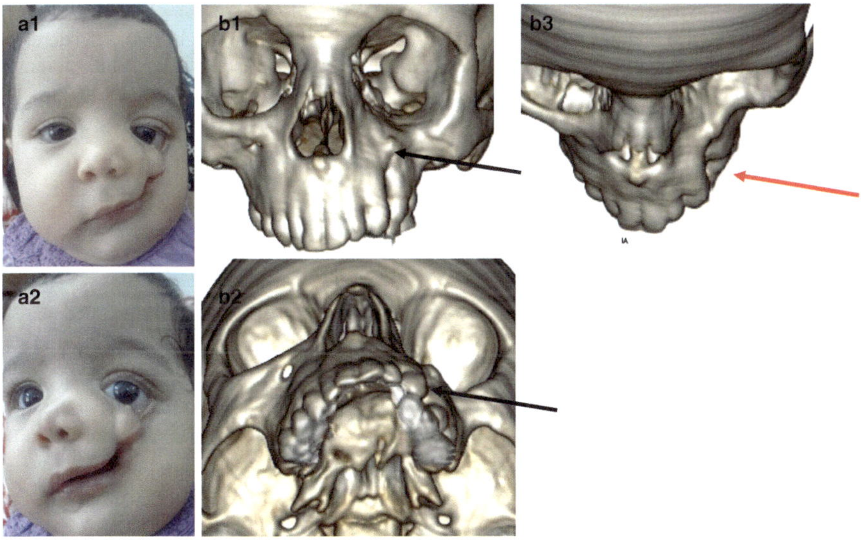

Fig. 9.3 Radiological findings. (**a**) Left TC5 front/oblique. (**b**) Left side TC5. Bone cleft lateral to infraorbital forame black arrow. Alveolar cleft between canine and molar deciduos, black arrow. Left maxilla hypoplastic red arrow

more like TC6 and the others. In TC4, most of our unilateral cases were incomplete regular cleft palate, and in TC3, complete cleft lip and palate with no difference from everyday cleft lip and palate. TC6 has a very short soft palate with a bone cleft in the deciduous molar, all muscles laterally placed (Fig. 9.6).

Understanding the embryology of facial development and what happened in oblique facial clefts needs to be clarified. Failed processes of craniofacial fusion need to be clearly explained. Some rare facial cracks may be related to fusion

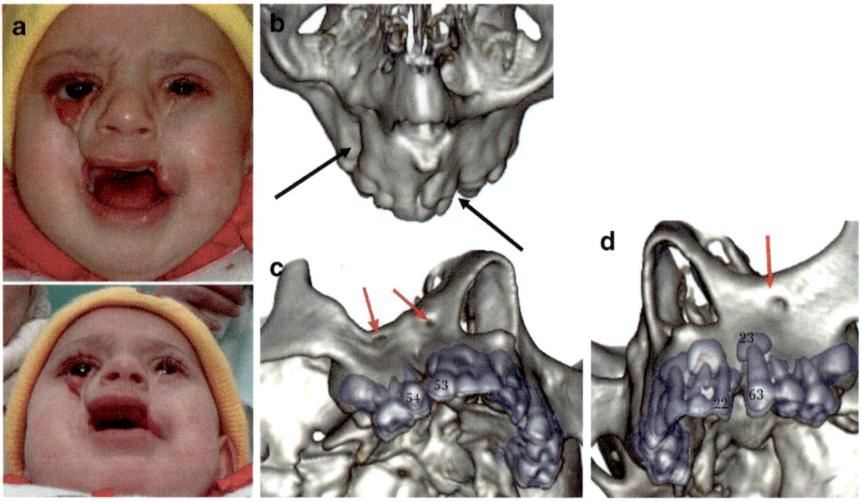

Fig. 9.4 Radiological findings. (**a**) Right TC5 left TC4 front inferior. (**b**) Right Tessier 5 lateral to infraorbital forame, between 53 and 54 teeth. (**c**, **d**) Left Tessier 4 medial to infraobital forame, between 22/23 and 63 red arrow

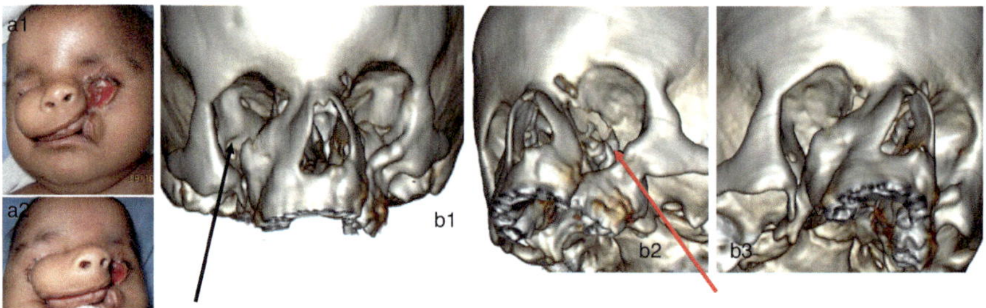

Fig. 9.5 Radiological findings. (**a**) Right TC5 and left TC4 front and inferior view. (**b**) 3D CT scan, (**b1**) right TC 5 right side with vertical orbital dystopia, black arrow. (**b2**) Left TC 4 left side enlargement of the orbit, red arrow. (**b3**) right TC5 maxillary hypoplasia

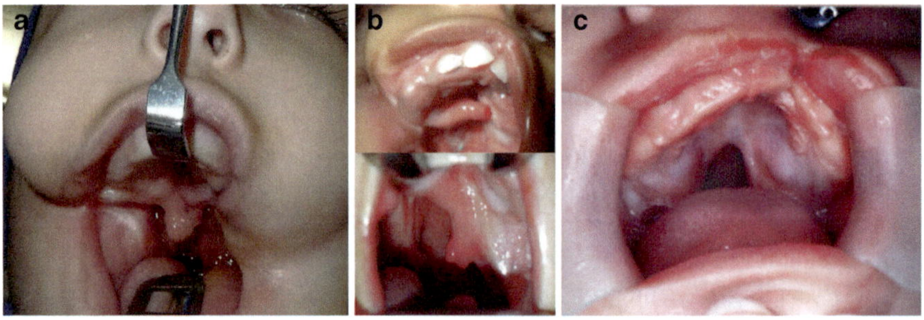

Fig. 9.6 palatal aspect of TC5 compared to TC4 and TC6. (**a**) TC6, (**b**) TC5, (**c**) TC4

problems of embryonic processes, but TC5 does not correspond to well-known embryologic grooves or planes of mesenchymal-supported epithelium. Possibly, it may be explained by the primary arrest of development, neurovascular insufficiency or necrosis, or a result of tears in the developing maxillary process [10, 11]. In only two patients, amniotic bands are observed in a few complex cases, and may act directly with tethered tissue migration and increased local pressure that produces cellular ischemia. Cannistrà et al. published an interesting study with a fetus with TC5. His case had agenesis of the maxillary nerve and the structures innervated by this nerve. The conclusion supports that some atypical facial clefts, such as TC5, can result from defects occurring late in development rather than during the period of primary facial morphogenesis [12].

9.2 Clinical Findings

In our series of patients, TC5 is the lower incidence among our facial clefts, only 26 patients, classified into two clinical types: type I—lateral orbital canthal displacement, lateral coloboma lower eyelid, the lateral facial cleft between oral commissure and infraorbital nerve, bone cleft lateral to infraorbital nerve. Type II—associated with other facial malformations and clefts. The only other facial malformations from those type II were Tessier's Cleft numbers 3, 4, 6, 7, 8, 9, and 03 anophthalmia and 01 OAVS. Five patients with Tessier Cleft 4 and 05 with Tessier 8 (Table 9.1). Only three patients had isolated TC5 bilateral; all the others were unilateral isolated or associated with other facial clefts. One patient with anophthalmia had a big orbital-alveolar cleft between the first and second deciduous molar. In this case, bone graft was done in the floor of the orbit and maxilla associated with orbital expansion (Fig. 9.7).

Table 9.1 Patients with TC5 anatomical findings

Type I lateral orbital canthus displacement, lateral coloboma lower eyelid, lateral facial cleft between oral commissure and infraorbital nerve, bone cleft lateral to infraorbital nerve
Type II associated with others facial malformations and clefts

Others Facial Malformation associated		
Tessier 3	01	patient
Tessier 4		**05**
Tessier 6	01	
Tessier 7	01	
Tessier 8		**05**
Tessier 9		**03**
OAV	01	
Anophtalmia/microphtalmia		**03**

Cleft 5	Number of patients
Type I	16
Type II	10
Total	**26**
Unilateral.	23
Bilateral	03

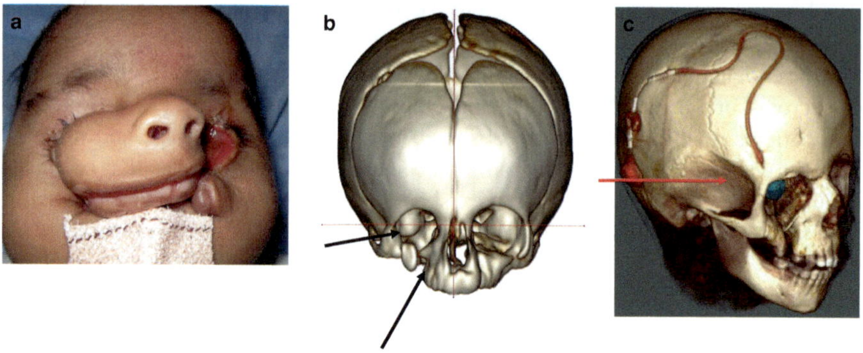

Fig. 9.7 Anophthalmia and TC5. (**a**) Right TC5 and left TC4, (**b**) R microphthalmia and lateral maxillary cleft black arrow, (**c**) right orbital expander red arrow

9.2.1 *Orbital*

The skeletal defect with an absence of orbital floor and rim does not support the eyeball, and vertical dystopia and enophthalmos can be present. A palpebral fissure can stay in antimongoloid inclination because of the lack of bony support for the lateral canthal ligament. Coloboma located on the lateral third of the lower eyelid may be mild with a small notch in the palpebral rim or severe with a big coloboma of the lower eyelid. The surgical objectives aim to close the eyelid cleft, elevate the lateral canthal ligament, maintain the dimensions of the palpebral fissure, support the eye with bony grafting of orbital floor, and achieve everything with good quality of scar and well positioned.

9.2.2 *Upper Lip*

The cleft, when present, is located near the oral commissure. The appearance is like macrostomia, with an upward direction. It is necessary to define the new commissure using the contralateral side as a pattern. In cases with an association of cleft lip or another oblique facial cleft, or even TC5 bilateral, it is possible to use a vertical line from the iris as a landmark. All the demarcations must be done with special care to have the proper measures.

9.2.3 *Jugal Area*

"Joker" appearance is due to the shortening of the middle third and the macrostomia due to a cleft lip. The cleft can be partial or complete, and facial muscles can be affected. During the repair, it is necessary to elongate the skin, and multiple Z-plasty is indicated in many cases. An incomplete cleft may be managed with less scar.

9.3 Surgical Treatment

The quality of results in treating all rare facial cleft is often far from those considered brilliant. Tessier suggested that the immediate results of surgery depend not only upon the technique used but also relative to the potential hypogenesis of the facial structures and the other associated anomalies [13]. This fact was found in our practice. Also, the result depends on tissue remodeling caused by the exerted pressure of scar contracture and muscle contraction. The objectives in these patients are to repair eyelid coloboma, reposition lateral canthal ligament, close the maxillary cleft, and bony grafting on the orbital floor and anterior face of the maxilla alveolar bridge. The repair of this malformation requires multiple staged procedures. Finally, urgency occurs to repair the lower eyelid and protect the remaining dystopic eye.

Patients may present a collapsed maxilla arch. Panoramic X-ray reveals that the alveolar ridge is broken on the molar area, and abnormalities of molar teeth may be evidenced. A computed tomography (CT) scan revealed an alveolar cleft and hypoplastic maxilla, with a deficiency in the buttress region. Orthopedic and orthodontic works are necessary for older patients, aiming for alveolar bone grafting, even for anterior maxilla defects.

Multiple Z-plasty was utilized by many surgeons, including our team [1, 14]. Each side received a Z-plasty; if necessary, others can be added in the middle of the maxilla. In addition, Pereira et al. proposed an interesting approach to repair, using a combination of Z-plasty and two rotational flaps. A flap from the inner aspect of the cheek is rotated superiorly, repositioning the lower eyelid, and another flap is rotated superiorly to reconstruct the upper eyelid [15] (Figs. 9.8, 9.9).

In our series, the myocutaneous flap, with a lateral pedicle transposed from the upper to lower eyelid, is an essential step for eyelid repositioning. This flap was initially indicated for secondary cases when the correction was not satisfied; more recently, this flap was used primarily (Figs. 9.8, 9.9).

Maxillary and orbital bony grafting were proposed to be done in the first surgery, together with soft-tissue repair, by many authors [13, 16]; however, there is a risk of bone exposure and loss of the bone field [16]. Secondary graft, around 4–6 years of age, is more accessible and safer. When the child is not so young, the donor area is more predictable and not a problem. Tessier postulated that orbital dystopia is essential to treat before 12 months of age [13]. We do not indicate bone grafting so early. Surgery must be undertaken for affected eyelids with corneal exposure as soon as the child can be stabilized. In the presurgical period, ophthalmic lubricant ointment is used for the exposed cornea.

The orbital bone defect may be corrected primarily at the soft-tissue closure or secondarily, after some months or years following soft-tissue repair, restoring the continuity of the orbital floor, anterior face of the maxilla, and alveolus. The options for donor area may be calvarium, iliac crest, or rib. We utilized bony grafting in four patients, two calvariae, and two iliac crests. The tissue expander is indicated for a secondary procedure involving refinements of scars. Menard et al. published their experience using a tissue expander to reconstruct several facial clefts [17]. Two of our patients were treated with a tissue expander, used to improve the position of the scars as a cosmetic refinement. Eye protection is the first attention when the child is

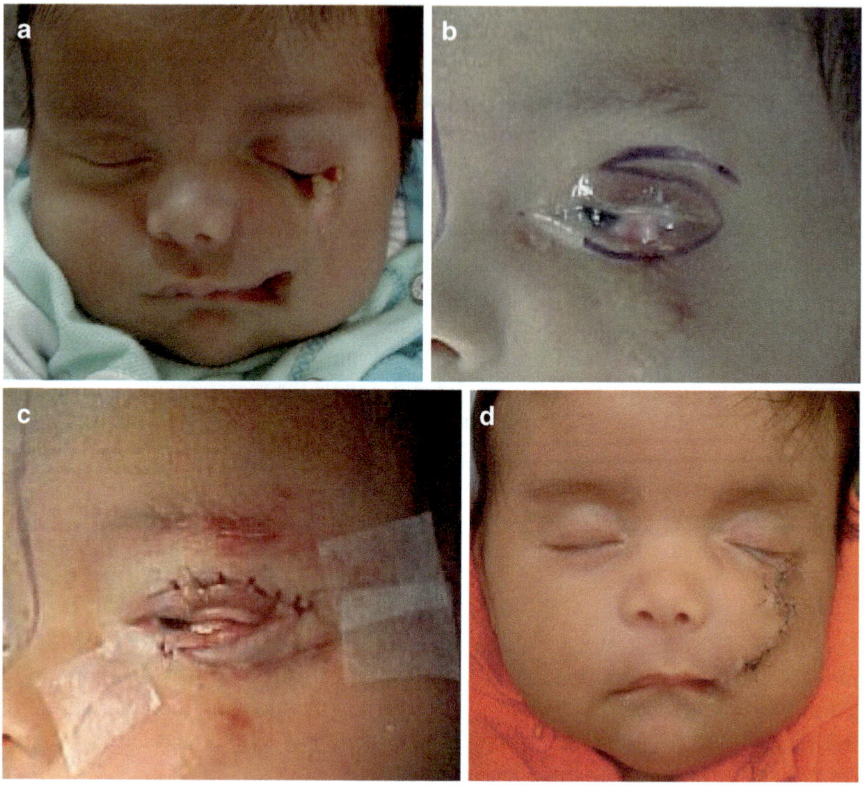

Fig. 9.8 (**a**) Surgical treatment—upper eyelid flap. (**a**) Left TC5 inferior orbit coloboma, (**b**) upper eyelid miocutaneous flap, (**c**) intra operative flap rotation, (**d**) final aspect of correction

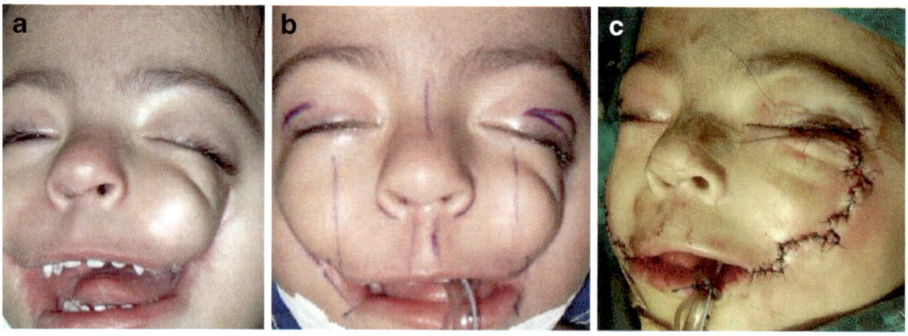

Fig. 9.9 Surgical treatment—multiple Z-plasty . (**a**) TC5 bilateral pre op macrostomia, (**b**) intra op markings, (**c**) multiple Z-plastie and upper eyelid flap

evaluated. Eye gel and surgery as soon as possible are essential to the treatment. If there is soft tissue to repair completely, it should be done. However, if it is necessary to have temporary management, tarsorrhaphy can help. Tonello et al. proposed a purse-string conjunctival suture to cover the severe corneal exposition as a temporary method [18].

9.4 Our Cases

A 7 year-old boy presented after a previous repair of a bilateral facial cleft. The patient had an initial picture with TC5 on the right side with an associated TC3/TC4, previously operated on in another service. Primary correction with small flaps had been once performed. There was a vertical orbital dystopia, lower position of the left eyeball and right lateral canthal ligament, coloboma in the inferior eyelid, and macrostomia on the right side. Surgery was done using a glabellar flap on the left side and a myocutaneous flap with a lateral pedicle from the upper eyelid to the inferior eyelid on the right side. Tomographic scan evidenced bilateral cleft, with bony depression on the right and real maxilla cleft, loose of the orbital floor, and alveolar cleft on the left side. 1 year later, a scar revision and bone grafting with the donor area in the iliac crest bone graft was performed. A tissue expander was used to resection the scars (Fig. 9.10).

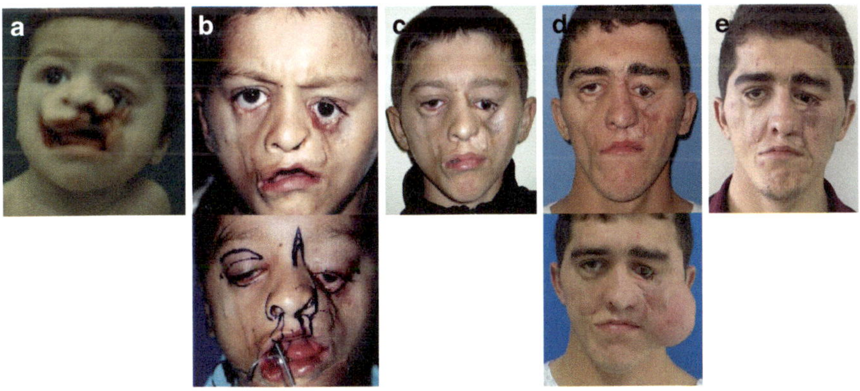

Fig. 9.10 Our cases of surgical treatment long term. (**a**) Picture send by parents, right TC5 and left TC4. (**b**) Patient first consultation proposed surgery. (**c**) After first surgery. (**d**) Tissue expander. (**e**) 20 years late

Our second case patient was born with a left TC5, presenting with a coloboma of the inferior eyelid with eyelashes extending over the cornea. The surgery was performed at 2 months of age using multiple Z-plasty. Secondary surgery was needed to reposition the lateral canthal ligament, and a myocutaneous flap was used—a follow-up of 8 and 12 years. Notice the choristoma on the cornea of the left eye (Fig. 9.11).

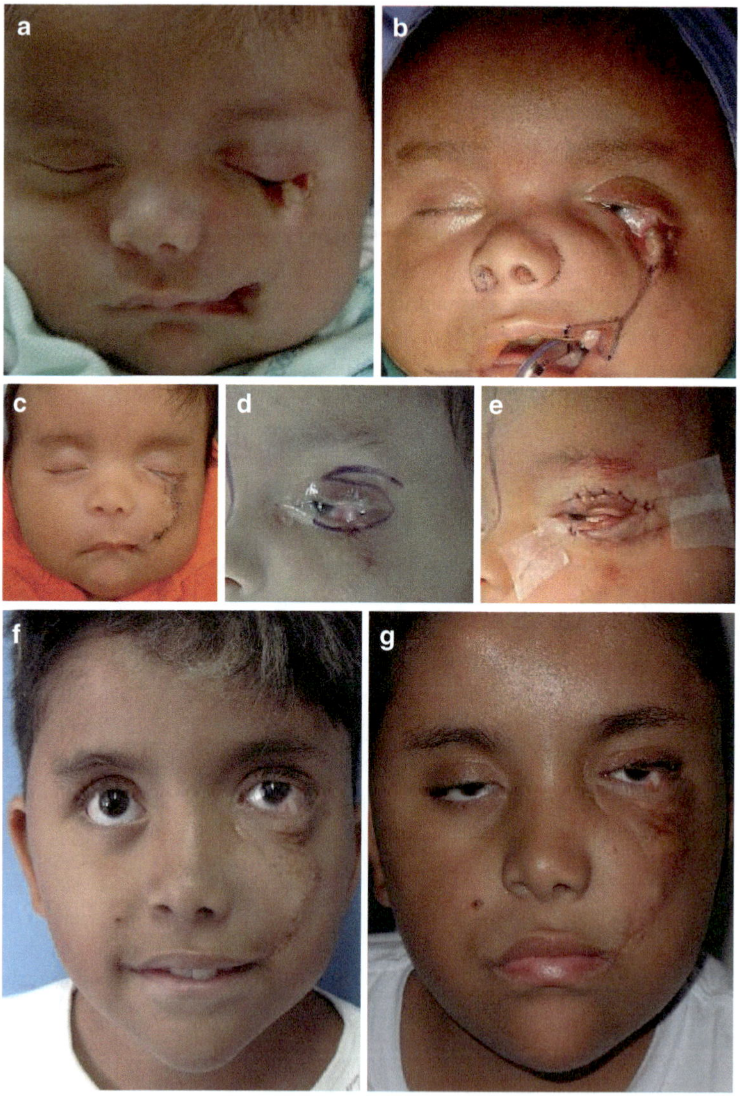

Fig. 9.11 Our cases surgical treatment long term. (**a**) Pre op TC5, (**b**) pre markings, (**c**) PO with ectropium, (**d**) secondary correction, (**e**) upper eyelid flap, (**f**) immediate PO, (**g**) late post operative view

The patient is a 1-year-old girl presenting with a TC5; the cleft begins on the right side running through the middle third of the inferior eyelid, 1 cm medial to the oral commissure, giving an appearance of macrostomia. On the left side, a more typical TC4 was identified. The first procedure was done with multiple Z-plasty over the right-side cheek and commissure utilizing the Tessier classic technique on the left—follow-up 14 late (Fig. 9.12).

In this patient with bilateral TC5, we can observe the surgical treatment done with straight-line correction and muscular reattachment with bilateral lip repair (Fig. 9.13).

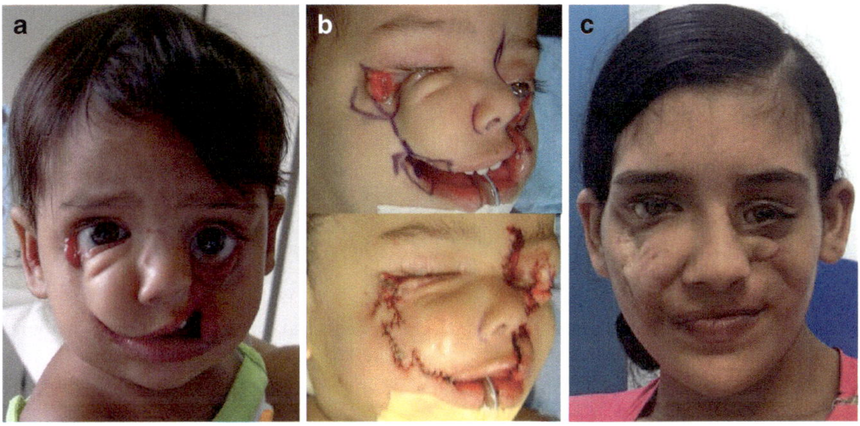

Fig. 9.12 Our surgical treatment for long-term severe cases with TC5 right side and TC4 left side. (**a**) Right TC5 left TC4, (**b**) correction right TC5, (**c**) 14 years late post operative

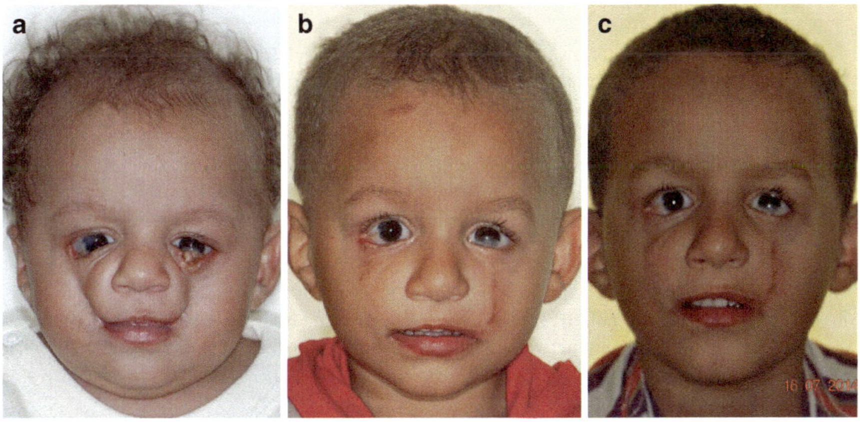

Fig. 9.13 Long-term follow-up straight-line correction. (**a**) Bilateral TC5, (**b**) 1 year late, (**c**) 6 years late

References

1. da Silva Freitas R, Alonso N, Busato L, Ueda WK, Hota T, Medeiros SH, et al. Oral-nasal-ocular cleft: the greatest challenge among the rare clefts. J Craniofac Surg. 2010;21(2):390–5. https://journals.lww.com/00001665-201003000-00024.
2. da Silva Freitas R, Alonso N, Shin JH, Busato L, Dall'Oglio Tolazzi A, e Cruz GA. The Tessier number 5 facial cleft: surgical strategies and outcomes in six patients. Cleft Palate Craniofac J. 2009;46(2):179–86. https://doi.org/10.1597/07-192.1.
3. Olasoji HO, Tahir C, Isa A. An unusual bilateral oblique facial cleft in a newborn. Int J Pediatr Otorhinolaryngol. 2005;69(7):999–1001. https://linkinghub.elsevier.com/retrieve/pii/S0165587605000686.
4. Kawamoto HK. The kaleidoscopic world of rare craniofacial clefts: order out of chaos (Tessier classification). Clin Plast Surg. 1976;3(4):529–72.
5. Alonso N, da Silva Freitas R. Craniofacial clefts and others related deformities. In: Plastic Surgery Indications and Practice. p. 455–71.
6. Alonso N, Tonello C. Rare facial clefts. In: Hamdan U, Rogers-Vizena C, Vyas R, Sommerlad B, Low D, editors. Interdisciplinary cleft care global perspectives. San Diego CA: Plural Publishing; 2023. p. 689–701. http://www.pluralpublishing.com.
7. Morian R. Über die schräge Gesichtsspalte (about oblique facial clefts). Arch Klin Chir. 1887;35:245–88.
8. van der Meulen JC, Mazzola R, Vermey-Keers C, Strieker M, Raphael B. A morphogenetic classification of craniofacial malformations. Plast Reconstr Surg. 1983;71(4):560–72. http://journals.lww.com/00006534-198304000-00022.
9. Tessier P. Anatomical classification of facial, cranio-facial and latero-facial clefts. J Maxillofac Surg. 1976;4:69–92. https://linkinghub.elsevier.com/retrieve/pii/S0301050376800136.
10. Johnston MC, Sulik KK. Some abnormal patterns of development in the craniofacial region. Birth Defects Orig Artic Ser. 1979;15(8):23–42.
11. Warkany J, Takacs E. Experimental production of congenital malformations in rats by salicylate poisoning. Am J Pathol. 1959;35(2):315–31.
12. Cannistrà C, Bontemps C, Valero R, Iannetti G, Barbet JP. Orbitofacial cleft number 5: radiographic, anatomical, and histologic study of a 24-week-old fetus. Plast Reconstr Surg. 2006;118(7):1538–42. http://journals.lww.com/00006534-200612000-00006.
13. Tessier P, Hervouet F, Lekieffre M. Plastic surgery of the orbit and eyelids. New York: Masson Publishing; 1981. p. 394.
14. Miyajima K, Natsume N, Kawai T, Iizuka T. Oblique facial cleft, cleft palate, and supernumerary teeth secondary to amniotic bands. Cleft Palate Craniofac J. 1994;31(6):483–6. https://doi.org/10.1597/1545-1569_1994_031_0483_ofccpa_2.3.co_2.
15. Pereira FJ, Milbratz GH, Cruz AAV, Vasconcelos JJA. Ophthalmic Considerations in the Management of Tessier Cleft 5/9. Ophthal Plast Reconstr Surg. 2010;26(6):450–3. https://journals.lww.com/00002341-201011000-00016.
16. Resnick JI, Kawamoto HK. Rare craniofacial clefts: tessier no. 4 clefts. Plast Reconstr Surg. 1990;85(6):843–9. http://journals.lww.com/00006534-199006000-00001.
17. Menard RM, Moore MH, David DJ. Tissue expansion in the reconstruction of Tessier craniofacial clefts: a series of 17 patients. Plast Reconstr Surg. 1999;103(3):779–86.
18. Tonello C, Paula RG, Paula IP, Nunes RB, Kokitsu-Nakata NM, Alonso N. Eyeball preservation with purse-string conjunctival closure for melting corneal ulcer in rare facial cleft. Cleft Palate Craniofac J. 2021;58(9):1195–200. https://doi.org/10.1177/1055665620980632.

Chapter 10
Cleft 6

Philippe Pellerin, Nivaldo Alonso, Renato da Silva Freitas, and Cristiano Tonello

10.1 Introduction

Pearls

- Cleft 6 is not part of Treacher Collins syndrome which is a separate entity.
- There are three separate phenotypes: (**a**) anterior toward the canthus, (**b**) intermediate toward the zygomatic arch, (**c**) posterior toward the external ear.
- High-resolution CT scan with 3D reconstruction is indispensable for the diagnosis.

Tessier's original description (Fig. 10.1).

In his original description [1] Tessier's opinion is:" *No. 6 belongs specifically to the so-called Treacher Collins – Franceschetti complex. It is very much like cleft no. 5. It is a maxillary-zygomatic (M.Z.) cleft with coloboma of the lower*

P. Pellerin (✉)
Plastic Surgery Department, University of Lille, Lambersart, France

N. Alonso
Department of Plastic Surgery, Universidade de São Paulo, São Paulo, Brazil
e-mail: nivalonso@usp.br

R. da Silva Freitas
Plastic Surgery Unit, Hospital de Clínicas, Universidade Federal do Paraná, Curitiba, Brazil

Craniofacial Surgery, Assistance Center for Cleft Lip and Palate (CAIF), Hospital do Trabalhador, Curitiba, Brazil

C. Tonello
Craniofacial Surgery Department, Universidade de São Paulo, Bauru, São Paulo, Brazil
e-mail: cristianotonello@usp.br

N. Alonso et al. (eds.), *Facial Reconstruction of Unusual Facial Clefts*,
https://doi.org/10.1007/978-3-031-40926-4_10

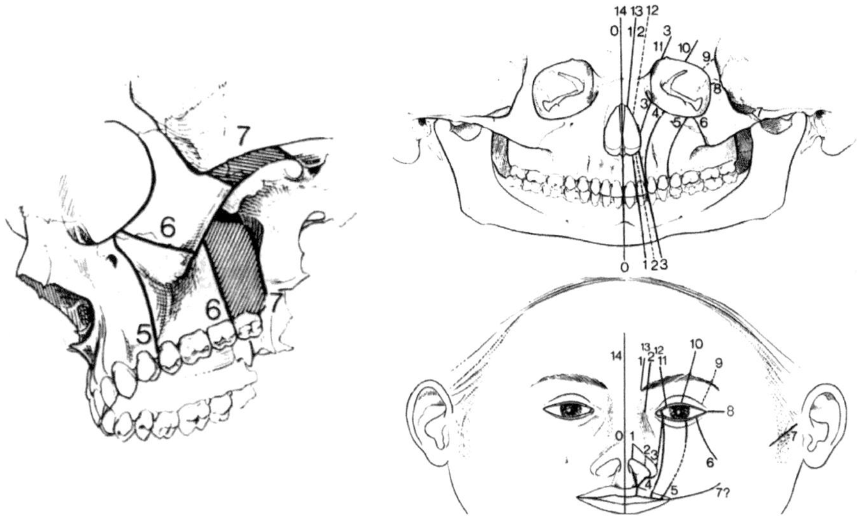

Fig. 10.1 Original Tessier's drawings for rare clefts (with permission from Me Tessier and Masson edit)

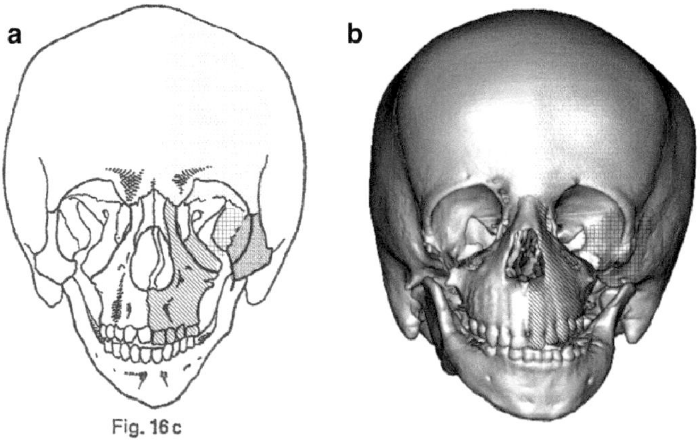

Fig. 10.2 Artist drawing of TCS in Tessier (**a**) compared to actual 3D CT scan of a TCS. (**b**) Oblique stripes pattern to the maxillary, Dotted pattern to the malar bone, Square pattern to the sphenoid bone. (with permission from Me Tessier and Masson edit)

eyelid". Nowadays, we know that Treacher Collins, as well as other syndromic mandibulofacial dysostoses, are consequences of specific mutations [2], the result of neural crest cells migration defects and of consecutive skeletal hypoplasia and not a clefting process, but still, there are patients without mandibulofacial dysostosis mimicking their clinical features, in his original publication the 16c drawing (Fig. 10.2) reprint thank Me Tessier permission) It is quoted as a case of Treacher

Collins-Franceschetti syndrome. Out of today's knowledge in macromolecular genetics and advanced medical imaging, we know that it could not be one.

On the other hand, Tessier's description of Cleft 7:" *No. 7 belongs in-common to Treacher Collins and hemifacial microsomia. It is a temporo-zygomatic cleft, usually with the absence of the zygomatic arch and concomitant deformities of the mandibular ramus, condyle and coronoid process.*" We understand that he did the same mistake with Cleft 7 that he did with Treacher Collins about Cleft 6. Cleft 7.

If we, as for Treacher Collins, consider hemifacial microsomia as hypoplasia, only macrostomia in the context of hemifacial microsomia should be left as a Cleft 7 (see Chap. 11) So the purpose of this chapter is to do an accurate description of what could be found between Cleft 5 and Cleft 7 and describe it as Cleft 6.

Since Cleft 5 involves the maxillary and Cleft 7 the mandible, Cleft 6 has to involve the zygomatic bone or zygomatic arch…

10.2 Materials and Methods

We have searched for patients presenting with symptoms belonging neither to Cleft 5 nor Cleft 7, meaning we have excluded Treacher Collins. From the patients affected by hemifacial microsomia (we will switch from hemifacial to craniofacial microsomia, as a preferred naming), we have considered the Cleft 7 diagnoses only for those who had a macrostomia which is then considered as a defective fusion between the maxillary bud and the mandibular bud probably because of the first and second branchial arches defect (see Chap. 11).

10.2.1 Literature Cases. (Table 10.1 with References)

The research for papers describing conditions matching the requirement has been challenging. At first look, very few Cleft 6 are published under this diagnosis. The first description we found was probably the one by Muralt in "éphémérides des curieux de la nature" 1715 p. 304, the drawing was reprinted in Ahlfeld Atlas [55], Table XXVII, Fig. 6 (Fig. 10.3a). Next was by Chavane, 1890 [28] as the description of a stillborn: "*malformation faciale (section par bande amniotique)*" (Fig. 10.3b).Then after came a case by Rushton and Walker [23] coming by the title of" *Unilateral Secondary Facial Cleft with Excess Tooth and Bone Formation*" They suggested calling this condition: polygnathus or paragnathus, in which a rudimentary half lower jaw with teeth occurs at the side of the principal jaw or in the cheek. A significant paper was from Hou [17], who found 23 patients with oblique facial clefts associated with the accessory maxilla, which we consider as facial #6 cleft. Most of the patients were misdiagnosed with Cleft 7, and we do not agree with the authors who confuse macrostomia and Cleft 7 as Woods [40] or Khorasani [56]. Some cases of patients with Cleft 6] have been published as Cleft 5.Most authors

Table 10.1 Cases of clefts number 6 found in the literature

Author	Reference number	Sex	Side	Macrostomia	Cheek	Sideburn	Palate	Malar cleft	Appendage	Bone appendage	Subtype	Associated rare cleft	Other anomalies
Hou et al. (2011)	[3]	M	Bilat.	Mid	Mid		Yes	Yes	Yes	Yes	6b		
Borzabadi-Farahani et al. (2013)	[4]	M	Bilat.	Mid	Mid				Yes	Yes	6b		Assymetric
Sun et al. (2020)	[5]	F	Bilat.	Minor	Minor			Yes	No	Yes	6b		Assymetric
Bilkay et al. (2000)	[6]	np	Left	Mid	Mid		Yes	Yes	Yes	No	6b	Cleft 5 right	Micro-anophtalmia left
Gleizal et al. (2007)	[7]	np	Bilat.	Severe	Severe	Yes	Yes				6a		
Chauhan and Guruprasad (2015)	[8]	M	Bilat.	Severe	Severe	Yes	Yes	Yes	Yes	Yes	6b		
Cheung et al. (1993)	[9]	M	Bilat.	Severe	Severe	Yes	Yes	Yes	No	Yes	6b		
Crespo Guerra et al. (2010)	[10]	F	Bilat.	Total	Total	Yes	Yes	Yes	No	No	6c		Mandibular hypoplasia but ascending ramus normal in shape
Özçelik et al. (2014)	[11]	F	Right	Total	Total	Yes	Yes	Hor.		Yes	6c		Condyle and coronoïd deformed and hypoplasic
Anantanarayanan et al. (2007)	[12]	M	Right	Mid	Mid	Yes		Yes	No	Yes	6b		

Buonocore et al. (2014)	[13]	M	Right	Total	Total			Hor.	No	Yes	6c		Condyle and coronoïd deformed and hypoplasic
		M	Left	Mid	Mid			Yes		Yes	6b		
		M	Bilat.	Minor	Minor			Not.		No	6a		
Uchikawa et al. (2011)	[14]	F	Right	Minor	Minor		Yes	Yes	No	Yes	6b	Cleft 5 left	Colobomatous cyst, microphtalmia
Sun et al. (2013)	[15]	F	Left	Mid	Mid	No		Yes	No	Yes	6b		Osseous appendage attached to the mandible, a transition b to c?
Kuriyama et al. (2008)	[16]	M	Bilat.	Severe	Severe	Yes	Yes	Yes	No	Yes	6b		
Hou et al. (2015)	[17]	F	Bilat.	Minor	Minor		No	Yes		Yes	6b		
Tharanon et al. (1998)	[18]	M	Bilat.	Minor	Minor		Yes	Yes	No	Yes	6b		
Jian and Chen (1995)	[19]	F	Right	Mid	Mid		No	Yes		Yes	6b		
DeGurse et al. (1995)	[20]	M	Left	Minor	Dimple			Yes		Yes	6b		
Stoneman (1978)	[21]	F	Left	Minor	Dimple		No	Yes	No	Yes	6b		
Miyajima et al. (1994)	[22]	M	Left	Mid	Mid		Yes	Yes		Yes	6b	Cleft 3 right	
Rushton and Walker (1936)	[23]	M	Right	Severe	Severe	Yes	Yes	Yes		Yes	6b		
Rintala et al. (1980)	[24]	M	Bilat.	Severe	Severe		Yes	Yes		Yes	6b	Cleft 2 right	
Ranta and Rintala (1988)	[25]	M	Right	Minor	Minor		Yes	Yes		Yes	6b	Cleft 5 left	
Sjamsudin et al. (2001)	[26]	F	Right	Severe	Severe		Yes	Yes		Yes	6b	Cleft 8 right	Microglossia
Saadi et al. (2011)	[27]	Np	Left	Severe	Severe		Yes				6b	Cleft 4 right	Mutation cytoskelatal protein SPCC1L

(continued)

Table 10.1 (continued)

Author	Reference number	Sex	Side	Macrostomia	Cheek	Sideburn	Palate	Malar cleft	Appendage	Bone appendage	Subtype	Associated rare cleft	Other anomalies
Chavane (1890)	[28]	Np	Right	Severe	Severe		Yes	Yes			6a	Cleft 5 left	Encephalocele, ABS
Mayou and Fenton (1981)	[29]	Np	Left	Total	Total		Yes	Yes			6b	Cleft 5 right	ABS
Morovic et al. (2004)	[30]	F	Bilat.	Severe	Severe		Yes				6b	Cleft 8 right	ABS
Obdeijn et al. (2010)	[31]	F	Bilat.	Severe	Severe					Yes	6b		ABS
Ramanathan et al. (2012)	[32]	M	Left	Severe	Severe		No	Yes	No	Yes	6b		
Walker (1961)	[33]	M	Left	Severe	Severe						6a	Cleft 8 left, 4 right	
		Np	Right	Severe	Severe						6a	Cleft 8 right, 4 left	
Balaji (2017)	[34]	M	Left	Severe	Severe	Yes	Yes	Yes			6c	Cleft 3 left,7 left	Hemifacial microsomia
Kanth et al. (2021)	[35]	F	Right	Mid	Mid		Yes	Yes	No	No	6a		
Fijałkowska and Antoszewski (2015)	[36]	M	Left								6	Cleft 4 right	
		F	Left								6a		
		F	Right								6a		
		M	Bilat.	Severe	Severe						6b	Cleft 8 right, 2 left	
Darzi and Chowdri (1993)	[37]	F	Right	Minor	Mid		Yes		Yes		6a	Cleft 3 and 9 left	ABS; microphtalmia
Morita et al. (2008)	[38]	F	Left	Minor	Minor		Yes	No	Yes		6b	Cleft 5 right	
Tiwari and Tapadar (2015)	[39]	M	Left	Severe	Severe		Yes	No	Yes		6b	Cleft 3 and 5 left	
Woods et al. (2008)	[40]	M	Bilat.	Mid	Severe			Yes	Yes	Yes	6b		
Mello and Jones (2009)	[41]	M	Bilat.	Mid	Mid		No	Yes	Yes	Yes	6a 6b		

Reddy et al. (2021)	[42]	M	Right	Severe	Severe						6a	Cleft 8 right, 5 Left	Right microphtalmia
		M	Left	Severe	Severe						6c		
		M	Left	Mid	Mid						6a		
Racz et al. (2017)	[43]	M	Left	Minor	Minor					Yes	6b	Cleft 4 right	
		M	Right	Mid	Mid			Yes			6a	Cleft 4 left	Right epibulbar epidermoid, left anophtalmia
Cameron et al. (1993)	[44]	F	Bilat.	Mid	Mid			Yes		Yes	6b	Right UCLP	
Bhattacharya et al. (1988)	[45]	F	Left	Severe	Mid			Yes	Yes	Yes	6b	Cleft 3 right	Right microphtalmia
Tripathy et al. (2013)	[46]	M	Right	Mid	Minor	No	No	Yes	Yes	Yes	6b		
Wang (2020)	[47]	F	Bilat.	Minor	Minor		No	Yes	No	Yes	6b 6c		
Xu et al. (2013)	[48]	M	Bilat.	Minor	Minor		No	Yes	No	Yes	6b		
Sutton (1888)	[49]		Bilat.	Total	Total	No					6b	Cutis aplasia-cleft9	ABS
Debout (1862)	[50]	M	Bilat.	Total	Severe		Yes				6b		
		M	Left	Total	Severe						6b		
Pelvet (1864)	[51]		Left	Severe	Severe	Yes					6b	Cleft 3 right	
Millard (1996)	[52]	M	Left	Total	Total						6c		
Pitanguy (1967)	[53]	M	Bilat.	Total	Total	No					6a	Cleft 8 bilat	
Converse (1974)	[54]									Yes	6c		
										Yes	6c		
											6c		
											6c		

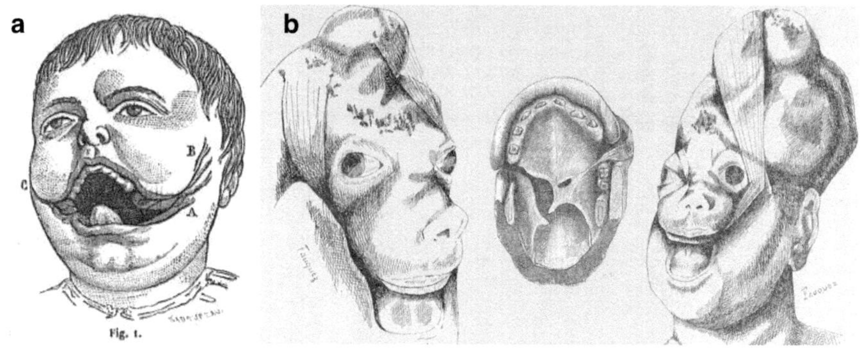

Fig. 10.3 Historic cases reported by Muralt 1715, (**a**) and Chavane 1890 in an ABS-affected stillborn (**b**)

have carefully used the generic adjective: latero-facial or oblique facial cleft to qualify their unusual observations.

In a large number of papers relating to what we now know as being Cleft 6, the authors emphasized the supernumerary osteo-dental material and as Hou did, named the condition: "maxillary duplication". As a whole, only five of the publications referred to their case as cleft number 6 [3, 6, 34, 36, 39].

This bibliographic research came with 52 publications. Most of them reported a single case except for Converse's [54] and Fijakolska's four cases [36], Buonocore's [13] and Gosla [42] series of three and two cases for Walker [33], Racz [43] and Debout [50]. The total of reported cases is 65 patients with Cleft 6, summarized in Table 10.1.

10.2.2 Clinical Series: (Table 10.2)

The book authors have merged their series of rare clefts and, after a cross-review, found a total of 36 patients. We here thank PR Anastasov from Plovdiv, Bulgaria; PR Brusati from Milan, Italy; PR Shi Bing from Chengdu; and Dr. Tang Xiao Jun from Beijing from PR of China for lending their cases to P. Pellerin.

In the first center, out of a series of 156 patients with rare clefts (we exclude 33 cases of syndromic mandibulofacial dysostosis and 187 craniofacial microsomia except for 16 patients affected by a true macrostomia which have been included as Cleft 7), we found 11 cases of number six cleft.

In the second center, out of 370 patients with rare clefts (Treacher Collins and craniofacial microsomia patients being excluded as well), we found 25 patients affected by Cleft 6, which makes a total series of 36 clinical cases.

Overall, 101 observations of Cleft 6 were considered for this description. Among Cleft 6 patients, 34 had a bilateral Cleft 6, which makes 135 clefts.

Table 10.2 Author's case series of clefts number 6

#	Sex	Side	Macrostomia	Cheek	Sideburn	Palate	Malar cleft	Cutaneous appendage	Super. Append	Subtype	Associated cleft	other anomalies
1	F	Bilat.	Mild	Mild	Yes	No	Yes	Yes	Yes	6b		
2	F	Bilat.	Severe	Severe	Yes	Yes	Yes	No	No	6a	Cleft 8 bilateral	
3	F	Right	Mild	Minor	Yes	Yes	Yes	No	No	6a	Cleft 4 left	
4	F	Bilat.	Mild	Mild	Yes	No	Yes	No	No	6a	Cleft 8 bilateral	
5	F	Right	Mild	Mild		Yes	Yes	No	No	6a	Cleft 5 and 8 right; 4 left	Right microphtalmia, left severe ocular malformation
6	F	Left	Minor	Minor	No	No	Yes	No	Yes	6ab	Left cleft 8	Combine both the caracteristics of a and b
7	F	Left	Mild	Minor		No	Yes	No	Yes	6b	Right cleft 5	
8	M	Bilat.	Severe	Severe	No	Yes			Yes	6b		
9	M	Bilat.	Severe	Severe		Yes	Yes	Yes	Yes	6b		Bilateral assymetric, left>right
10	F	Bilat.	Severe	Severe		Yes	Yes	No	Yes	6b		
11	M	Bilat.	Severe	Severe		Yes		No		6a	8 bilat	
12	F	Unilat.	Severe	Severe						6a	8 bilat.; 5 and 2 right; 4left	ABS
13	F	Left	Severe	Severe						6c		Coronoïd process,condyle, pterygoïd process hypoplasic
14	M	Right	Severe	Severe		Yes	Yes	No		6c	7 right	Aplasia right ascending ramus
15	F	Right	Severe	Severe		Yes				6a	8 and 5right; 4left	Left anophtalmia
16	F	Left	Severe	Severe	Yes					6a	10 bilat; 4 and 2 right	Right anophtalmia
17	F	Right	Severe	Severe	Yes	Yes				6a	2 bilat.; 8 Right; 4 left	

(continued)

Table 10.2 (continued)

#	Sex	Side	Macrostomia	Cheek	Sideburn	Palate	Malar cleft	Cutaneous appendage	Super. Append	Subtype	Associated cleft	other anomalies
18	M	Left	Minor	Minor		Yes				6a		The cleft is mainly pterygo-palatal
19	F	Right	Severe	Severe			Yes	Yes		6c	7 right	Left hemifacial microsomia
20	F	Right	Mild	Mild		Yes				6c		Interesting since it is a partial cleft in all of its aspects
21	F	Right	Severe	Mild			Yes	Yes	Yes	6b		
22	F	Left	Severe	Mild		Yes	Yes	No	Yes	6b	Cleft 4 right	
23	M	Right	Mild	Mild			Yes		Yes	6c		Facial palsy, coronoid and pterygoid process hypoplastic
24	M	Right	Severe	Severe		Yes	Yes	No	Yes	6c	Cleft 2 right	Coronoid and pterygoid process hypoplastic
25	M	Left	Minor	Mild					Yes	6b	Cleft 4 right	
26	F	Left	Minor	Minor		Yes	Yes		Yes	6c		Pure osseous appengage (no tooth bud)
27	M	Left	Minor	Minor			Yes		Yes	6b	Cleft 4 right	
28	M	Right	Severe	Mild			Yes		Yes	6b	Cleft 4 left	

10.2.3 *Method*

A qualitative analysis of cases was done on a PowerPoint presentation. For literature cases, we managed to procure all the publication.pdf, the text was thoroughly reviewed, and any valuable data was highlighted in the text. Pictures from the.pdf were copied and pasted into a series of slides for each case.

The clinical series were analyzed similarly from their medical chart, pictures, and medical imaging. When available, the native DICOM data have been re-post processed to get more information.

The authors shared the PowerPoint files to be analyzed and discussed during web meetings.

The data are gathered in Table 10.2.

10.3 The Spectrum of Cleft 6

We found out from the analysis of those 101 patients that they could be sorted into three subtypes.

All Clefts 6 have common symptoms medially, but they differ by their distal part.

10.3.1 *Symptoms Common to all the Cleft 6: (Fig. 10.4)*

The medial (to the midline and frontal direction) part of the cleft is common to the three, and it affects both the soft tissue and the bone.

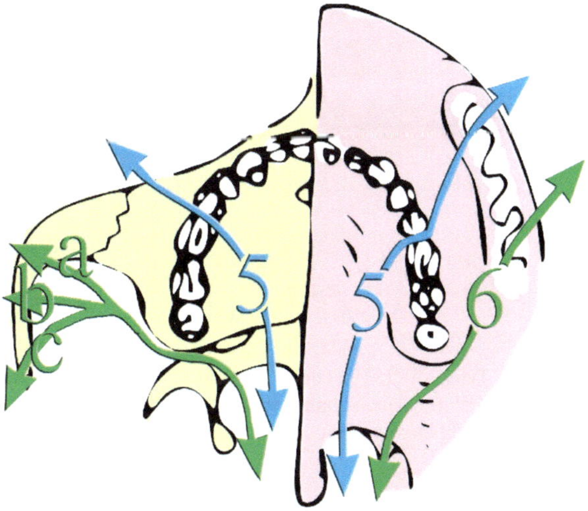

Fig. 10.4 Part of the cleft 6 common to the three subtypes compared with the trajectory of others rare clefts

10.3.1.1 Soft Tissue

Macrostomia (Fig. 10.5) is common to all the Clefts 6, it ranges from the minor form to the complete splitting of the cheek up to the pterygomaxillary sulcus. We found it as total (9/101); severe (43/101), mild (21/101) and minor (22/101); in six cases, the severity could not be assessed.

The cleft palate (Fig. 10.6) related to Cleft 6 is only a lateral cleft of the soft palate. It is not present in all cases, depending on the severity of the cleft. When present, it could be a simple furrow running from the sulcus behind maxillary tuberosity up to a bifid uvula or a complete oblique cleft leaving the lateral half-uvula close to the lateral pharyngeal wall; the tonsil is missing in some cases (mostly subtypes 6c). When there is a bilateral cleft of the soft palate, it is left attached to the hard palate in the midline, a uvula-like stump (described by Tessier as a feature of Treacher Collins) mimicking a narrow soft palate which is not always recognized for a cleft. Cleft palate was present in 42 patients; in 11 patients, no cleft palate was found, and it has not been checked in 38 cases.

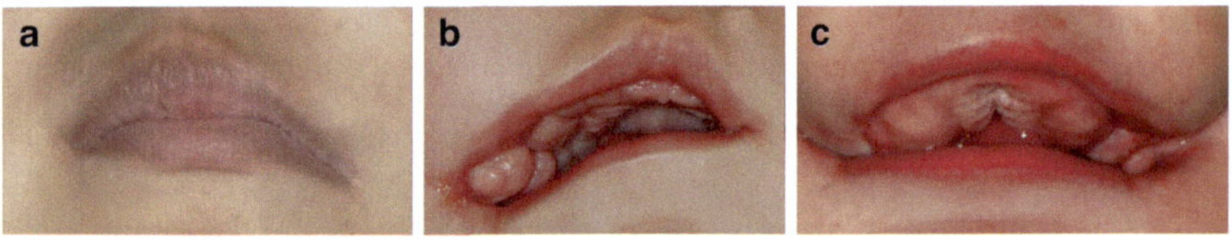

Fig. 10.5 The degree of macrostomia: (**a**) minor; (**b**) mild: (**c**) severe

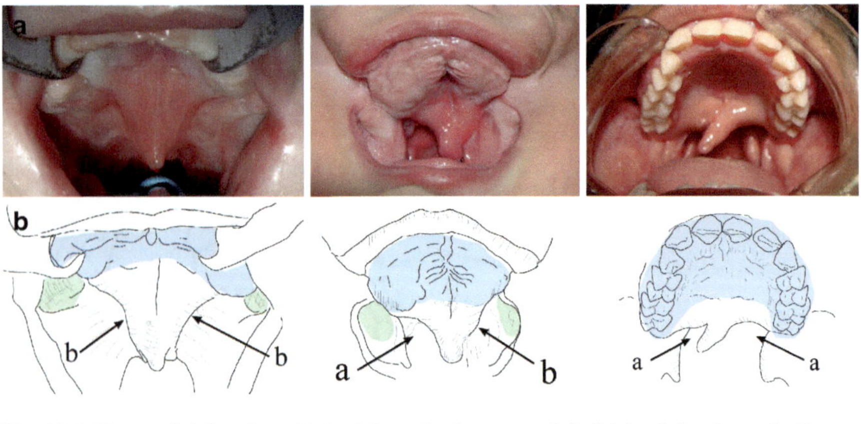

Fig. 10.6 Types of cleft palate: Right; bilateral submucous cleft (**b**) in cleft subtype b. Center; assymetrical cleft palate, submucous (**b**) left side, total (**a**) right side. Left; bilateral total cleft palate (**a**).Colored blue: maxilla; colored green: osteo-dental appendage

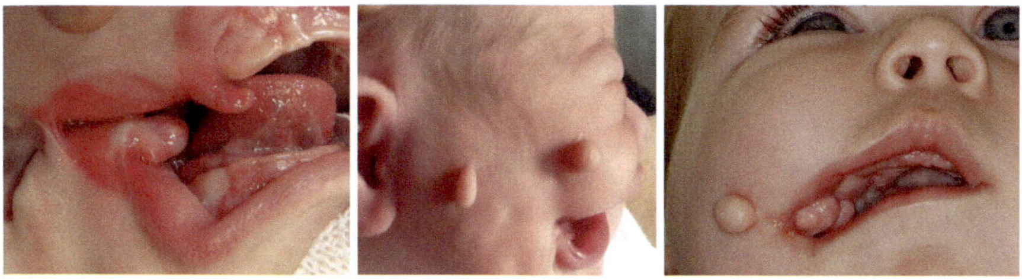

Fig. 10.7 Several types of soft tissue appendages that could be found in cleft 6

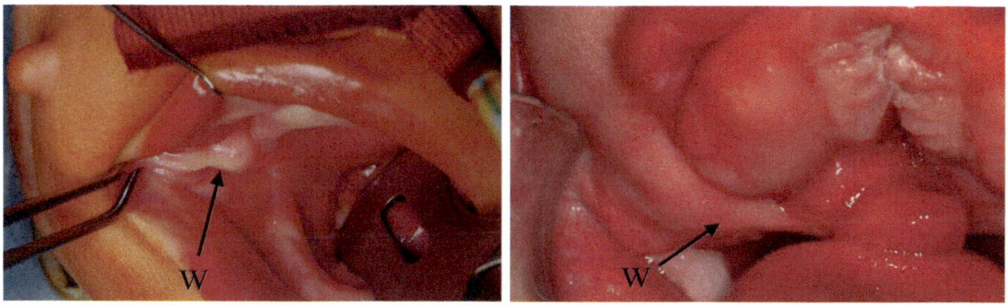

Fig. 10.8 Webs attaching the oral commissure to the retro-maxillary sulcus: ***w*** arrow

Soft Tissue Appendages: (Fig. 10.7)

Some cases display appendages close to the edges of the macrostomia, either cutaneous external or mucous in the oral cavity. We found such appendages in 18 cases. There was no appendage ten times, and the information was unavailable in 52 patients.

Webbing: (Fig. 10.8)

There is frequently a web covered with epithelium between the distal end of the macrostomia and the retro-maxillary sulcus attached to the soft palate when it is cleft.

10.3.1.2 Skeleton: (Fig. 10.9)

The skeletal part of Cleft 6 is as in Tessier's original description (Fig. 6.1). It is a cleft between the maxillary tuberosity and the pterygoid process. This cleft often presents itself as a gap between the tuberosity and the pterygoid process, but it is frequently accompanied by hypoplasia of the pterygoid process. When in subtype b, there is an osteo-dental appendage externalized to the oral cavity, one has to be careful not to confuse the condition with an alveolar cleft through the molar area, which, if true, would be a Cleft 5. Here again, the CT scan is very useful. In subtype c, the pterygoid process is constantly hypoplastic, and even if the mandibular

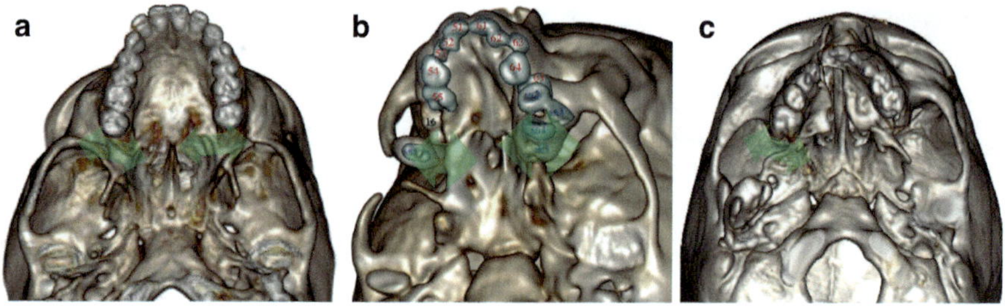

Fig. 10.9 Pterygomaxillary skeletal cleft in the subgroup of Cleft 6: green arrow, notice that in subtype b the cleft should not be confused with the space between the ectopic bone and teeth appendage in b the normal teeth (colored in blue) are numbered to demonstrate the difference with the supernumerary teeth

condyle keeps a standard shape, the coronoid process is missing, all the most if there is ectopic bone and teeth in the infratemporal fossa (cf. infra).

10.3.2 Symptoms are Specific to Subtypes. (Figs. 10.10 and 10.11)

If all the clefts number 6 have the same mesial part, we found that they diverge in three possible subtypes that we elected to name from mesial to distal: a, b, and c.

10.3.2.1 Subtype 6a

Subtype 6a is the most mesial. There were 25 cases of this subtype in the series. The macrostomia prolongates itself with a more or less deep furrow running across the cheekbone, bulging toward the lateral canthus. From most of the surgical dissection, we found that it interrupts the superficial muscle layer. It could join a cleft number eight, the complementary number to six in Tessier's cleft rule (see Chap. 12). The sideburn peek was evident only in one published patient [9]; it is not a usual part of this subtype.

The skeletal cleft (Fig. 10.11) is a more or less deep notch usually located at the root of the zygomatic process of malar bone.

10.3.2.2 Subtype 6b

Subtype 6b is intermediate. It is the most frequent, with 52 cases. The furrow, which prolongates the macrostomia, is oriented more posteriorly to the zygomatic arch bulging. The sideburn peak is less unusual and was reported five times (in other patients, authors did not pay attention to this symptom, and the condition could not be checked out of the displayed documents).

The skeletal condition (Fig. 10.12) is highly evocative since it not only includes an osseous defect to the zygomatic process of malar bone but in almost all of the cases (40 at the less, and the data were missing in historical cases), an appendage of

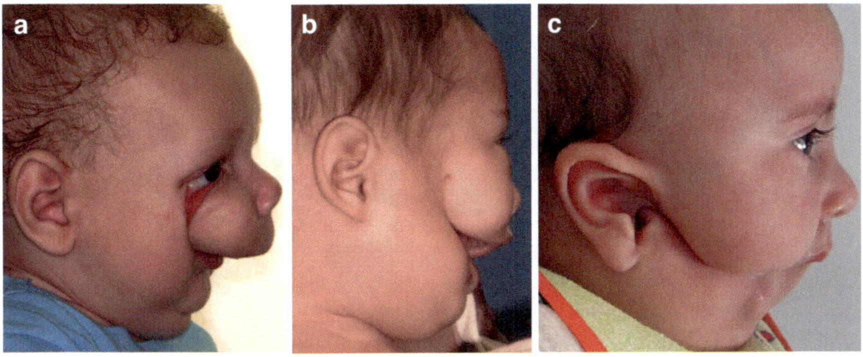

Fig. 10.10 The three paths of Cleft 6 though the cheek: (**a**) Toward the lateral canthus. (**b**) Toward the zygomatic arch (notice the sideburn peak). (**c**) Toward the external ear

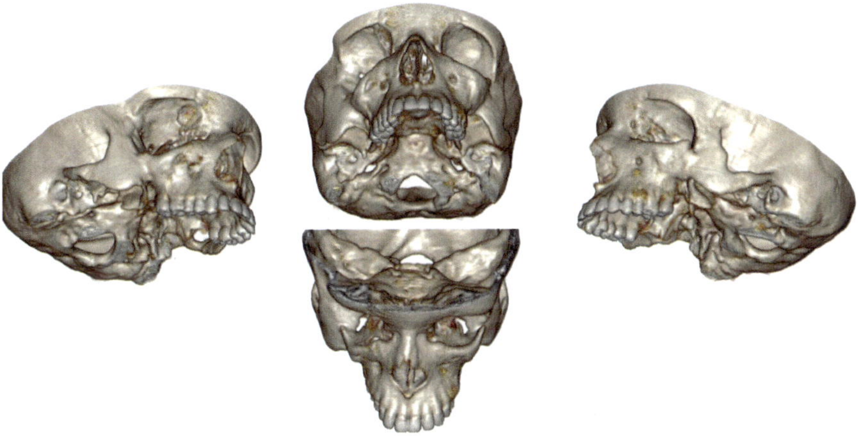

Fig. 10.11 Craniofacial skeleton in cleft 6a associated with cleft 8: notice the defect of the lateral orbital rim dues to cleft 8

bone including supernumerary teeth buds is found attached to the edges of the cleft. This appendage goes downward and exteriorizes itself in the oral cavity. It could be found behind and laterally to the maxillary tuberosity, which is usually displaced but contains a normal number of teeth or buds.

This specificity has been considered by many authors as a maxillary duplication and led them to publish the cases under this appellation. But in fact, the condition is so specific that it could be considered as a pathognomonic sign of Cleft 6b.

10.3.2.3 Subtype 6c

The subtype 6c is the rarest, with 20 observations. It is the most distal type and is frequently confused with Cleft 7. The macrostomia is usually severe and is prolonged by a furrow almost horizontal heading toward the external ear ending

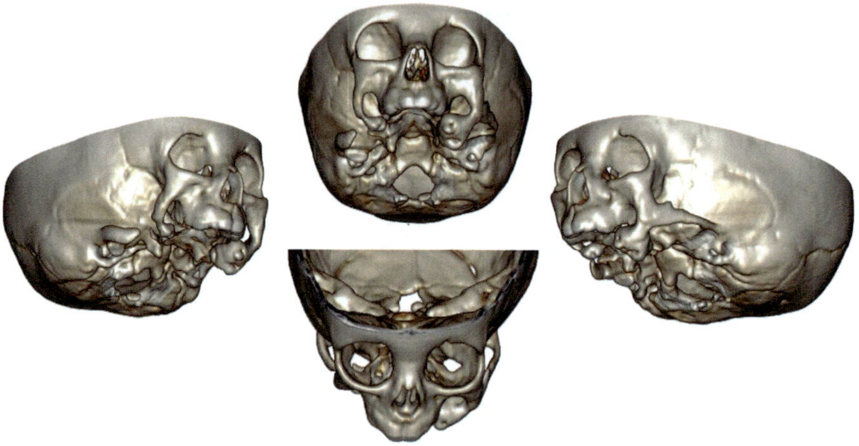

Fig. 10.12 Craniofacial skeleton in bilateral Cleft 6b, club shape appendages on both sides, though asymmetric

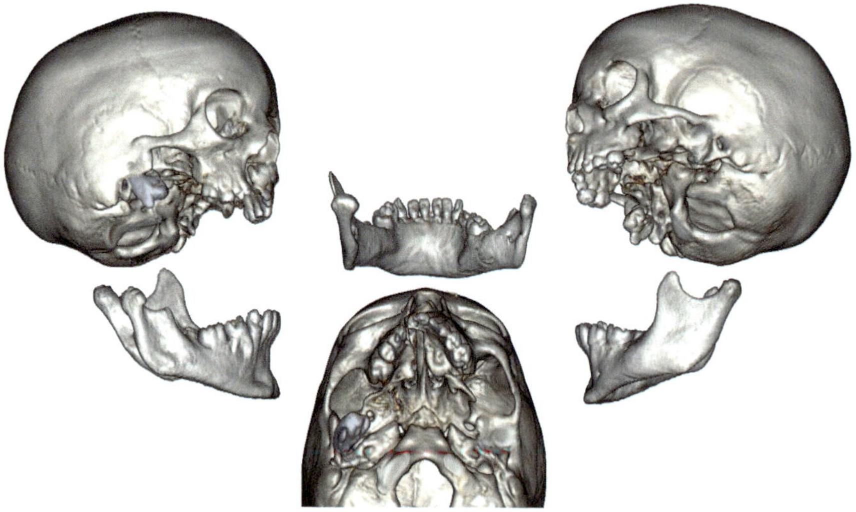

Fig. 10.13 Craniofacial skeleton in Cleft 6c. The root of the zygomatic process of temporal bone is split. Supplementary bone and teeth appendage is accentuated in blue color. The coronoid process is hypoplastic, but the condylar process is about normal

between the anterior helix root and the tragus above the auditory meatus, defect of the parotid gland and facial nerve has been observed.

The hairline is directly involved by the cleft which left no room for a sideburn peak.

The skeletal cleft (Fig. 10.13) splits the transversal root of the temporal, zygomatic process above the osseous auditory conduct, which is usually displaced downward. We found some time, as for Cleft 6b subtype, an osseous appendage with supernumerary tooth buds.

The ascending ramus could be impaired but not as in craniofacial microsomia: (Fig. 10.14) the condyle and temporomandibular joint are less concerned than the coronoid process. The pterygoid process is usually hypotrophic, sometimes completely absent.

In this subtype, we found a most hypoplastic soft palate where it has been difficult to find some muscles belonging to the veli palatini muscles.

Figures 10.14 and 10.15 summarize the path of those different subtypes.

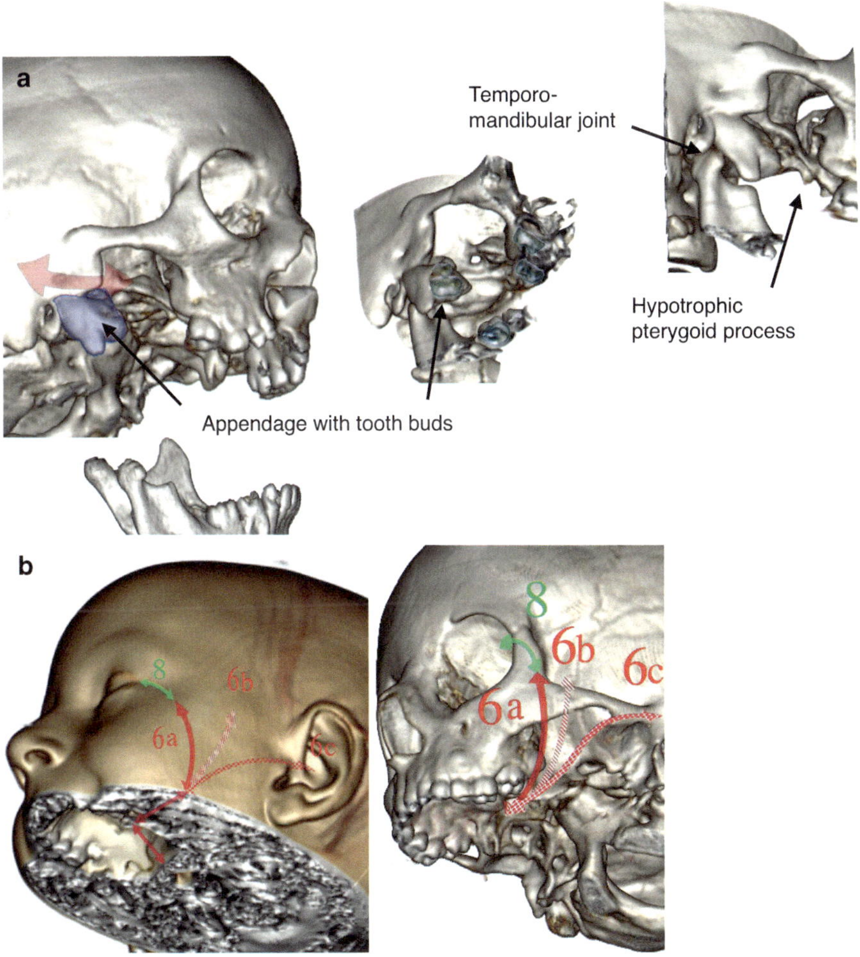

Fig. 10.14 (**a**) Details of the temporo-zygomatic area in Cleft 6c (**b**) Schematic drawing of cleft 6

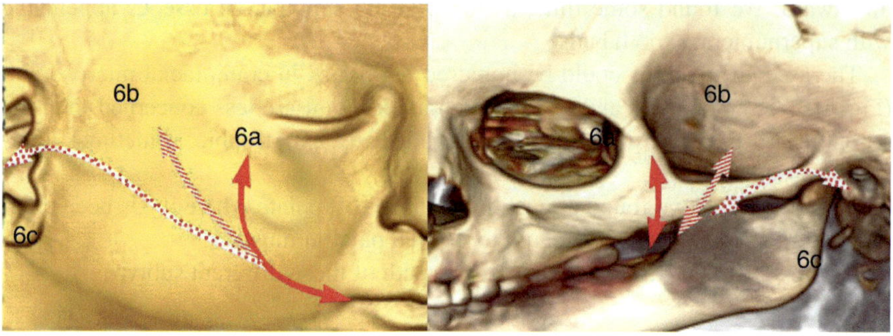

Fig. 10.15 Schematic drawing of cleft 6

10.4 Associated Malformations

10.4.1 Cleft 8

According to Tessier's rule, the clefts are arranged as diameters whose centers are at the orbit, and the sum of upper and lower clefts is 14. In this way, Cleft 8 is complemental to Cleft 6. This is true for subtype a. We found this association to Cleft 6 in 19 of the 25 subtypes a and none in other subtypes. The spectrum of Cleft 8 associated with Clefts 6 was, for the less severe, a lateral epibulbar dermoid and, for the most severe, a complete cleavage at the lateral palpebral commissure between the two eyelids. It is then in continuity with the macrostomia. Millard, in "cleft craft" [57], reported a case from Pitanguy [53] and called it oculo-lateral cleft.

10.4.2 Other Rare Clefts

Multiple facial clefts are a frequent occurrence since we found it 51 times out of the 101: the most frequent association is with Cleft 4 (43), then after with Cleft 5 (3); Cleft 2 are associated six times; Cleft 3 six times; Cleft 7 two times; Clefts 9 and 10 one time.

10.4.3 Mandibular Malformation. (Fig. 10.16)

In many patients with subtypes a and b, the mandible could be small but not malformed. Even in patients presenting noticeable mandibular hypoplasia, the shape of the ascending ramus is conserved, contrary to the condition met in craniofacial microsomia. Except in the two cases of association with Cleft 7.

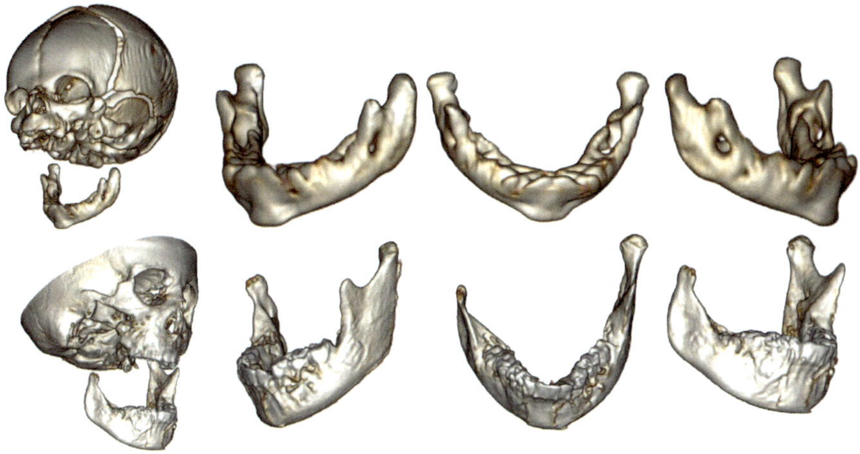

Fig. 10.16 Comparison between the mandible in cleft 6 and in CMF. Top row: bilateral cleft 6a, the mandible is small, but the general ascending ramus is conserved. Bottom row: cleft 6c, coronoid process absent but the shape of condyle conserved

In the Cleft 6 subtype c, there is a specific malformation of the coronoid process; the ascending ramus is small, but the condyle is subnormal, again contrary to the condition in craniofacial microsomia.

10.4.4 Ocular Malformations

Ocular malformations are pretty frequent. We found nine patients with micro-anophthalmia. Epibulbar dermoid is frequently associated with Cleft 8. (see Chap. 12).

10.4.5 Amniotic Band Sequence

The amniotic band sequence (ABS) was reported seven times in the whole series and will be discussed below.

10.5 Differential Diagnosis

As seen from the review of the literature, Cleft 6 is, most of the time, the object of misdiagnosis. In order to avoid it, we thought it useful to lay stress on the differences with close conditions.

10.5.1 Mandibulo Facial Dysostosis

In 1976 Tessier's opinion was that Cleft 6 belonged to Treacher Collins syndrome [1], but we have learned from that time that Treacher Collins, as well as another mandibulofacial dysostosis [58–60] syndromes, were specific entities related to known mutations (TCO1 mutation for Treacher Collins [2]). We think it better to remove those syndromes from the list of rare clefts and put them as differential diagnoses. The skeletal anomalies are global hypoplasia of mandible, maxillary, and malar bone; the aspect of the cleft is due to the inability of hypoplastic processes of malar bone to reach the orbital process of the frontal bone, and the zygomatic process of the temporal bone itself, hypoplastic. The whole of the mandible is hypoplastic when normal in subtype 6a and 6b and only locally concerned in subtype 6c. In the meantime, the external ear is either normal or partially split in subtype 6c. Tessier published an artist's drawing (Fig. 10.2a) as TCS, a misinterpretation of old medical imaging and intra-operative findings. We can see in a modern high-resolution 3D CT scan (Fig. 10.2b) that what has been interpreted as a cleft between the maxillary and the malar bone was the failure to reach the frontal, the sphenoid, and temporal orbital processes of a very hypoplastic malar bone attached to the maxillary itself hypoplastic.

10.5.2 Rare Clefts

10.5.2.1 Cleft 7 (Fig. 10.17)

Cleft 7 is a macrostomia supposedly due to a fusion defect between maxillary and mandibular buds from the pharyngeal arch One (PA1).

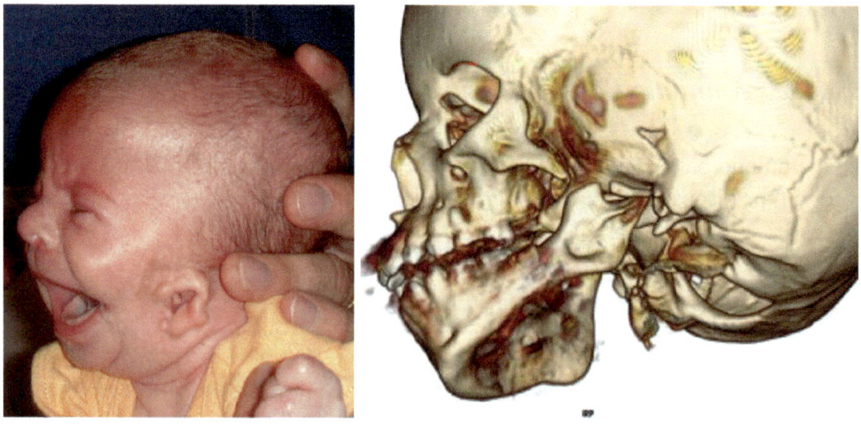

Fig. 10.17 Cleft 7 in the setting of craniofacial microsomia

In Tessier's opinion, Cleft 7 belongs to hemifacial microsomia [1], but since it features macrosomia as all of Clefts 6, the most common mistake has been to diagnose them as Cleft 7 nine times: [3–5, 8, 10, 14, 16, 40, 61].

We prefer to state that Cleft 7 is a macrostomia occurring in the setting of first and second branchial syndrome or craniofacial microsomia, as quoted by Tessier [62] and Poswillo [63]. We have to notice that in Cleft 7, everything is due to hypoplasia: the craniofacial microsomia as well as the mechanism of macrostomia. When for Cleft 6, at least 6b and 6c, there are supernumerary organs.

As a consequence, we would say that the diagnosis mostly lies in the presence of any sign of the oculo-auriculo-vertebral spectrum that we prefer to name craniofacial microsomia (CFM) associated with the macrostomia: not so much as for "oculo-" since choristoma and other ocular malformations could be associated to Cleft 6 as well as to Cleft 7. Any degree of auricular malformation with the exception of the auricular cleft of Cleft 6c. Preauricular tags and any degree of CFM. Medical imaging is here again of the utmost importance.

10.5.2.2 Cleft 5

Cleft 5 (Fig. 10.18) has too to be differenced from Cleft 6. Historically, Van Huysse named "macrostome" a case initially published by Remedy and reported in Ahlfeld Atlas [55] (Tal. XXV, Fig. 5). This case is, in fact, a Cleft 5. Racz [43], as others and even ourselves, before sorting our cases during this book redaction, made the same error. The external aspect is quite similar to Cleft 6a. Two points nevertheless could help: the eyelid coloboma is on the inferior lid and lets a part of the inferior palpebra

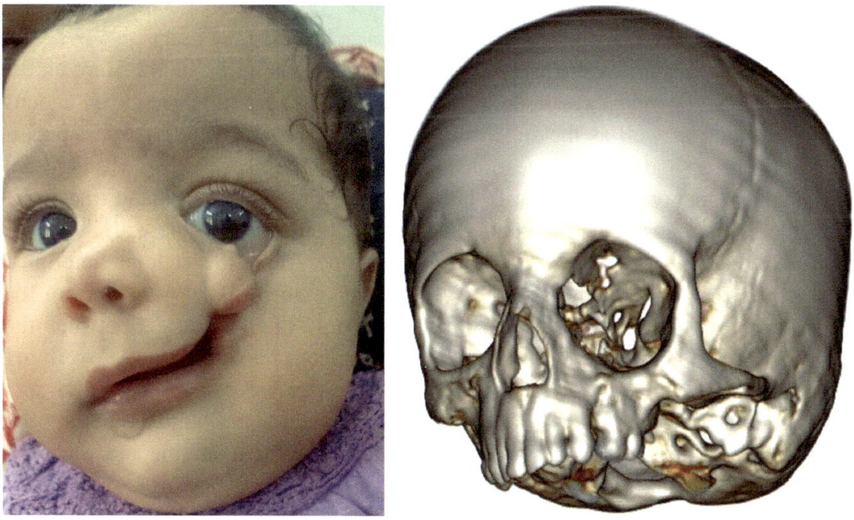

Fig. 10.18 Cleft 5: the cleft path runs across the molar alveolar area, involve the hard palate, the inferior orbital rim is split outside the infra-orbital foramen

lateral to the cleft. The macrostomia could be a superior cleft lip, leaving the oral commissure intact, but it is not constant, and this leftover could be hidden in the macrostomia.

The intra-oral aspect of Cleft 5 is very different: the cleft runs through the alveolar ridge at the molar level, while Cleft 6 runs across the retro-maxillary sulcus. Someone may confuse Cleft 6a with Cleft 5 when the sulcus between the tuberosity and the exteriorized osteo-dental appendage is interpreted as a cleft through the molar alveolar area. In this case, looking at the 3D CT scan is the only way to differentiate the supernumerary material in babies before the eruption of any deciduous teeth.

10.6 Discussion

10.6.1 Macrostomia

Macrostomia is a common symptom of Clefts 5, 6, and 7.

It appears that for many clinicians such as Woods [40] or Khorasani [56] and others macrostomia would be considered Cleft 7. This conception misleads most of them. The point is discussed in the specific chapter devoted to Cleft 7, but just let us remember that all of Cleft 6 as well as most of Cleft 5, present macrostomia as their most prominent symptom.

10.6.2 Significances of Supernumerary Skeletal Material

There are concerns about the significance of appendages in the field of rare clefts. The soft tissue appendages seen on the edges of some clefts either on the cutaneous or mucous side as well as the supernumerary skeletal and dental material specifically in Clefts 6b and 6c pose questions. Rushton and Walker (1937) [23] suggested that the phenomenon of dual manifestation of the accessory maxilla and transverse facial cleft is perhaps not coincidental but rather a distinct syndrome with its pathogenesis different from either of the deformities alone. About the skeletal material, a theory proposed by Cheung [9] states that a late compensatory growth from the embryonic temporal bone could have penetrated into the deep tissue between the embryonic maxilla and mandible before the complete breakdown of the overlying ectoderm.

We found in the literature reported cases with anatomical features quite similar to Cleft 6b, but the skeletal appendage was attached to the mandible and was published as mandibular duplication [15].

As part of Klippel–Feil syndrome, two cases have been published of skeletal formation, including tooth buds, without attachment to the mandible nor to the maxilla but located in the infratemporal fossa [64, 65].

But among the different theories, one looks very interesting since it could explain most of the findings in our research. The Ds. Mutation in mice since it could at the same time explain the frequency of ABS syndrome-like conditions, the explanation of cutaneous appendage, and mainly the excess of bone and teeth material, which is considered by many as duplication. Since it is a genetics matter, we will discuss it below.

10.6.3 ABS and Cleft 6 (Fig. 10.19)

Chavane's case published of that we call Cleft 6 [28] was a still born with ABS. In this series, we found seven cases of ABS associated with Cleft 6. All of them were observations of multiple rare clefts.

John M. Opitz, who prefers the term ADAM sequence to ABS in a comprehensive review [66], definitively relates ("apodictically") the ADAM sequence as proposed by Streeter [67] to an intrinsic cause: of genetic origin and propose as first candidates: Sincytin genes, placenta growth factor 2 but quote too the hypothesis of an homologous to disorganizing mutation in mice (Ds.) See below.

10.6.4 Genetics and Cleft 6

There have been many tremendous progresses in the understanding of ontogeny genetic control. Among the forest of those new knowledges there are a few paths which deserve to be explored for the understanding of Cleft 6 etiology.

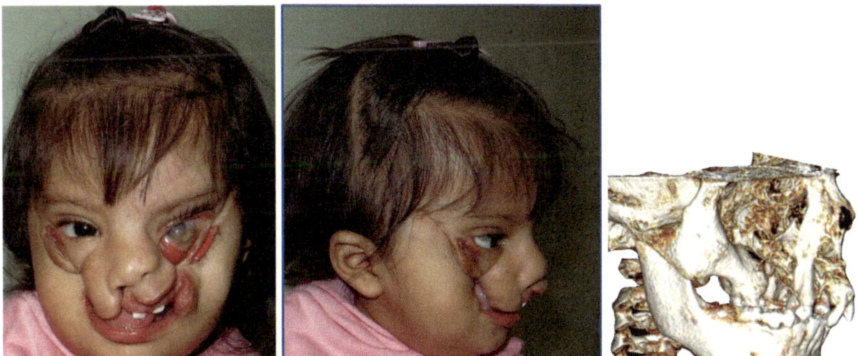

Fig. 10.19 Multiple clefts in the setting of ABS

10.6.4.1 SPEEC1L Mutation

Some rare clefts are directly related to known mutations.

Genetics are discussed more thoroughly in a specific chapter, and we must cite SPEEC1L mutation as a specific cause for Cleft 6 [27] [68]. This mutation is known for affecting the cytoskeleton in neural crest cells (NCC), affecting their migration ability.

10.6.4.2 Origin of Maxillary NCC

The neural crest cells (NCC) intended for the maxillary have a specific origin.

It has been recently demonstrated in Lee's research [69] that NCC migrating to the maxillary came from the postoptic area when it was previously admitted that they were from the first pharyngeal arch (PA1). Since all the symptoms of Cleft 6 exclusively affect the maxillary component, we could surmise that it is a place to look for the specific mechanism of dysmorphology.

10.6.4.3 Segregation between Maxillary and Mandibular NCC

The sorting between maxillary and mandibular NCC is under specific genetic control.

Coming from the research in phylogenesis, we know that there is a patterning of NCC sorting upper and lower jaw components [70]. The acquisition of this function has determined the apparition of jaw articulation in vertebrates. The hampering of these functions could be an explanation for the supernumerary bone and teeth material, and we may quote Beverdam [71]," null mutations in Dlx5/6 result in mirror image duplications of the upper jaw" and Sato [72], "An endothelin-1 switch specifies maxillomandibular identity".

10.6.4.4 The Hypothesis of Disorganization Mutation in Mice (ds)

As quoted above, the hypothesis of an equivalent in man of the disorganization mutation in man is a highly interesting one. This mutation was discovered in 1958 by Ms. Hammel [73] in a new mice species. An equivalent of this mutation in man was suspected in 1989 by Winter [74]. Hammel quoted the observed malformations found in the affected mice population as presenting an "extensive pleiotropy and generalized polymeria". She found the nature of inheritance autosomal dominant but with a variety of expressions of the mutation in heterozygotes, the mutation being lethal in homozygotes.

The anomalies affected both skeletal and visceral structures at any place of the body. The pleiomorphism was high, and no two similar inbred strains having the same phenotype could be found. The most frequent and significant malformations were cranioschisis (53%), Hamartomas (40%), reduction of the mandible, macrostomia, and maxillary duplication.

Winter [74] was the first to bring the report of a case that could be a homolog of Ds. In man. Crosby [75] established that the Ds. mutation was a gain of function. He then established [76] that the malformations came from a two-hit model explaining the pleiomorphism of manifestations. It was another of his conclusions that sporadic, nonheritable congenital malformations could be related to somatic mutations at Ds-like loci.

Purandare [77] raised the hypothesis that some patients displaying the features of ABS but with some symptoms unusual in ABS could, in fact, be Ds. homolog.

10.7 Treatment

Several defects have to be addressed in Cleft6: macrostomia, cheek defect, cleft palate, and supernumerary appendages.

The palpebral defect does not belong to Cleft 6 but to Cleft 8 and will be discussed in the specific Cleft 8 chapter (Chap. 12).

10.7.1 Technics

10.7.1.1 Macrostomia

Many technics have been published for macrostomia repair. All of them agree on the utmost importance of careful muscle repair.

In the same way, common to all of the techniques is the landmark to locate the new oral commissure, a vertical line through the pupil, the eyeball being in a neutral position.

The differences come with the mucosal and cutaneous flap design.

As noticed in Woods's paper [40], it could be used straight line, w-w plasty, local flaps, or Z plasty. As Bütow [78], we prefer the Z plasty; our technique of predilection is a double opposition Z plasty (Fig. 10.20).

The cutaneous and mucosal flaps undermining give extensive access to the muscle layer of orbicularis oris, triangular labia, and facilitates a precise repair of this layer, specifically rebuilding a modiolus. The double opposite Z plasty shifts the suture lines, decreasing the scar retraction tendency. The Z plasty lengthened the distance between the tragus and oral commissure, which is usually reduced.

The positioning of the triangular flap medially based on the upper lip vertically after its downward rotation reconstructs the area of skin located between the oral commissure and the nasolabial fold. The oblique suture line between the two cutaneous flaps reconstructs the nasolabial fold and, being oriented according to Langers's lines, has a better healing quality with a less conspicuous scar. The

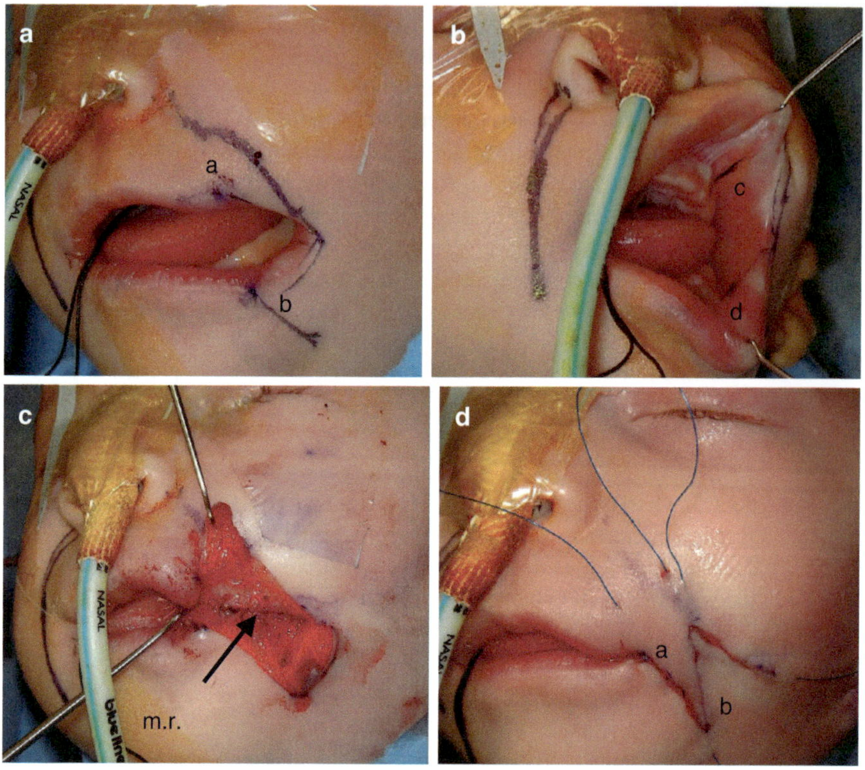

Fig. 10.20 Double opposite Z plasty: (**a**) upper lip flap, its base toward the midline; (**b**) lower lip flap, its base toward the cheek; (**c**) mucous flap from the upper lip, its base is distal; (**d**) mucous flap from the lower lip the base is to the midline. The muscle repair ***m.r.*** is of the outmost importance

"dog-ear" effect when rotating the flap brings some volume and participates in correcting the flattened cheek.

In the worst forms, when the macrostomia is in continuity through the whole cheek, a first Z plasty could be combined either with a straight closure or a second Z plasty (Fig. 10.20).

10.7.1.2 Cheek Defect

When existing, the soft tissue cheek defect could be repaired, as said above, through different cutaneous approaches, but the most logical is after the Z plasty for macrostomia to go along with a W plasty (Fig. 10.21) as for the orbicularis oris the buccinator muscle should be repaired carefully, but the idea brought by Gleizal [79] that mandible elevator muscles could be repaired as well, is a pure invention: we have carefully exanimated on CT scan of Cleft 6c, those which are going through

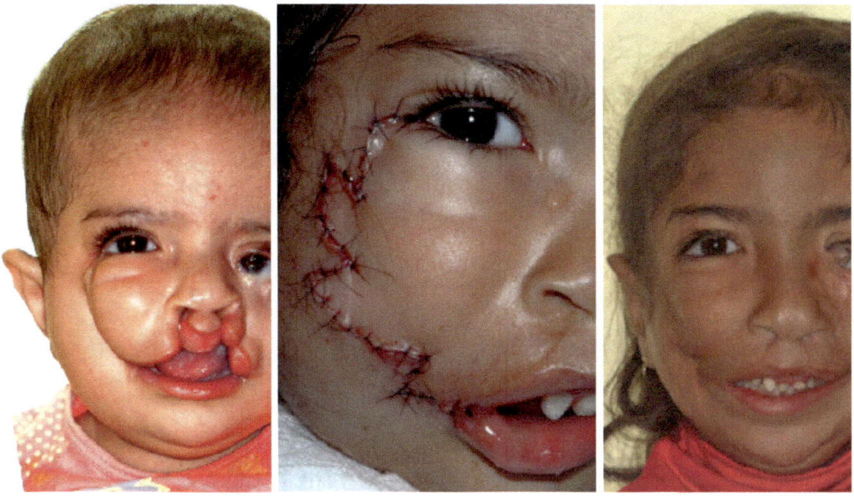

Fig. 10.21 Cheek repaired by association of W plasty to Z plasty macrostomia repair in a case of cleft 6a associated with cleft 8

the temporal and masseter trajectory: the masseter, hypoplastic is inserted to the inferior edge of the osseous cleft or to the appendage when existing, lateral pterygoid muscle does the same and is partially inserted on the hypoplastic coronoid process. The temporal muscle is absent and cannot be repaired.

The most conspicuous sequel of Cleft 6 to the cheek is the flattening of the zygomatic prominence. Many ways to address this problem are available; lipofilling has increasing popularity these days, but from our ancient experience with this technique in the field of craniofacial microsomia, we would be careful keeping it for the final touch-up and refinements cause massive lipofilling in other fields have shown themselves unstable by the long term and tend to droop.

Our preferred technique (Fig. 10.22) to correct the malar bulging when related to the cleft of the zygomatic bone is grafting a piece harvested by cortical splitting in the parietal area. Those pieces could be precisely designed preoperatively with the help of a CT scan; even a template could be used. It is particularly useful when coping with sequels of Cleft 6 plus Cleft 8 because it allows a robust lateral canthopexy.

10.7.1.3 Appendages

The appendages in soft tissues and the club shape appendage with bone and teeth buds have to be resected. As underlined by many authors even in their paper [22] and [32], this is supernumerary material that tampers with the positioning and growth of adjacent structures. Bone and teeth appendage resection is easily performed through an intra-oral approach.

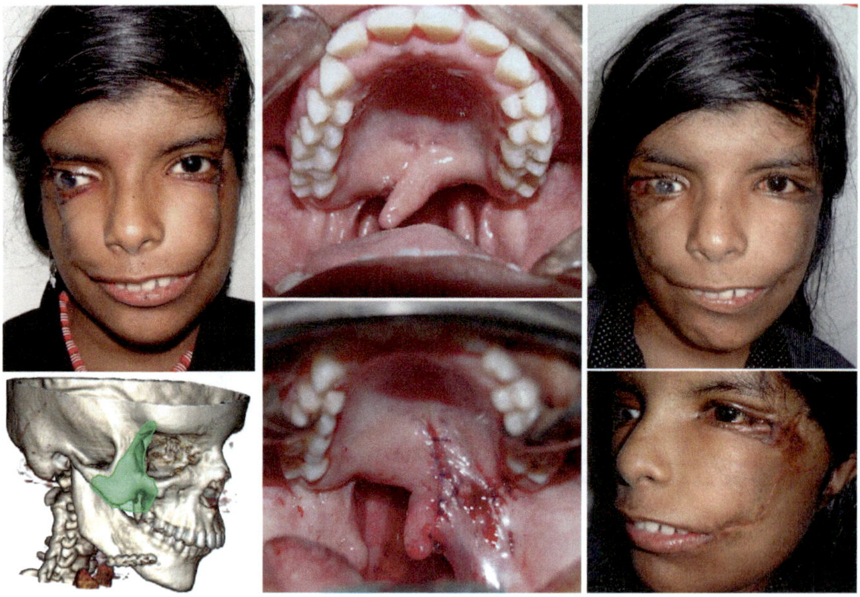

Fig. 10.22 Case 1: treatment sequence for a cleft 6a associated with cleft 8. Skull split malar graft. Double opposite Z-veloplasty on the left side

10.7.1.4 Cleft Palate

Pure cleft 6 involves only the soft palate. In subtype c, the pterygoid is frequently hypotrophic, as well as the part of the soft palate lateral to the cleft, and the repair could be tricky under such conditions. Still, in most subtypes a and c, the lateral part of the cleft could be found when carefully searched and is worth trying to perform a staphyloraphy. Doing a double opposite Z plasty, as in Furlow's technique, was a good solution. Figures 10.22 and 10.23 or an intra-velar veloplasty more or less associated with a local mucosal flap.

10.7.2 Surgical Planning

10.7.2.1 Stages for Primary Repair

Primary repair should be better done in large craniofacial centers. Unfortunately, many nonspecialized surgeons think those are apparent macrostomia conditions that are easy to fix, and they address this part of the problem.

In our experience, it is better when there are intra-oral anomalies to fix to start with that part; this is the reason why it matters so much to have an appropriate diagnosis and a full check-up of all the deformities thanks to the CT scan. All the same, to recognize the malformations, one needs to know them in the first place.

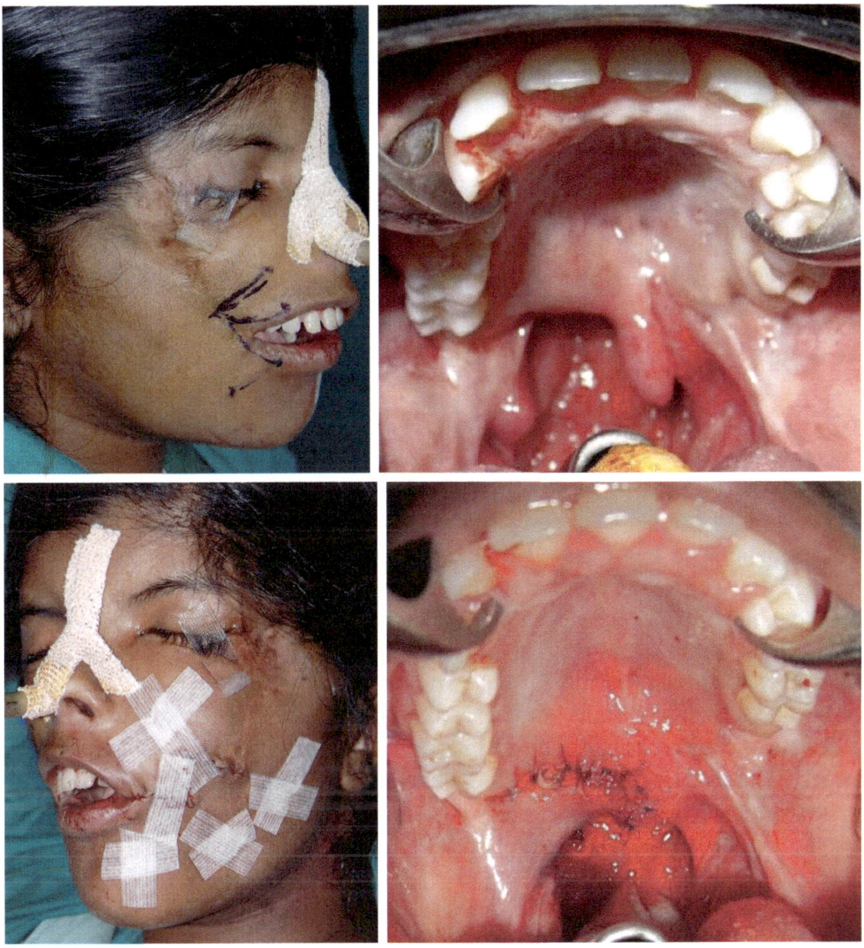

Fig. 10.23 Case 1: second time. Double Z veloplasty right side. Z plasty both sides of macrostomia

As long as the macrostomia is not repaired, the intra-operative access to the palatal and oro-pharyngeal area is facilitated, so we advise postponing its repair until after fixing the palatal condition.

Persisting nasality after primary staphyloraphy would need any technic of pharyngoplasty according to local conditions and the operator's habits.

10.7.2.2 Orthognathic Surgery

Many of those patients have a primary Angle class II occlusion. Most severe cases should be tested for obstructive apnea syndrome (OAS), and if positive, early mandibular distraction would be considered.

Otherwise, orthognathic surgery in the case of maxillo-mandibular disharmony would be performed as usual after a presurgical orthodontic treatment at the end of growth.

10.7.2.3 Oculoplastic Surgery

The associated oculo-palpebral malformations must be addressed at the same time. Cleft 8, when associated with Cleft 6, is obviously repaired in the same procedure (see Chap. 12).

10.7.3 Surgical Cases

10.7.3.1 Case 1 (Figs. 10.22 and 10.23)

This patient, who has received primary care elsewhere, was misdiagnosed and referred as a TCS to our institution. The retrospective diagnosis was bilateral Cleft 6 subtype a with bilateral left 8. She undergoes a two-step surgery. The first step (Fig. 6.19) is through a bi-coronal approach dissection of the orbital and malar cleft area, harvesting of split cortical bone from the parietal area to be grafted to the malar bone. Under the same anesthesia, double opposite Z plasty was to repair the left cleft of the soft palate. The second step (Fig. 6.20) occurred 6 months later: repair of the right cleft palate by a double opposition Z plasty. Correction of the bilateral macrostomia by the Z plasty technic.

10.7.3.2 Case 2 (Fig. 10.24)

The patient was affected by a bilateral Cleft 6b, asymmetric, cutaneous appendage to the right cleft palate to the left. The first step (Fig. 6.21a) is resectioning the cutaneous appendage and macrostomia, and cheek cleft by a W plasty. The second step (6.21b): intra-velar veloplasty and local mucous flap, resection of the osteo-dental appendage and lipofilling to the cheek.

10.7.3.3 Case 3 (Fig. 10.25)

Patient with a right Cleft 6 subtype c sequels, facial palsy. Primary treatment elsewhere. We performed first, after orthodontic presurgical treatment, a bimaxillary osteotomy (Fig. 10.25a), revision of the macrostomia repair (Fig. 10.25b), and gold plate to the superior eyelid (Fig. 10.25c).

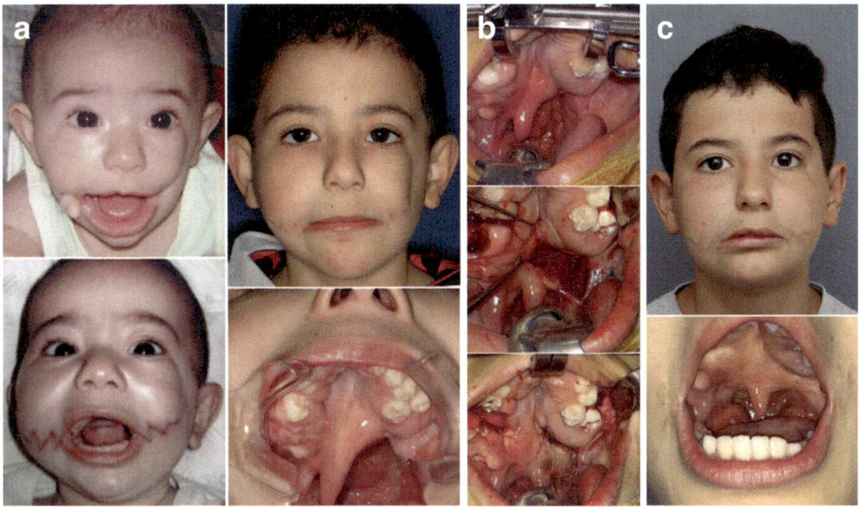

Fig. 10.24 Case 2 Treatment sequence: primary case of cleft 6b. (**a**) first step Z plasty on macrostomia completed as a W to the cheek and resection of cutaneous appendages. (**b**) Second step, veloplasty and resection of osteo-dental appendage. (**c**) Third step, cheek lipofilling, pharyngoplasty. Final result

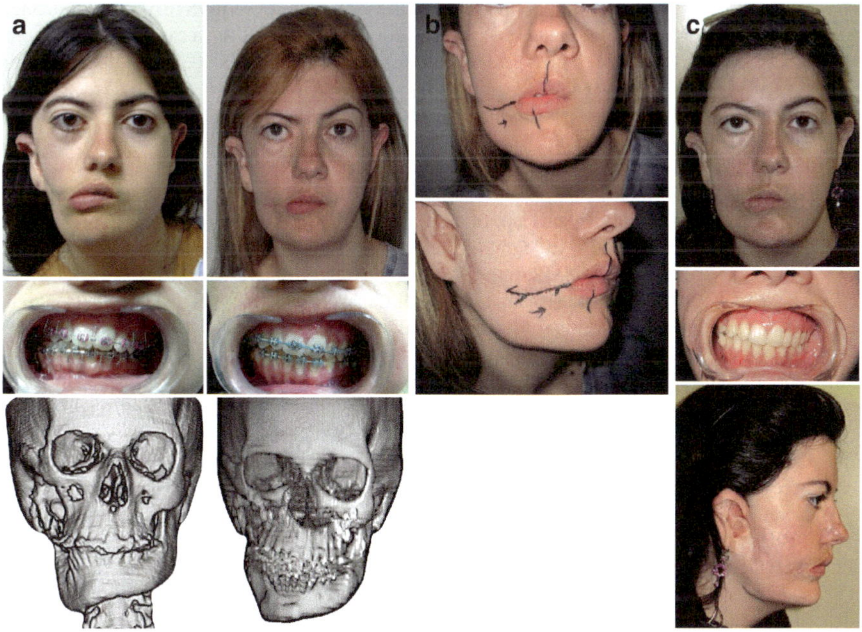

Fig. 10.25 Case 3 treatment sequence: Cleft 6c, primary treatment in another institution, sequels mandibulo-maxillary disharmony, facial palsy. Preoperative orthodontics. (**a**) lengthening the vertical ramus and maxillary osteotomy. (**b**) macrostomia scar revision. (**c**) gold plate to the superior eyelid for facial palsy

10.8 Conclusions

The Cleft 6 was probably in Tessier's description the less precise with a misleading confusion with Treacher Collins syndrome.

It could be well understood if you consider the time when Tessier did this tremendous description. He had neither modern medical imaging nor macromolecular genetic studies for syndromes. So, we are proud for having, in his honor, completed his research and recognized the three subtypes of Cleft 6.

References

1. Tessier P. Anatomical classification of facial, cranio-facial and latero-facial clefts. J Maxillofac Surg. 1976;4:69–92. https://linkinghub.elsevier.com/retrieve/pii/S0301050376800136.
2. Vincent M, Geneviève D, Ostertag A, Marlin S, Lacombe D, Martin-Coignard D, et al. Treacher Collins syndrome: a clinical and molecular study based on a large series of patients. Genet Med. 2016;18(1):49–56. http://www.nature.com/articles/gim201529.
3. Hou R, Feng X, Zhang J, Lu B, Liu G, Wang L, et al. A rare bilateral Tessier no. 6 and 7 clefts. J Cranio-Maxillofac Surg. 2011;39(2):93–5. https://linkinghub.elsevier.com/retrieve/pii/S1010518210001952.
4. Borzabadi-Farahani A, Yen SL-K, Francis C, Lara-Sanchez PA, Hammoudeh J. A rare case of accessory maxilla and bilateral Tessier no. 7 clefts, a 10-year follow-up. J Cranio-Maxillofac Surg. 2013;41(6):527–31. https://linkinghub.elsevier.com/retrieve/pii/S1010518212002582.
5. Sun M, Lv N, Xiao Y, Li J, Guan G. A rare case of accessory maxilla: a case report and literature review of Tessier no. 7 clefts. J Int Med Res. 2020;48(5):030006052092568. https://doi.org/10.1177/0300060520925680.
6. Bilkay U, Gundogan H, Ozek C, Gurter T, Akin Y. A rare craniofacial cleft: bilateral tessier no. 5 cleft accompanied by no. 1 and no. 6 clefts. Ann Plast Surg. 2000;45(6):654–7. http://journals.lww.com/00000637-200045060-00016.
7. Gleizal A, Wan DC, Picard A, Lavis J-F, Vazquez M-P, Beziat J-L. Bilateral Macrostomia as an isolated pathology. Cleft Palate Craniofac. 2007;44(1):58–61. https://doi.org/10.1597/05-106.
8. Chauhan DS, Guruprasad Y. Bilateral Tessier's 7 cleft with maxillary duplication. J Maxillofac Oral Surg. 2015;14(S1):108–12. https://doi.org/10.1007/s12663-012-0346-x.
9. Cheung LK, Samman N, Tideman H. Bilateral transverse facial clefts and accessory maxillae—variant or separate entity? J Cranio Maxillofac Surg. 1993;21(4):163–7. https://linkinghub.elsevier.com/retrieve/pii/S1010518205801064.
10. Crespo Guerra MC, López del Castillo CA, Agüero Díaz Á, Bastian ML. Fisura tipo 7 de Tessier: presentación de un caso. Rev Arch Méd Camagüey. 2010;14:0. http://scielo.sld.cu/scielo.php?script=sci_arttext&pid=S1025-02552010000500013&nrm=iso.
11. Özçelik D, Toplu G, Türkseven A, Şenses DA, Yiğit B. Lateral facial cleft associated with accessory mandible having teeth, absent parotid gland and peripheral facial weakness. J Cranio-Maxillofac Surg. 2014;42(5):e239–44. https://linkinghub.elsevier.com/retrieve/pii/S1010518213002576.
12. Anantanarayanan P, Manikandhan R, Thomas T, Satish KM. Lateral facial cleft, accessory maxilla and hemifacial microsomia: an uncommon triad. J Oral Maxillofac Pathol. 2007;11(2):80. http://www.jomfp.in/text.asp?2007/11/2/80/37389.
13. Buonocore S, Broer PN, Walker ME, da Silva FR, Franco D, Alonso N. Macrostomia: a Spectrum of deformity. Ann Plast Surg. 2014;72(3):363–8. https://journals.lww.com/00000637-201403000-00022.

14. Uchikawa Y, Ogata H, Hattori N, Miyamoto J, Nakajima T. Palatoplasty for bilateral oblique cleft of the soft palate accompanied by Tessier number 5–7 cleft. Cleft Palate Craniofac. 2011;48(2):231–5. https://doi.org/10.1597/09-068.
15. Sun L, Sun Z, Ma X. Partial duplication of the mandible, parotid aplasia and facial cleft: a rare developmental disorder. Oral Surg Oral Med Oral Pathol Oral Radiol. 2013;116(3):e202–9. https://linkinghub.elsevier.com/retrieve/pii/S2212440313000060.
16. Kuriyama M, Udagawa A, Yoshimoto S, Ichinose M, Suzuki H. Tessier number 7 cleft with oblique clefts of bilateral soft palates and rare symmetric structure of zygomatic arch. J Plast Reconstr Aesthet Surg. 2008;61(4):447–50. https://linkinghub.elsevier.com/retrieve/pii/S1748681506004529.
17. Hou M, Liu C, Wang J, Zhang L, Gao Q. Lateral or oblique facial clefts associated with accessory maxillae: review of the literature and report of a case. J Cranio-Maxillofac Surg. 2015;43(5):585–92. https://linkinghub.elsevier.com/retrieve/pii/S101051821500030X.
18. Tharanon W, Ellis E, Sinn DP. A case of maxillary and zygomatic duplication. J Oral Maxillofac Surg. 1998;56(6):770–4. https://linkinghub.elsevier.com/retrieve/pii/S0278239198908175.
19. Jian X-C, Chen X-Q. Neurocristopathy that manifests right facial cleft and right maxillary duplication. Oral Surg Oral Med Oral Pathol Oral Radiol Endod. 1995;79(5):546–50. https://linkinghub.elsevier.com/retrieve/pii/S1079210405800927.
20. DeGurse K, Chung H, Pharoah M. Facial dimple with accessory bone and teeth. Dentomaxillofac Radiol. 1995;24(2):135–8. https://doi.org/10.1259/dmfr.24.2.9515386.
21. Stoneman DW. Congenital facial fistula with formation of accessory bone and teeth. Oral Surg Oral Med Oral Pathol. 1978;45(1):150–4. https://linkinghub.elsevier.com/retrieve/pii/0030422078902384.
22. Miyajima K, Natsume N, Kawai T, Iizuka T. Oblique facial cleft, cleft palate, and supernumerary teeth secondary to amniotic bands. Cleft Palate Craniofac. 1994;31(6):483–6. https://doi.org/10.1597/1545-1569_1994_031_0483_ofccpa_2.3.co_2.
23. Rushton MA, Walker FA. Unilateral secondary facial cleft with excess tooth and bone formation. Proc R Soc Med. 1936;30(1):79–82. https://doi.org/10.1177/003591573603000119.
24. Rintala A, Leisti J, Liesmaa M, Ranta R. Oblique Facial Clefts. Scand J Plast Reconstr Surg. 1980;14(3):291–7. https://doi.org/10.3109/02844318009106724.
25. Ranta R, Rintala A. Oblique lateral oro-ocular facial cleft. Int J Oral Maxillofac Surg. 1988;17(3):186–9. https://linkinghub.elsevier.com/retrieve/pii/S0901502788800298.
26. Sjamsudin J, David DJ, Singh GD. An Indonesian child with orofacial duplication and neurocristopathy anomalies: case report. J Cranio-Maxillofac Surg. 2001;29(4):195–7. https://linkinghub.elsevier.com/retrieve/pii/S1010518201902215.
27. Saadi I, Alkuraya FS, Gisselbrecht SS, Goessling W, Cavallesco R, Turbe-Doan A, et al. Deficiency of the cytoskeletal protein SPECC1L leads to oblique facial Clefting. Am J Hum Genet. 2011;89(1):44–55. https://linkinghub.elsevier.com/retrieve/pii/S0002929711002163.
28. Chavane A. Malformation faciale (section par bride amniotique). Bull Société Anat Paris. 1890;5(4):137–41. https://gallica.bnf.fr/ark:/12148/bpt6k6327302h/f159.item#.
29. Mayou BJ, Fenton OM. Oblique Facial Clefts Caused by Amniotic Bands. Plast Reconstr Surg. 1981;68(5):675–81. http://journals.lww.com/00006534-198111000-00001.
30. Morovic CG, Berwart F, Varas J. Craniofacial anomalies of the amniotic band syndrome in serial clinical cases. Plast Reconstr Surg. 2004;113(6):1556–62. http://journals.lww.com/00006534-200405000-00003.
31. Obdeijn MC, Offringa PJ, Bos RRM, Verhagen AAE, Niessen FB, Roche NA. Facial clefts and associated limb anomalies: description of three cases and a review of the literature. Cleft Palate Craniofac. 2010;47(6):661–7. https://doi.org/10.1597/09-033.
32. Ramanathan M, Parameswaran A, Jayakumar N, Sneha P, Sailer HF. A rare case of multiple oblique facial clefts with supernumerary teeth: case report. Craniomaxillofac Trauma Reconstr. 2012;5(4):239–42. https://doi.org/10.1055/s-0032-1329541.

33. Walker G. Malformations of the face. Edinburgh and London: E&S Livingstone Ltd.; 1961. p. 202.
34. Balaji S. Two-stage corrections of rare facial tessier's cleft - 3,4,5,6,7. Ann Maxillofac Surg. 2017;7(2):287. http://www.amsjournal.com/text.asp?2017/7/2/287/218986.
35. Kanth AM, Krevalin M, Adetayo OA. Surgical approach to Hemipalatal discrepancy in Tessier 7 reconstruction: review of literature and case series. Cleft Palate Craniofac. 2021;58(9):1094–101. https://doi.org/10.1177/1055665620984045.
36. Fijałkowska M, Antoszewski B. Rare facial clefts. Pol J Surg. 2015;87(8):389–94. https://www.degruyter.com/view/j/pjs.2015.87.issue-8/pjs-2015-0077/pjs-2015-0077.xml.
37. Darzi MA, Chowdri NA. Oblique facial clefts: a report of Tessier numbers 3, 4, 5, and 9 clefts. Cleft Palate Craniofac. 1993;30(4):414–5. https://doi.org/10.1597/1545-1569_1993_030_0414_ofcaro_2.3.co_2.
38. Morita K, Iwasa T, Imaizumi F, Negishi A, Omura K. A case of maxillary duplication with a soft palate reconstruction using a forearm flap. Int J Oral Maxillofac Surg. 2008;37(9):862–5. https://linkinghub.elsevier.com/retrieve/pii/S0901502708001665.
39. Tiwari P, Tapadar J. Partial duplication of maxilla associated with Tessier 3 and incomplete Tessier 6 cleft: a new entity. IOSR J dent. Med Sci. 2015;14(5tessier):4.
40. Woods RH, Varma S, David DJ. Tessier No. 7 cleft: a new subclassification and management protocol. Plast Reconstr Surg. 2008;122(3):898–905. http://journals.lww.com/00006534-200809000-00028.
41. Mello et Jorge - Fissura número 5 de Tessier relato de caso.pdf.
42. Gosla Reddy et Acharya - 2021 - Rare Facial Clefts.pdf.
43. Racz C, Dakpé S, Kadlub N, Testelin S, Devauchelle B, Rachwalski M, et al. Phenotypic spectrum of Tessier facial cleft number 5. J Cranio-Maxillofac Surg. 2018;46(1):22–7. https://linkinghub.elsevier.com/retrieve/pii/S1010518217303517.
44. Cameron AC, McKellar GMW, Widmer RP. A case of neurocristopathy that manifests facial clefting and maxillary duplication. Oral Surg Oral Med Oral Pathol. 1993;75(3):338–42. https://linkinghub.elsevier.com/retrieve/pii/003042209390147V.
45. Bhattacharya S, Tripathi A, Pradhan KL, Bhatnagar SK, Chandra R. Rare craniofacial clefts with duplication of alveolar arch. Eur J Plast Surg. 1988;11(2):83–6. https://doi.org/10.1007/BF00299218.
46. Tripathy R, Mishra S, Sabhlok SS. Accessory maxilla with a lateral cleft lip: a rare case report. J Oral Maxillofac Surg Med Pathol. 2013;25(3):238–40. https://linkinghub.elsevier.com/retrieve/pii/S2212555812000993.
47. Wang Y, Liu H, Zhang N, Luo E. Partial duplication of the jaw: case reports and review of relevant publications. Br J Oral Maxillofac Surg. 2020;58(1):34–42. https://linkinghub.elsevier.com/retrieve/pii/S0266435619307077.
48. Xu C, Zhang Y, Yang Y, Liang Y. Malformations of the zygomatic and maxillary regions. J Craniofac Surg. 2013;24(4):1465–9. https://journals.lww.com/00001665-201307000-00102.
49. Sutton B. On some cases of congenital fissures of the mouth. Trans Odontol Soc G B. 1888;20 new series(November 1887–June 1888):97–115. https://archive.org/details/s6777id1399047/page/116/mode/2up.
50. Debout. Coup d'oeil sur une des formes les plus rares du bec de liévre, les fissures horizontales. Remarques et observations. Bull Général Thérapeutique Médicale Chir. 1862;(N° 63):13–22. https://services.biusante.parisdescartes.fr/medica-pdf/main.php?key=cGFydGlhbHw5MDAxNHgxODYyeDYzfDEyfDIz.
51. Pelvet. Mémoire sur les fissures congénitales des joues. Gaz Médicale Paris. 1864;19:418–23. https://services.biusante.parisdescartes.fr/medica-pdf/pdf.php?key=cGFydGlhbHw5MDE4MngxODY0eDE5fDQxOHw0MjI&f=OTAxODJ4MTg2NHgxOS00MTgtNDIy&one=1.
52. Millard R. Lareral facial clefts. In: Cleft craft. Boston: Brown and Co.; 1996. p. 769–79.
53. Pitanguy I, Franco T. Nonoperated Facial Fissures in Adults. Plast Reconstr Surg. 1967;39(6):569–77. http://journals.lww.com/00006534-196706000-00005.

54. Converse JM, Wood-Smith D, Mccarthy JG, Coccaro PJ, Becker MH. Bilateral facial microsomia: diagnosis, classification, treatment. Plast Reconstr Surg. 1974;54(4):413–23. http://journals.lww.com/00006534-197410000-00005.
55. Ahlfeld F. Atlas, Die Missbildungen des Menschen-Taf. XXIV-XLIX, vol. III. Leipzig: Fr. Wilh. Grunow; 1882. p. 31. https://archive.org/details/BIUSante_44232x04/page/n7/mode/2up.
56. Khorasani H, Boljanovic S, Knudsen MAK, Jakobsen LP. Surgical management of the Tessier 7 cleft: a review and presentation of 5 cases. JPRAS Open. 2019;22:9–18. https://linkinghub.elsevier.com/retrieve/pii/S2352587819300300.
57. Millard R. oblique facial clefts. In: In: cleft craft. Boston: Little, Brown and Cie; 1996. p. 781–807.
58. Bernier FP, Caluseriu O, Ng S, Schwartzentruber J, Buckingham KJ, Innes AM, et al. Haploinsufficiency of SF3B4, a component of the pre-mRNA Spliceosomal complex, causes Nager syndrome. Am J Hum Genet. 2012;90(5):925–33. https://linkinghub.elsevier.com/retrieve/pii/S0002929712002054.
59. Gordon CT, Weaver KN, Zechi-Ceide RM, Madsen EC, Tavares ALP, Oufadem M, et al. Mutations in the endothelin receptor type a cause mandibulofacial Dysostosis with alopecia. Am J Hum Genet. 2015;96(4):519–31. https://linkinghub.elsevier.com/retrieve/pii/S0002929715000233.
60. Guion-Almeida ML. Apparent Malpuech syndrome: report on three Brazilian patients with additional signs. Am J Med Genet. 1995;58(1):13–7. https://doi.org/10.1002/ajmg.1320580104.
61. Gosla Reddy S, Acharya AP. Rare facial clefts. In: Bonanthaya K, Panneerselvam E, Manuel S, Kumar VV, Rai A, editors. Oral and maxillofacial surgery for the clinician. Singapore: Springer Singapore; 2021. p. 1735–68. https://doi.org/10.1007/978-981-15-1346-6_77.
62. Tessier P. Introduction aux dysplasies oto-mandibulaires (D.O.M.) ou «Vingt ans après ». Ann Chir Plast Esthet. 2001;46(5):381–4. https://linkinghub.elsevier.com/retrieve/pii/S029412600100053X.
63. Poswillo D. The pathogenesis of the first and second branchial arch syndrome. Oral Surg Oral Med Oral Pathol. 1973;35(3):302–28. https://linkinghub.elsevier.com/retrieve/pii/0030422073900704.
64. Durmus Kocaaslan N, Satır T, Celebiler O, Numanoğlu A. Duplication of the mandible in Klippel–Feil syndrome. J Plast Reconstr Aesthet Surg. 2013;66(4):e107–10. https://linkinghub.elsevier.com/retrieve/pii/S1748681512007371.
65. Al-Ani SA, Rees M, de Chalain TM. Our experiences managing a patient with mandibular duplication and cervical spinal fusion. J Craniofac Surg. 2009;20(6):2118–22. https://journals.lww.com/00001665-200911000-00032.
66. Opitz JM, Johnson DR, Gilbert-Barness EF. ADAM "sequence" part II: hypothesis and speculation. Am J Med Genet A. 2015;167(3):478–503. https://doi.org/10.1002/ajmg.a.36937.
67. Bamforth JS. Amniotic band sequence: Streeter's hypothesis reexamined. Am J Med Genet. 1992;44(3):280–7. https://doi.org/10.1002/ajmg.1320440304.
68. Gfrerer L, Shubinets V, Hoyos T, Kong Y, Nguyen C, Pietschmann P, et al. Functional analysis of SPECC1L in craniofacial development and oblique facial cleft pathogenesis. Plast Reconstr Surg. 2014;134(4):748–59. http://journals.lww.com/00006534-201410000-00032.
69. Lee S-H, Bédard O, Buchtová M, Fu K, Richman JM. A new origin for the maxillary jaw. Dev Biol. 2004;276(1):207–24. https://linkinghub.elsevier.com/retrieve/pii/S0012160604006165.
70. Cerny R, Lwigale P, Ericsson R, Meulemans D, Epperlein H-H, Bronner-Fraser M. Developmental origins and evolution of jaws: new interpretation of "maxillary" and "mandibular". Dev Biol. 2004;276(1):225–36. https://linkinghub.elsevier.com/retrieve/pii/S0012160604006177.
71. Beverdam A, Merlo GR, Paleari L, Mantero S, Genova F, Barbieri O, et al. Jaw transformation with gain of symmetry afterDlx5/Dlx6 inactivation: Mirror of the past? Genesis. 2002;34(4):221–7. https://doi.org/10.1002/gene.10156.

72. Sato T, Kurihara Y, Asai R, Kawamura Y, Tonami K, Uchijima Y, et al. An endothelin-1 switch specifies maxillomandibular identity. Proc Natl Acad Sci. 2008;105(48):18806–11. https://doi.org/10.1073/pnas.0807345105.
73. Hummel KP. The inheritance and expression of disorganization, an unusual mutation in the mouse. J Exp Zool. 1958;137(3):389–423. https://doi.org/10.1002/jez.1401370303.
74. Winter RM, Donnai D. A possible human homologue for the mouse mutant disorganisation. J Med Genet. 1989;26(7):417–20. https://doi.org/10.1136/jmg.26.7.417.
75. Crosby JL, Varnum DS, Washburn LL, Nadeau JH. Disorganization is a completely dominant gain-of-function mouse mutation causing sporadic developmental defects. Mech Dev. 1992;37(3):121–6. https://linkinghub.elsevier.com/retrieve/pii/092547739290074T.
76. Crosby JL, Varnum DS, Nadeau JH. Two-hit model for sporadic congenital anomalies in mice with the disorganization mutation. Am J Hum Genet. 1993;52(5):866–74.
77. Purandare SM, Ernst L, Medne L, Huff D, Zackai EH. Developmental anomalies with features of disorganization (ds) and amniotic band sequence (ABS): a report of four cases. Am J Med Genet A. 2009;149A(8):1740–8. https://doi.org/10.1002/ajmg.a.32716.
78. Bütow K-W, Botha A. A classification and construction of congenital lateral facial clefts. J Cranio-Maxillofac Surg. 2010;38(7):477–84. https://linkinghub.elsevier.com/retrieve/pii/S1010518210000302.
79. Gleizal A, Wan DC, Kwan MD, Beziat J-L. Myoplasty for congenital Macrostomia. Cleft Palate Craniofac. 2008;45(2):179–86. https://doi.org/10.1597/05-190.1.
80. Converse JM, Coccaro PJ, Becker M, Wood-Smith D, On hemifacial microsomia. The first and second branchial arch syndrome. Plast Reconstr Surg. 1973;51(3):268–79.

Chapter 11
Cleft 7

Philippe Pellerin, Cristiano Tonello, Renato da Silva Freitas, and Nivaldo Alonso

> **Pearls**
> Cleft 7 is a macrostomia occurring in the craniofacial microsomia spectrum setting.

11.1 Introduction to Cleft 7

The diagnosis of Cleft 7 is one of the most controversial diagnoses among rare clefts since there is frequent confusion between macrostomia and cleft 7. Many authors did not understand that macrostomia is a common symptom in Cleft 5, 6, and 7.

It is striking in Woods's paper "Tessier No. 7 Cleft: A New subclassification and Management Protocol" [1]. His paper excludes oculoauriculovertebral sequences (OAV) cases, far from Tessier's opinion.

P. Pellerin (✉)
Plastic Surgery Department, University of Lille, Lambersart, France

C. Tonello
Craniofacial Surgery Department, Universidade de São Paulo, Bauru, São Paulo, Brazil
e-mail: cristianotonello@usp.br

R. da Silva Freitas
Plastic Surgery Unit, Hospital de Clínicas, Universidade Federal do Paraná, Curitiba, Brazil

Craniofacial Surgery, Assistance Center for Cleft Lip and Palate (CAIF), Hospital do Trabalhador, Curitiba, Brazil

N. Alonso
Department of Plastic Surgery, Universidade de São Paulo, São Paulo, Brazil
e-mail: nivalonso@usp.br

N. Alonso et al. (eds.), *Facial Reconstruction of Unusual Facial Clefts*,
https://doi.org/10.1007/978-3-031-40926-4_11

Excluding OAV (we prefer to use the term Craniofacial microsomia) means excluding what Tessier named Cleft 7 from the field of Tessier's rare Cleft 7. At the same time, Woods described the Cleft 6 as a Cleft 7, as did Vermeij-Keers [2] L. 1–3.

In his original publication [3], Tessier described Cleft 7: "No. 7 belongs in common to Treacher Collins and hemifacial microsomia." Tessier confirmed this point later, [4] in a preface to the French Society of Plastic Surgery congress report in 2001. We have already explained why we prefer to exclude Treacher Collins syndrome (TCS), but excluding the macrostomia occurring in OAV makes no sense. In the OAV setting, macrostomia could be related to a default of fusion between the maxillary and mandibular buds of the first pharyngeal arch. This default of fusion could be due to those buds' hypoplasia, which is very specific to first and second branchial arch defects and justifies the name of craniofacial microsomia frequently used in place of OAV. Such default of fusion is one of the rare embryological explanations for the etiology of rare clefts.

Woods were misled to exclude the actual Cleft 7 as proposed in Tessier's classification and shifted Cleft 6 to Cleft 7.

A common mistake other than confusing Cleft 6 with Cleft 7 is confusing with Cleft 5; we will discuss the point below.

11.2 History

The term macrostomia comes front the ancient Greek: μακρο-, which means big and στόμα for the mouth. It was used, by Langenbeck, in 1822 about a case in which the drawing was formerly reported in Förster [5], with the spelling "makrostomia". Along with Langenbeck's patient, Förster reported the cases of others authors in the XXV and XXVII planches of his atlas (Fig. 11.1). Among those cases, Kraske's patient, displayed in Fig. 9 of the planchet XXVII, was the only one with a Cleft 7.

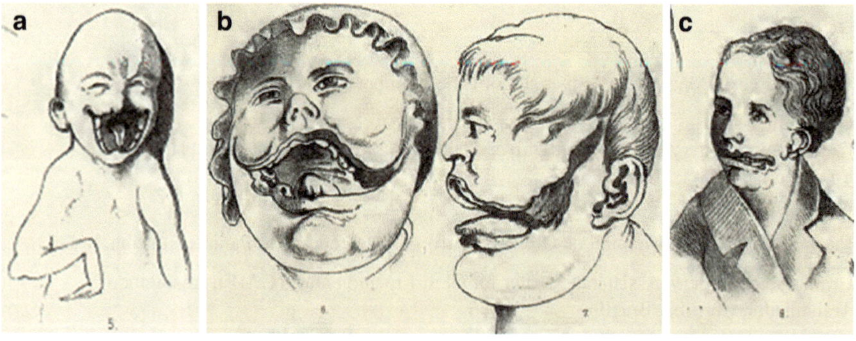

Fig. 11.1 History. Table XXV and XXVII From Ahlfeld atlas: Human deformities 1880. (**a**) Table XXVII, figure 5, after Muralt 1715, Ephemides Academiae Caes. Leopold, Obs. 134. (**b**) Table XXVII, figures 6 and 7 after Langenbeck 1818, Neue Bibliothek für Ophthalmologie und Chirurgie. (**c**) Table XXVII, figures 9, Kraske's patient, after Lesser, Deutsche Zeitschrift für Chirurgie, 2. Band, S. 311

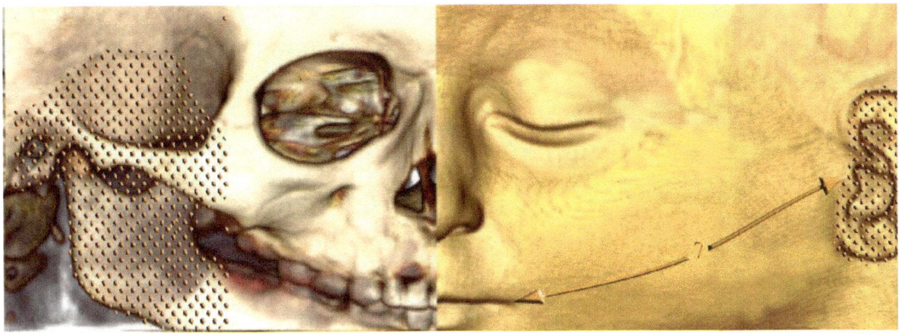

Fig. 11.2 Clef 7 schematic drawing. Double end arrow shows the path of cleft, pits, and fistulas, appendages, and enchondromas. Dotted area shows areas of hypoplasia related to CFM

Debout, in 1862, [6] used the term macrostomia to name the latero-facial cleft.

Henceforth, it will be used for this purpose most of the time. It will be used as a general term to name conditions in which the transversal size of the mouth is enlarged.

Van Duyse, in 1882 [7], 70 years before Goldenhar, was the first to systematically describe the association between macrostomia and epibulbar hamartomas. He credited Muraut (*J. Murault. Ephem. Acad. Caes. Leopold.*, 1715, cent. III et IV, obs. 134, p. 304) for the inaugural naming with macrostomia.

Then came Tessier's classification (Fig. 11.2), in which a distinction was made between Cleft 7, Cleft 6, and some cases of Cleft 5 as causes for macrostomia.

11.3 Etiology

The relation between macrostomia and craniofacial microsomia (CFM) makes it one of the few facial clefts that could result from a failure in the fusion of primordial facial processes, which many consider as the process of "true clefts." In this occurrence, macrostomia could be understood as an imperfect fusion between the maxillary and mandibular processes issued out of the first pharyngeal arch. Associated anomalies such as sinus and appendages or tags being on the same line suggest a perturbation of the fusion process. Poswillo's research in experimental teratogenesis [8] suggested a disruption related to the stapedial artery when he reproduced the spectrum of CFM in mice and observed that hematomas in its area could be the reason for the defect. This hypothesis was widely shared for years. A careful reading of Poswillo's research finds that in the same paper, he mentioned the teratogenic action of retinoic acid, which is nowadays known to act on a specific gene pathway by binding to the retinoic acid receptor family that disrupts the expression of Hox genes and perturbs the morphogenic movements during gastrulation [9–11].

Poswillo's vascular theory, even if found attractive at the time and even could be related to a genetic mechanism of vascular disruption [12] loses more and more room for the benefit of straighter genetic explanations. Thanks to the tremendous

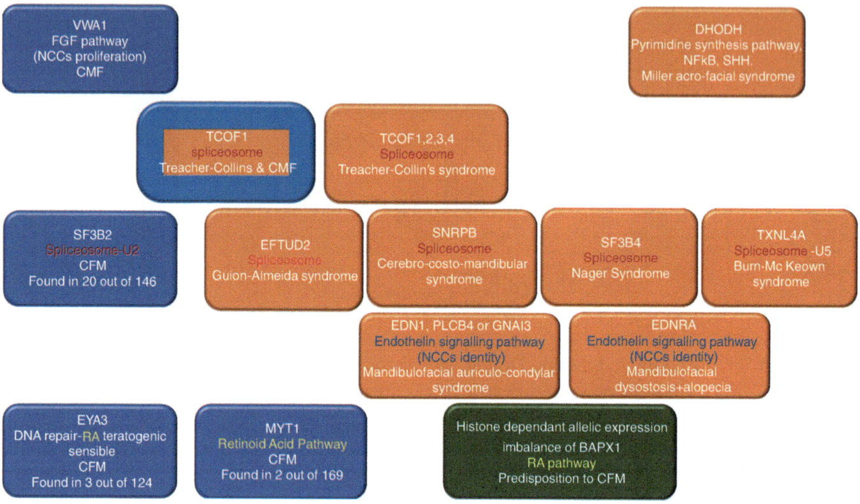

Fig. 11.3 Known mutations involved in CFM. Blue shapes are known mutation found in CMF. Orange shapes are known mutation found in mandibulofacial dysostosis. Green shape is an epigenetic condition associated with CMF

progress in macromolecular genetics, many explanations have been found to explain teratogenic mechanisms (see above) or gene involvements. The gene involvements could be related to chromosomal anomalies (deletion, polysomy.) or mutations. The number of mutations being proven to be the cause of CFM is rapidly increasing. The most frequent gene involved is SF3B2, found by Timberlake et al.in 20 out of 138 CMF patients who benefited from a whole exome sequencing [13]. It is striking that this gene codes for a protein that is a component of the U2 itself, a component of the spliceosome, the same involved in many of the mandibulofacial dysostotic syndromes. A specific TCOF1 mutation, the same gene involved in Treacher-Collin's syndrome, has been found accountable for cases of CMF [14]. Mutations to TCOF1, TCOF2, TCOF3, and TCOF4 are responsible for Treacher-Collin's syndromes, several phenotypes related to different perturbations in the same path. To our knowledge, the main path involves mutations affecting different components of the spliceosomal complex, either responsible for syndromic mandibulofacial dysostosis or CFM. A second path involves the endothelin signaling pathway, and the third concerns the retinoic acid pathway (Fig. 11.3).

11.4 Literature Series

It is impressive that there has been such a mess in the appellation of Cleft 7 after the publication of Tessier's classification of rare Clefts. Quoting Kawamoto [15], one could say that Tessier's classification has sorted the order out of the chaos. Still, it did not work well for macrostomia, probably because there was confusion between Cleft 5, 6, and 7. Thanks to the progress in medical imaging, we now have a precise visualization of pathologic anatomy to clear this confusing area.

This is the first reason bibliographic research has been difficult; we probably missed many cases.

The second reason is that the nomenclature of malformations affecting simultaneously the external ear and the mandible is confused. Hemifacial Microsomia (HFM) has been very popular, but what when it is bilateral?

Cohen put the problem clearly in 1989 [16] and cast a table (Table 11.1) that summarizes the different names given to the condition, a table which we augmented of Tessier's appellation, which sounds good but is, unfortunately, a French acronym.

Cohen's proposal has been Oculoauriculovertebral spectrum (OAVS). The Fourth edition of Gorlin's book: Syndromes of head and neck [17] sided with this opinion, and the acronym OAVS is widely used. OAVS is often used to include a wider spectrum than CFM and is eagerly used by geneticists, but vertebral involvement is not constant. McCarthy solved this dilemma with the introduction of the term Craniofacial microsomia (CFM), which could be unilateral or bilateral and considers the fact that not only the ear and mandible are involved but that there are associated defects of the temporal bone. CMF is a term that Joseph McCarthy claimed for his paternity and was used in 1977 in Converse's book "Reconstructive Plastic Surgery" [18].

It has been considered the most appropriate for craniofacial teams by the European working group in the craniofacial microsomia [19].

Table 11.1 Left column: given appelation, right column: authors of this appelation

Varied names given to malformations affecting both first and second branchial arches. After Cohen	
Hemifacial microsomia	Gorlin and Pindborg (1964)
Oculoauriculovertebral dysplasia	Gorlin et al. (1963)
Goldenhar syndrome	Sugar (1966)
Goldenhar-Gorlin syndrome	Aleksic et al. (1975)
First arch syndrome	McKenzie (1958)
First and second branchial arch syndrome	Grabb (1965)
Lateral facial dysplasia	Ross (1975)
Familial facial dysplasia	Ide et al. (1970)
Otomandibular disostosis	Francois and Haustrate (1954)
Oral-mandibular-auricular syndrome	Stark and Saunders (1967)
Unilateral mandibulofacial dystosis	Wilson (1958)
Unilateral intrauterine facial necrosis	Walker (1961)
Auriculo-branchiogenic dysplasia	Caronni (1967)
Facio-auriculo-vertebral malformation spectrum	Smith (1982)
Oculoauriculovertebral spectrum (OAVS)	Cohen (1989)
Dysplasie oto mandibulaire (DOM)	Tessier (2001)
Cranio facial microsomia (CMF)	McCarthy (1977)

As craniofacial surgeons, we will side with McCarthy and use CFM. Depending on statistics, with frequent bias because of different criteria for inclusion of patients (minimal set of symptoms present in a patient to include him in the series.), the CFM frequency ranges from 1/3500 to 1/5600, which makes it the second most frequent malformation after the cleft lip and palate. Among patients with CFM, only a few have macrostomia and could be considered Cleft 7. Tasse, 2005, found 9 out of 53 [20]; Beleza-Meneles 13 out of 86 [21]; Birgfield [22] 6 patients out of 39; Caron, 2017 [23] in a multicentric study found 142 macrostomia out of 641 CMF (21%). As a whole, we could agree to a frequency of around 15% ± 5%.

11.5 Authors' Series

Lille series is of 22 macrostomia out of 132 CFM, which makes 16,6%. In Sao Paulo research, in 2008 out of 163 patients with CFM, 24 were found to have macrostomia, which makes 14,7%. More recently, Cristiano Tonello found 57 cases of macrostomia out of his series of 465 CMF, thus 12,25%.

11.6 The Full Spectrum of Cleft 7

11.6.1 Soft Tissue Symptoms

The soft tissue features are of two kinds: those strictly related to the cleft itself; the macrostomia and those related to the CFM and associated symptoms met in syndromic CMF.

11.6.1.1 The Macrostomia in Cleft 7

Macrostomia presents itself as an enlargement of the buccal slit. The considered normal position of the oral commissure has to be appreciated when the patient is at rest without smiling or having any facial mimic. It has at the same time to be in a neutral ocular position looking to the far, straightforward. Then, the buccal commissure has to be on the same vertical as the center of the pupil. When the commissure is medial to this vertical, we have a microstomia, and when it is lateral, we have a macrostomia (Fig. 11.4).

Unfortunately, it could be more difficult when in severe unilateral CFM, the lower face is shifted far from the midline since it could displace the commissure lateral to the pupilar vertical, yet the buccal slit is standard. Then we would measure the distance from the midline to the commissure if the macrostomia affects only one

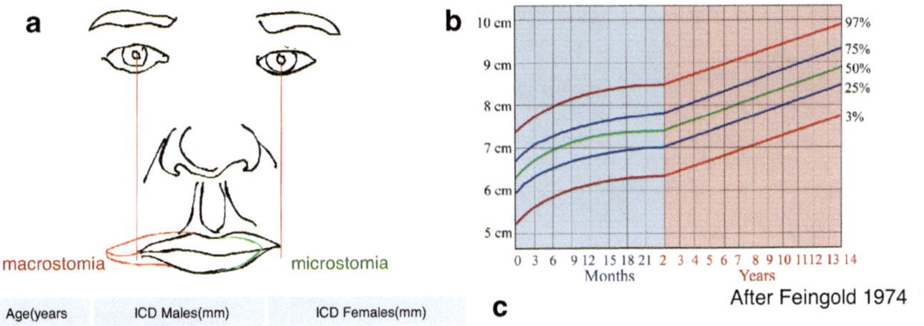

Age(years	ICD Males(mm)	ICD Females(mm)
0-1	32	27
2-3	35	30
4-5	39	36
6-7	42	40
8-9	44	42
10-11	46	43
12-13	48	45
14-15	50	47
18	55	52

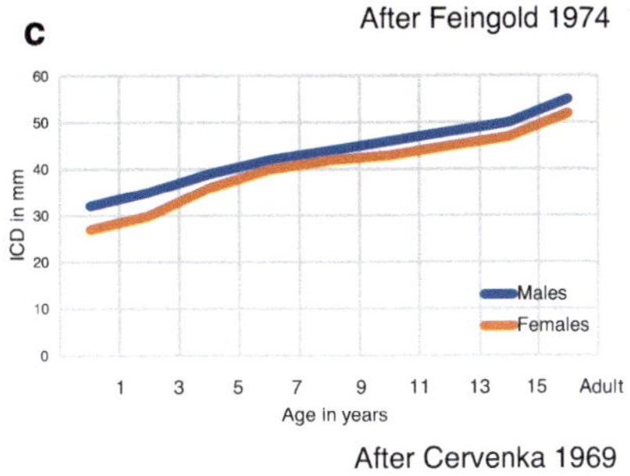

Fig. 11.4 Buccal commissure landmarks. (**a**) Grossly the pupils and buccal commissures are on the same line. (**b**) Chart of inter-pupilar distance, after Feingold. (**c**) Table and chart of buccal inter-commissural distances. We can see that in fact inter-pupilar distance grow larger than buccal inter-commissural distance

side or report the bi-pupilar distance if the position of both orbits is expected; in a few cases of complex craniofacial malformation when no normal landmark is left, we would have to rely upon charts.

The macrostomia in Cleft 7, left aside from the specific signs of CFM or association with other malformation is isolated. That means the cleft reaches either the orbit or the external ear. No alveolar cleft nor cleft palate is in continuity with the cleft commissure. Which, we will see below, is essential for the differential diagnosis.

The macrostomia affects the three layers of the cheek, skin, and muscle by splitting the modiolus and mucosa.

The commissure itself could be either that of a displaced but normal one or an abnormal one when the cutaneous-mucous line is disrupted, then, ever symmetrically. Usually, in that occurrence, the skin takes over the mucosa. The extent of the macrostomia goes from light to severe in a pure subjective appreciation (Fig. 11.5).

11.6.1.2 Associated CMF Symptoms

The full spectrum of CMF could be met in the setting of Cleft 7, and it could be combined with other craniofacial malformations, including other rare Clefts.

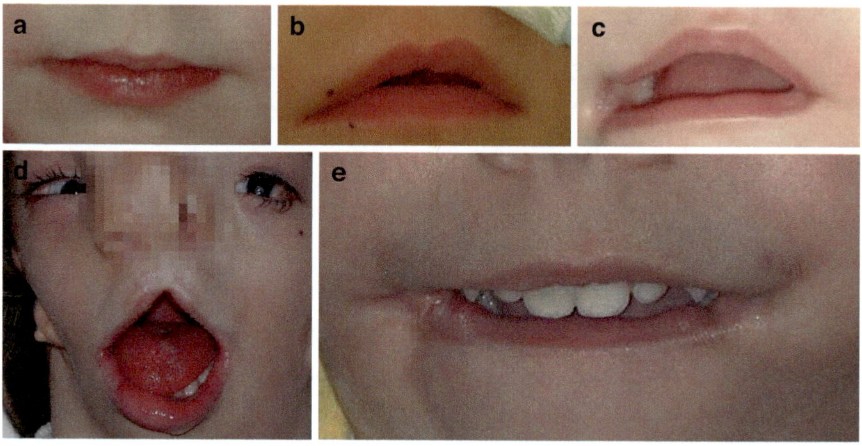

Fig. 11.5 Macrostomia. (**a**) Light. (**b**) Mild. (**c**) Severe. (**d**) In the setting of poly-malformations. (**e**) Bilateral

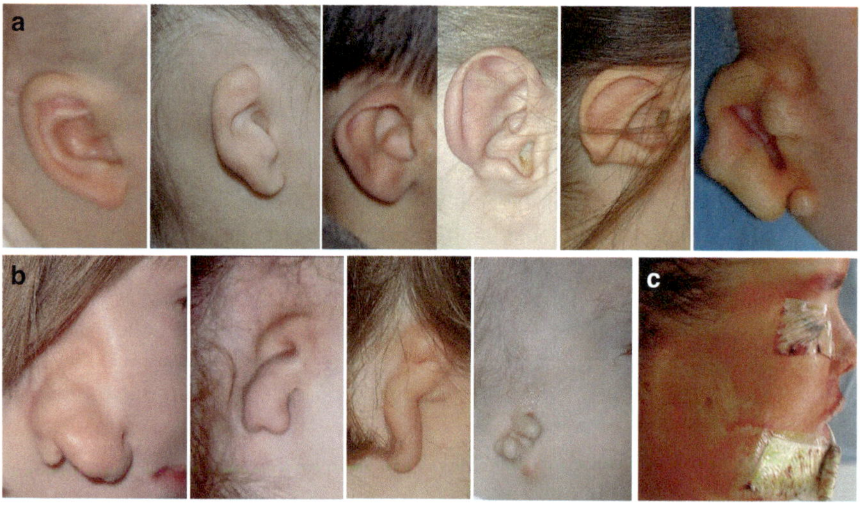

Fig. 11.6 Microtia of increasing severity. (**a**) Smaller ear compared to normal side but normal shape. (**b**) Lobular type the most frequent. (**c**) Total anotia (exceptional)

Microtia (Fig. 11.6)

The severity of microtia could range from a simple size reduction compared to the normal side to a complete anotia (which is quite rare). Most of the time, there are some remnants; most frequently, the lobule is conserved with a small amount of hugely deformed cartilage. Sometimes, the concha is conserved in normal or reduced size, and then the meatus is usually patent.

Many classifications have been proposed, but they are not important for our purpose.

Appendages (Fig. 11.7)

Skin appendages are frequent symptoms of CFM. They range along a line running from the tragus toward the commissure, considered the virtual line of embryonic fusion between the maxillary and mandibular processes of the facia primordia. Lipo-conjunctival tissue could fill those appendages covered by skin or include some cartilage then, they could be called enchondromas. Some huge and complex are called auricular ectopias. On the other hand, the smaller one could be called a tag. Syndromologists call "preauricular tags" the most dorsal, preauricular ones, but they could be found all the same on the cheek or at the commissure.

Some complex appendages, including a cartilaginous frame, are called auricular ectopia.

Sinus (Fig. 11.8)

Dermoid sinus could be associated; the most common are marginal helicine. They must be carefully dissected to reach the temporomandibular joint. Atypical localizations could be either isolated or messed up with the remnants of microtia.

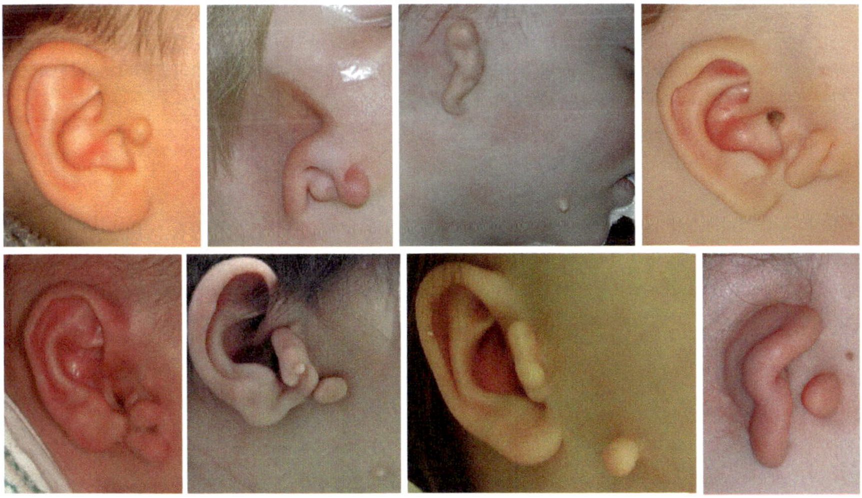

Fig. 11.7 Several types of preauricular and jugal appendages

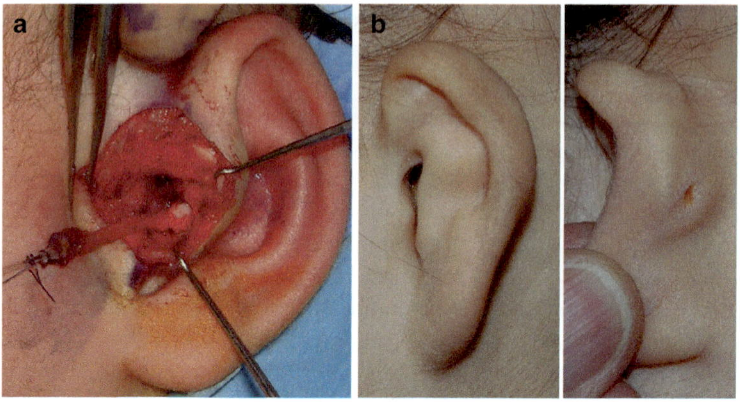

Fig. 11.8 Dermoid sinus. (**a**) Typical marginal helicine sinus. (**b**) Atypical retro-auricular sinus

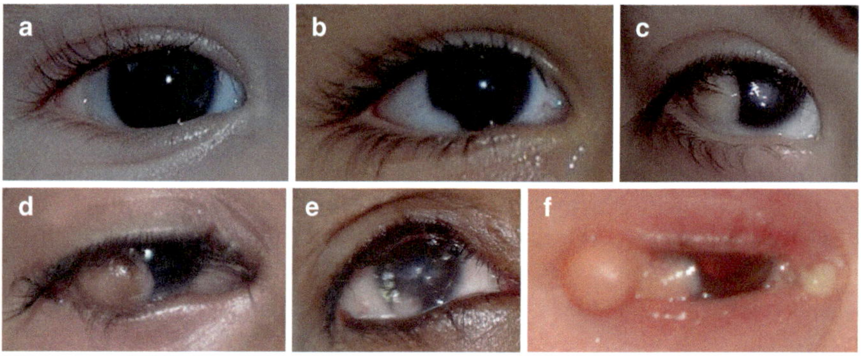

Fig. 11.9 Ocular hamartoma. (**a**) Lipoma subconjunctival. (**b**) Sclero-corneal lipoma. (**c**) Sclero-corneal dermoid. (**d**) Sclero-corneal lipo-dermoid. (**e**) Multiple hamartoma. (**f**) Dermoid hamartoma and Cleft 8

Ocular Hamartoma (Fig. 11.9)

They are part of Goldenhar syndrome and gave rise to the appellation of Oculoauriculovertebral (OAV) syndrome to this specific form of CFM.

They could be histological lipoma or dermoid, as topography subconjunctival or epibulbar.

Soft Tissue Defects

The hypoplasia of soft tissues could affect the muscles, the fat, subcutaneous, and Bichat's pad. Among the superficial muscles, the triangular labii is the most frequently affected, and one could discuss this symptom as facial palsy or muscular aplasia.

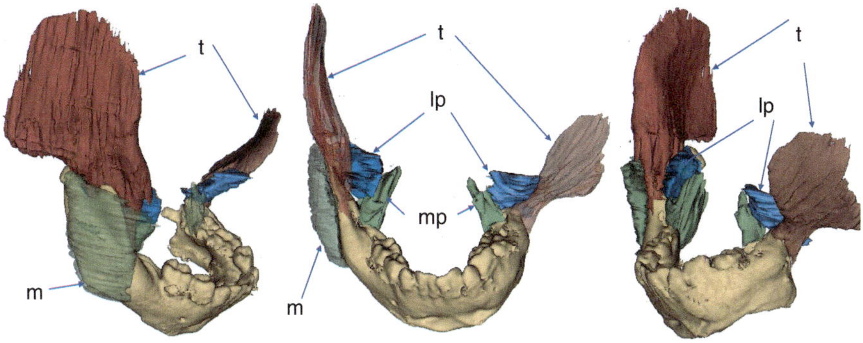

Fig. 11.10 Muscles hypoplasia in CFM, segmentation from a CT scan. *t* temporal muscle, *lp* lateral pterygoid muscle, *mp* medial pterygoid muscle, *m* masseter muscle

The levator muscles of the mandible have a development proportional to the mandibular involvement. A more or less severe muscular hypoplasia is always associated with mandibular hypoplasia and is proportional to it (Fig. 11.10).

Facial Palsy

Facial palsy is a concomitant defect of part of the facial nerve and the corresponding muscle, as said above, the triangular oris is the most frequently affected one.

11.6.2 Skeletal Symptoms

11.6.2.1 Mandibular Hypoplasia (Fig. 11.11)

Most craniofacial surgeons use Pruzansky's classification, which sorts the malformation in three degrees: Type I, when the mandible is decreased in size but has a standard shape, and type II when the size is decreased. The condyle and coronoid processes are still present but deformed, Type III when the ascending ramus is almost absent without discernable remnant of processes. Later, Kaban split type II into two subtypes, A and B [24] Type IIA: The mandibular ramus, condyle, and TMJ are present but hypoplastic and abnormal in shape. Type IIB: The mandibular ramus is hypoplastic and markedly abnormal in form and location, being medial and anterior. There is no articulation with the temporal bone. This led to the so-called "Pruzansky-Kaban classification". But Kaban's ascertainment that in type IIB, there is no muscular insertion to the mandible is untrue since segmentation found the attachment of temporo-masseteric muscle mass and both pterygoid muscles to the stump even in the case of Cleft III (Fig. 11.12).

The diagnosis is, nowadays, easier thanks to 3D CT scan analysis.

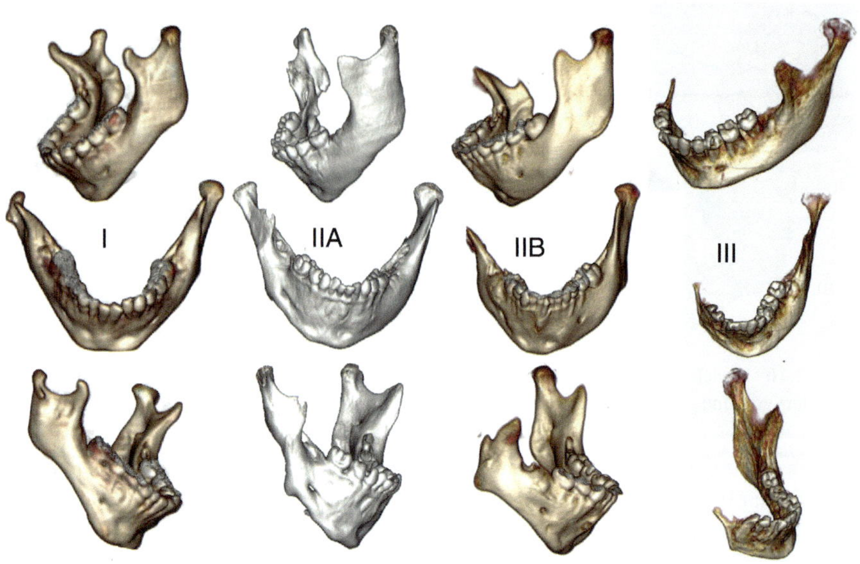

Fig. 11.11 Pruzansky-Kaban classification. I: Prudzansky-Kaban I. IIA: Prudzansky-Kaban IIA. IIB: Prudzansky-Kaban IIB. III: Prudzansky-Kaban III

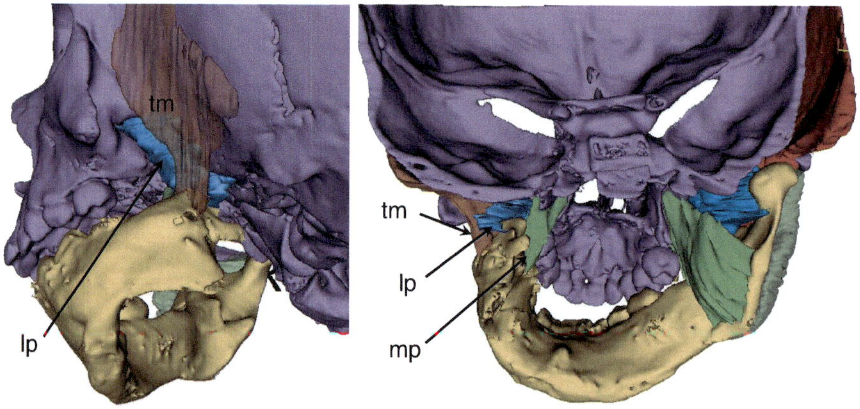

Fig. 11.12 Muscular insertion on Prudzansky's type III. ***tm*** temporo-masseteric muscle, ***lp*** lateral pterygoid muscle, ***mp*** medial pterygoid muscle

11.6.2.2 Craniomaxillary Hypoplasia (Fig. 11.13)

The hypoplasia of the maxilla and temporal bone is not mandatory for the diagnosis. Still, it is more frequent in cases where there is some setting of Goldenhar, which means when there is an association with ocular anomalies such as conjunctival hamartoma.

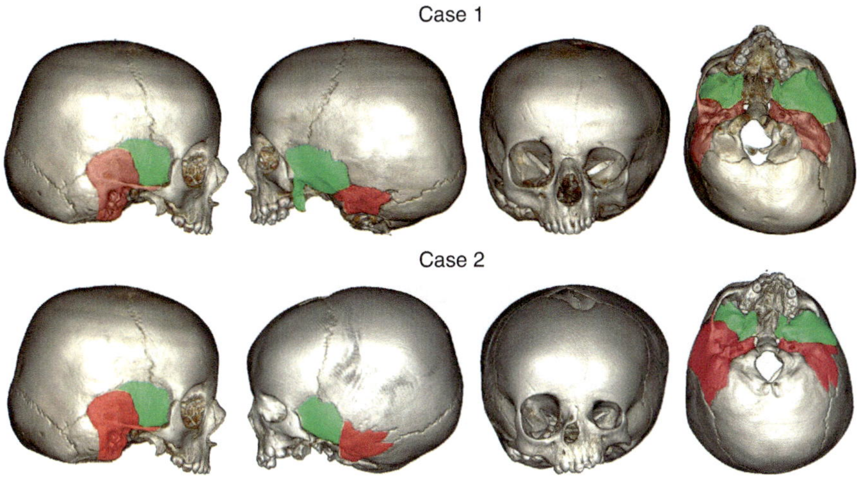

Fig. 11.13 Cranial hypoplasia. Two cases of cranio-maxillary hypoplasia, Green: sphenoid greater wing, Red: temporal bone, Notice that the sphenoid compensates the lack of temporal bone

When the temporal and malar bones are involved, most of the time, there is a gap in the zygomatic arch. hypoplasiaThe temporal bone's involvement mainly affects the squamous part and the zygomatic process. The petrous bone is less severely concerned, and if the external and middle ears are involved in the regional hypoplasia, leading to conductive deafness, it is infrequent that the cochlea itself would be defective, leaving some room for a treatment with a bone-anchored hearing aid.

11.7 Differential Diagnosis (Fig. 11.14)

As seen in the precedent chapter, macrostomia is not exclusively the consequence of Cleft 7 and is a common symptom of other rare Clefts that are grouped under the general term of oblique facial Clefts.

11.7.1 Cleft 5

Cleft 5 is typically an oro-ocular cleft in its complete form, which is then easily distinguished but could be partial and missing the coloboma. It is usually considered that onto the upper lip, the cleft lets intact a segment of the upper lip between the cleft itself and the commissure. Still, it frequently unwraps itself into the lower lip, and the last commissure could be no more discerned. We have then to rely upon the maxillo-palatal components to assess the diagnosis.

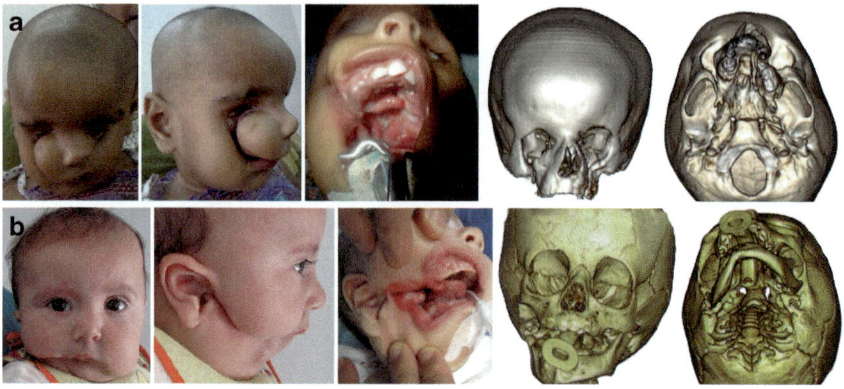

Fig. 11.14 Differential diagnosis. (**a**) Cleft 5 to the right (Cleft 4 to the left). (**b**) Cleft 6C

The maxillary part of Cleft 5 runs across the maxillary lateral to the infra-orbital foramen. The alveolar cleft is in the premolar-molar area, and a mucosal web attaches the apparent commissure to the edge of the alveolar cleft.

When a palatal cleft exists, it is lateral from the alveolar cleft, through the palatal shelve, laterally, the soft palate is cleft in two asymmetric parts by this lateral cleft.

Hence, the intra-oral examination is of the utmost importance to establish the diagnosis.

Remember that Cleft 7 includes neither alveolar nor palatal cleft, save for random association.

11.7.2 Cleft 6

Cleft 6 is an even more difficult diagnosis. When looking at the literature for Cleft 6, we found most published under the erroneous diagnosis of Cleft 7 [25]. We have described above, in detail, the features of Cleft 6, which could head through three different paths.

Clefts 6A, when associated with Cleft 8, are clear even if they could be misdiagnosed for Cleft 5. Cleft 6C has most of the time been confused with Cleft 7, all the most since they impair the external ear, but it is a cleft reaching the concha and not a microtia; the coronoid process of the mandible is hypoplastic, but the condylar process is normal, and we can observe the very specific osseous cleft through the transverse root of the zygomatic process of the temporal bone associated with the supernumerary bone appendage.

Cleft 6B is the most difficult to differentiate since even the CT scan could be confusing, with the gap between the maxillary and the bone and teeth appendage being interpreted as a cleft at the molar alveolar level. This mistake occurred to us before the review of our own cases.

Fortunately, here again, the intra-oral examination is the key: cleft palate, when present, is a most lateral cleft that respects the hard palate and involves the soft palate, from the retro maxillary furrow, obliquely toward the uvula.

The furrow between supplemental teeth from the appendage, in Cleft 6B, must not be interpreted as an alveolar cleft, which is very confusing in transitional dentition patients and needs to be assessed with a CT scan.

11.8 Treatment

11.8.1 Technic (Figs. 11.15, 11.16, and 11.17)

Literature is full of publications dedicated to the repair of macrostomia, whatever is related to clefts 7 or 6 that could be both causes for macrostomia. We have described above, in the Cleft 6 chapter, our preferred technique for macrostomia repairs and the reason for our choice, so we refer the reader to this place for the detailed technical description.

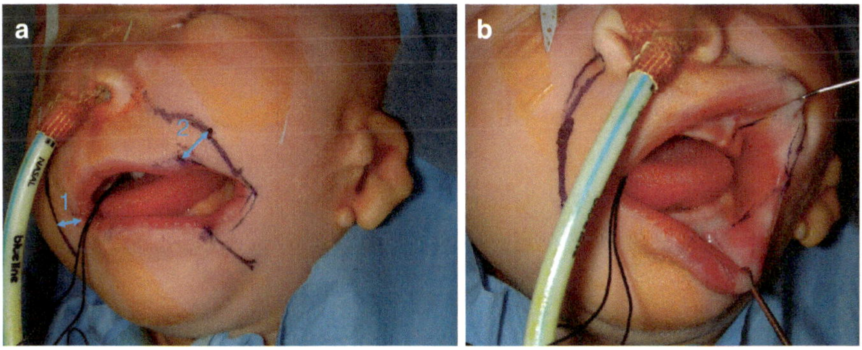

Fig. 11.15 Repair of a Cleft 7 by Z-plasty: flap design: (**a**) the width of the superior flap (2) has the same size that the distance from the commissure to the naso-labial sulcus (1). (**b**) The mucous flaps are opposite to the cutaneous ones

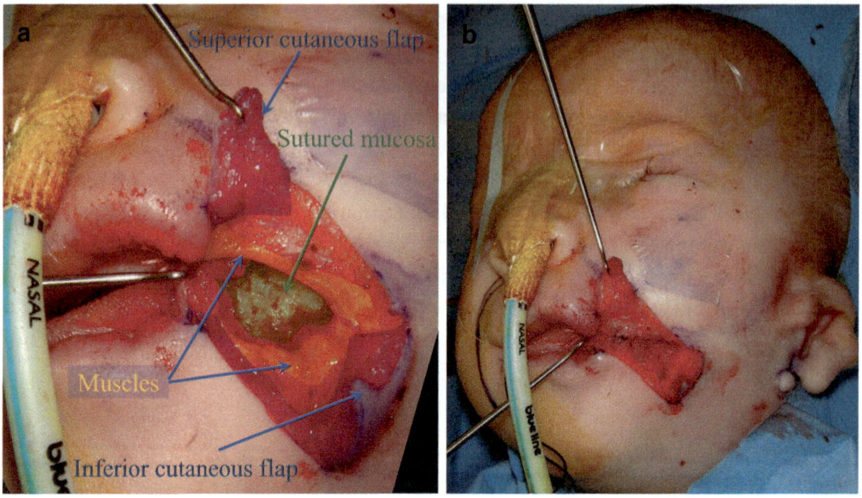

Fig. 11.16 (**a**) dissection showing the muscular defect. (**b**) Accurate repair of muscles

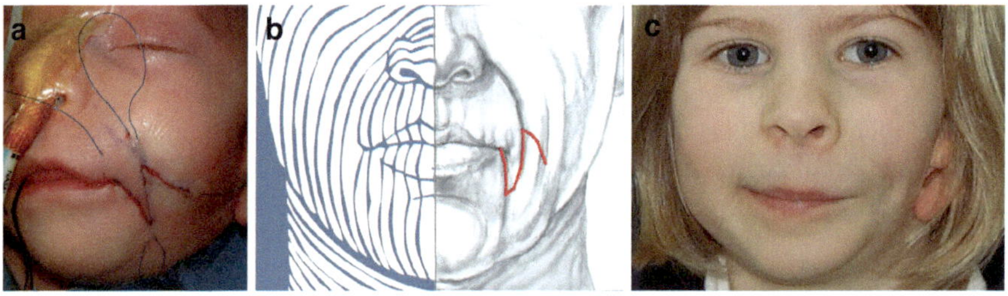

Fig. 11.17 (**a**) suture. (**b**) Relationship with Langer's lines. (**c**) Late result

11.8.2 Indications

Indications could be discussed about the choice of a technique and the timing of the surgery.

11.8.2.1 The Choice of the Technic

At any time, we would avoid complex drawings such as w-w or multiple S [26] because in case of bad results or inappropriate scarring, there is no way to attempt a redo without tissue loss.

Straight-line closure looks simple and could be easily changed to Z-plasty if necessary. Unfortunately, the technique leads to an unnatural commissure, a reason why such techniques as the triangular [27], square mucosal flap [28], or double triangular flap [29] have been advised to fix that problem.

We, personally, side in most of the time with the Z-plasty, and it is only in the most discreet forms of macrostomia that we should consider performing a straight closure since very small Z-plasty are as conspicuous as the ill-located straight scar and do not give the benefit of positive and negative dog ear effect to the 3D correction of the malformation.

11.8.2.2 Timing of Surgery

In patients where macrostomia is the main feature without any massive malformation associated, the treatment of macrostomia could be performed at any time.

But, where the macrostomia is a side aspect of a complex and difficult condition that needs to be addressed, the macrostomia will be postponed to the last stage for two reasons.

When extensive procedures of intra-oral surgery are required, a large mouth opening facilitates the approach. For instance, in patients requiring a mandibular distraction for Prudzansky-Kaban's mandibular hypoplasia type IIB and III, we use it to treat the macrostomia at the time of the device removal.

In patients with complex craniofacial malformation with orbital dystopia, the microstomia surgery is as well postponed as a final touch to give it the optimal imbalance in facial features.

11.8.2.3 Associated Procedures

The quality of the final aesthetical result in a patient affected by macrostomia depends not only on the quality of the macrostomia repair but also on the resolution of associated malformations in the setting of CFM. Skeletal deformity bears a heavy responsibility in facial asymmetry, which is, in turn, of the utmost importance for a balanced mouth position in the face. But correcting skeletal anomalies, even when perfect, does not fix everything. The soft tissue hypoplasia is still present; some skeletal overcorrection could hide a part of it, but lipostructure is a much more effective technique (Figure 7.16d), which at the same time improves the symmetry and could fix some scar adherence when present [30].

11.9 Authors' Cases

11.9.1 Case 1: (Fig. 11.18)

Case of CMF, the first surgery combined a mandibular distraction and a local flap to reconstruct the tragus with an auricular ectopia, to the Z-plasty repair of the macrostomia.

A second mandibular distraction with overcorrection was performed. The last step was a lipostructure.

11.9.2 Case 2: (Fig. 11.19)

In this case of CFM in the setting of Goldenhar's syndrome, associating to CMF an epibulbar hamartoma and vertebral anomalies, the mandibular hypoplasia, Pruzansky-Kaban type III required a mandibular distraction; thus, we decided to combine the macrostomia repair at the time of removing the device. The wide opening allowed, thanks to macrostomia facilitated intra-oral surgery.

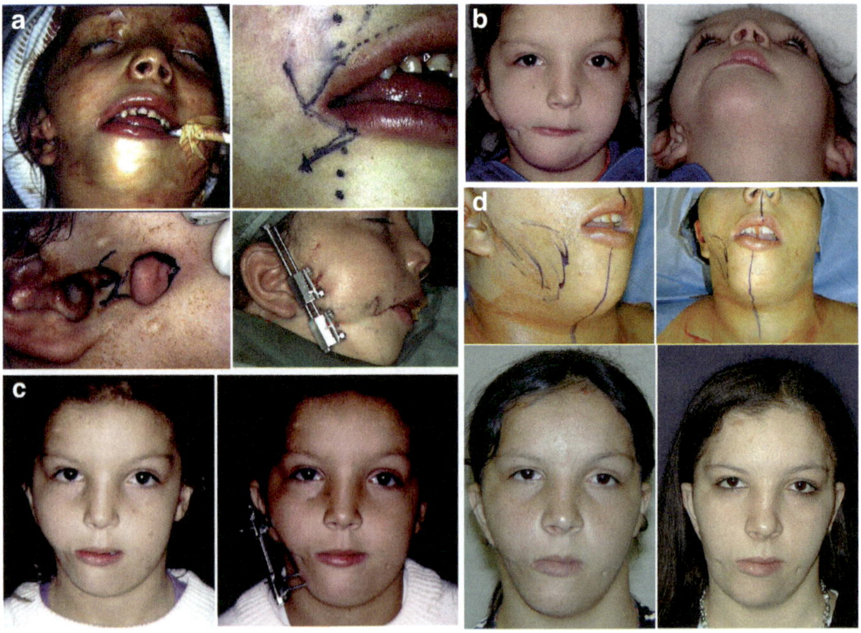

Fig. 11.18 Author's case 1. (**a**) 1993, macrostomia repair, tragus reconstruction with auricular ectopia, mandibular distraction. (**b**) 1994. (**c**) 1995, iterative mandibular distraction. (**d**) 2001, lipostructure, and the final result

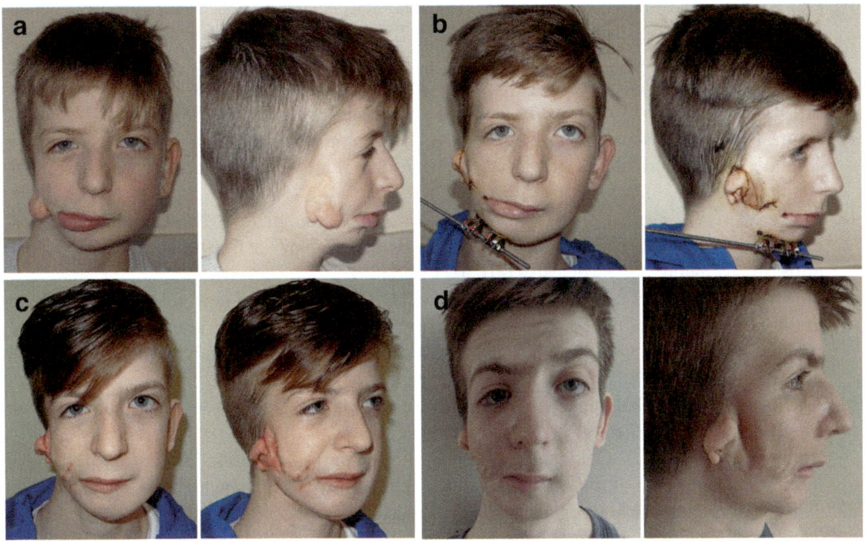

Fig. 11.19 Author's case 2. (**a**) Patient's initial condition. (**b**) Auricular plasty at the time of starting mandibular distraction. (**c**) Macrostomia correction at the time of distraction device removal. (**d**) After laying costal bone graft on the mandible and malar bone

References

1. Woods RH, Varma S, David DJ. Tessier No. 7 cleft: a new subclassification and management protocol. Plast Reconstr Surg. 2008;122(3):898–905. http://journals.lww.com/00006534-200809000-00028.
2. Vermeij-Keers C, Mazzola RF, Van der Meulen JC, Strickler M. Cerebro-craniofacial and craniofacial malformations: an embryological analysis. Cleft Palate J. 1983;20(2):128–45.
3. Tessier P. Anatomical classification of facial, cranio-facial and latero-facial clefts. J Maxillofac Surg. 1976;4:69–92. https://linkinghub.elsevier.com/retrieve/pii/S0301050376800136.
4. Tessier P. Introduction aux dysplasies Oto-mandibulaires (D.O.M.) ou «Vingt ans après ». Ann Chir Plast Esthet. 2001;46(5):381–4. https://linkinghub.elsevier.com/retrieve/pii/S029412600100053X.
5. Förster A. Die Missbildungen des Menschen, systematisch dargestellt, text and atlas. Vol. Text & Atlas. Jena; 1861. 168.
6. Debout. Coup d'oeil sur une des formes les plus rares du bec de liévre, les fissures horizontales. Remarques et observations. Bull Général Thérapeutique Médicale Chir. 1862;(N° 63):13–22. https://services.biusante.parisdescartes.fr/medica-pdf/main.php?key=cGFydGlhbHw5MDAxNHgxODYyeDYzfDEyfDIz.
7. Van Duyse, D. Macrostomes congénitaux avec tumeurs préauriculaires et dermoïdes de l'oeil. Ann Société Médecine Gand. 1882 Aout;36. https://archive.org/details/b2163774x.
8. Poswillo D. The pathogenesis of the first and second branchial arch syndrome. Oral Surg Oral Med Oral Pathol. 1973;35(3):302–28. https://linkinghub.elsevier.com/retrieve/pii/0030422073900704.
9. Fan WS, Mulliken JB, Padwa BL. An association between hemifacial microsomia and facial clefting. J Oral Maxillofac Surg. 2005;63(3):330–4. https://linkinghub.elsevier.com/retrieve/pii/S0278239104015307.

10. Gur M, Edri T, Moody SA, Fainsod A. Retinoic acid is required for Normal morphogenetic movements during gastrulation. Front Cell Dev Biol. 2022;10:857230. https://doi.org/10.3389/fcell.2022.857230/full.
11. Ghyselinck NB, Duester G. Retinoic acid signaling pathways. Dev Camb Engl. 2019;146(13):dev167502. https://www.ncbi.nlm.nih.gov/pmc/articles/PMC6633611/.
12. Naora H, Kimura M, Koizumi T, Tanaka S. Transgenic mouse model of hemifacial microsomia: cloning and characterization of Insertional mutation region on chromosome 10. Genomics. 1994;23(3):515–9.
13. Timberlake AT, Griffin C, Heike CL, Hing AV, Cunningham ML, Chitayat D, et al. Haploinsufficiency of SF3B2 causes craniofacial microsomia. Nat Commun. 2021;12(1):4680. https://www.nature.com/articles/s41467-021-24852-9.
14. Su PH, Yu JS, Chen JY, Chen SJ, Li SY, Chen HN. Mutations and new polymorphic changes in the TCOF1 gene of patients with oculo–auriculo–vertebral spectrum and Treacher–Collins syndrome. Clin Dysmorphol. 2007;16(4):261–7. https://journals.lww.com/00019605-200710000-00008.
15. Kawamoto HK. The kaleidoscopic world of rare craniofacial clefts: order out of chaos (Tessier classification). Clin Plast Surg. 1976;3(4):529–72.
16. Rollnick BR, Kaye CI. Oculoauriculovertebral Spectrum: An Updated Critique. Cleft Palate J. 1989;26(4):276–86. http://cleftpalatejournal.pitt.edu/ojs/cleftpalate/article/view/1287.
17. Gorlin RJ, Cohen MM, Hennekam RCM. Syndromes of the head and neck. 4th ed. Oxford [England]; New York: Oxford University Press; 2001. p. 1283. (Oxford monographs on medical genetics).
18. Converse JM, McCarthy JG, Wood-Smith D, Coccaro PJ. Craniofacial microsomia. In: Marquis J, Joseph MC, editors. Reconstructive plastic surgery. Philadephia: Saunders. http://www.sudoc.abes.fr/cbs//DB=2.1/SET=2/TTL=1/PRS=HOL/SHW?FRST=1&HLIB=940432101#940432101.
19. Renkema RW. European Guideline Craniofacial Microsomia. J Craniofac Surg. 2020;31(8):2385–484. https://doi.org/10.1097/SCS.0000000000006691.
20. Tasse C, Majewski F, Böhringer S, Fischer S, Lüdecke HJ, Gillessen-Kaesbach G, et al. A family with autosomal dominant oculo-auriculo-vertebral spectrum. Clin Dysmorphol. 2007;16(1):1–7. https://journals.lww.com/00019605-200701000-00001.
21. Beleza-Meireles A, Clayton-Smith J, Saraiva JM, Tassabehji M. Oculo-auriculo-vertebral spectrum: a review of the literature and genetic update. J Med Genet. 2014;51(10):635–45. https://doi.org/10.1136/jmedgenet-2014-102476.
22. Birgfeld CB, Heike CL, Saltzman BS, Leroux BG, Evans KN, Luquetti DV. Reliable classification of facial phenotypic variation in craniofacial microsomia: a comparison of physical exam and photographs. Head Face Med. 2016;12(1):14. https://doi.org/10.1186/s13005-016-0109-x.
23. Caron CJJM, Pluijmers BI, Wolvius EB, WN LC, Bulstrode N, Evans RD, et al. Craniofacial and extracraniofacial anomalies in craniofacial microsomia: a multicenter study of 755 patients. J Cranio-Maxillofac Surg. 2017;45(8):1302–10. https://linkinghub.elsevier.com/retrieve/pii/S1010518217302007.
24. Kaban LB, Moses MH, Mulliken JB. Surgical correction of hemifacial microsomia in the growing child. Plast Reconstr Surg. 1988;82(1):9–19.
25. Pellerin P, Tonello C, Freitas DS, Tang XJ, Alonso N. Tessier's cleft number 6 revisited: a series of 26 new cases and literature review of 44: the. Cleft Palate Craniofac J. 2022;60:938. https://doi.org/10.1177/10556656221086459.
26. Bauer BS, Wilkes GH, Kernahan DA. Incorporation of the W-plasty in repair of macrostomia. Plast Reconstr Surg. 1982;70(6):752–6. http://journals.lww.com/00006534-198212000-00019.
27. Hikosaka M, Nakajima T, Ogata H, Miyamoto J. Refined simple line closure for macrostomia repair: designing a mucosal triangular flap on the commissure region. J Cranio-Maxillofac Surg. 2009;37(6):341–3. https://linkinghub.elsevier.com/retrieve/pii/S1010518209000432.

28. Eguchi T, Asato H, Takushima A, Takato T, Harii K. Surgical repair for congenital macrostomia: vermilion square flap method. Ann Plast Surg. 2001;47(6):629–35. http://journals.lww.com/00000637-200112000-00009.
29. Tsumoto J, Imai K, Masuoka T, Sakahara D, Kawamoto K, Kang S, et al. Our surgical repair for Macrostomia with two novel small triangular flaps: long-term follow-up and results. Plast Reconstr Surg. 2018;142(1):63e–7e. http://journals.lww.com/00006534-201807000-00032.
30. Abduch LSF, da Rocha PB, Nasser IJG, Ono MCC, da Freitas RS. Dermal-fat graft for facial contouring in patients with craniofacial microsomia. J Craniofac Surg. 2019;30(7):2134–7. http://journals.lww.com/00001665-201910000-00054.

Chapter 12
Cleft 8

Philippe Pellerin, Nivaldo Alonso, Renato da Silva Freitas, and Cristiano Tonello

> **Pearls**
> Cleft 8 is usually part of a syndrome.
> It is more a symptom than a surgical challenge.

12.1 Original Tessier's Description (Fig. 12.1)

We will quote Tessier himself [1]" *Number eight is a fronto-zygomatic (F. Z.) cleft; it belongs to both the Treacher Collins and the Goldenhar syndromes. However, bony defects predominate in the Treacher-Collins syndrome, while soft tissue malformations are more severe in the Goldenhar syndrome. In the Treacher-Collins syndrome, because of the lack of malar bone, the lateral orbital rim is formed by the greater wing of the sphenoid, whim develops forward and medially. Dermatocele*

P. Pellerin (✉)
Plastic Surgery Department, University of Lille, Lambersart, France

N. Alonso
Department of Plastic Surgery, Universidade de São Paulo, São Paulo, Brazil
e-mail: nivalonso@usp.br

R. da Silva Freitas
Plastic Surgery Unit, Hospital de Clínicas, Universidade Federal do Paraná, Curitiba, Brazil

Craniofacial Surgery, Assistance Center for Cleft Lip and Palate (CAIF), Hospital do Trabalhador, Curitiba, Brazil

C. Tonello
Craniofacial Surgery Department, Universidade de São Paulo, Bauru, São Paulo, Brazil
e-mail: cristianotonello@usp.br

N. Alonso et al. (eds.), *Facial Reconstruction of Unusual Facial Clefts*,
https://doi.org/10.1007/978-3-031-40926-4_12

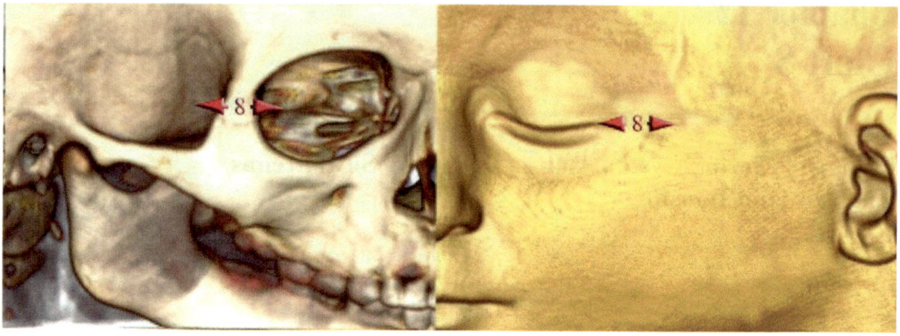

Fig. 12.1 Paths of Cleft 8 on the soft tissues (left) and skeleton (right)

and true cleft of the lateral canthus is part of the Goldenhar syndrome Cleft no. 8 seems to be the cranial correspondent to facial cleft no. 6."

In the Cleft 6 chapter (Chap. 10), we have already discussed the belonging of Treacher Collins's syndrome to the category of rare clefts and dismissed it. We prefer, with others, to remove TCS from this group.

In Tessier's publication, there is nothing more in the text than what is quoted above, so we have to look at the figures. On the general sketch of rare clefts, we can see the line crossing on the skeleton in the middle of the lateral orbital rim at about the level of the frontozygomatic suture. On the skin, the line crosses the lateral canthus.

There is also Fig. 19, in the same text [1], which displays the picture of a cleft 8 splitting the lateral canthus in the setting of Goldenhar's syndrome.

12.2 Cleft 8 in the Literature (Table 12.1)

Cleft 8 seems to be a rare occurrence: Moore [31] did not find a case in the Adelaide series of 170 patients with rare clefts in 1996, and Monasterio, in his 1987 series [32], found only 4 patients out of 176 patients. The only two large series are from Fuente del Campos [28]; he collected 8 cases in 1990, probably including the 3 cited above Monasterio's patients. The second series of 6 cases comes from Lessa [33]. Other publications are reports of a single case. Our research found, as a whole, only 42 published cases, but there is a bias when some reviews of ophthalmological papers speak of coloboma without precision, so the cases of lateral canthus could not be counted.

Table 12.1 Literature cases

Case #	Authors	References	Sex	Side	Epibulbar choristoma	Lateral rim bone defect	Associated cleft	Associated craniofacial pathology	Miscellaneous
1	McMullen (1920)	[2]	M	Left	Yes	No			
2	PS keys (2021)	[3]	M	Left	Yes	No	1–13 right, uclp		
3	Thesun (2021)	[4]		Right	No	No	5 right, 4 left	Bilateral anophtalmia	ABS
4	Muraskas (2003)	[5]	M	Left	No	No	4 left		ABS
5	forum_facmedecine	[6]	F	Left	Yes	No		Zygomatic choristoma, auricular appendage	
6	Sharifi (2016)	[7]		Bilat.	Yes	No			Encephalocraniocutaneous lipomatosis
7	Moog (2009)	[8]	M	Left	Yes	No		Alopecia, zygomatic lipoma	Encephalocraniocutaneous lipomatosis
8	Chandravanski (2014)	[9]	M	Right	Yes	No		Cutaneous dysplasia	Encephalocraniocutaneous lipomatosis
9	Lessa (2020)	[10]	F	Right	Yes	No			
10	Lessa 2020	[10]	F	Left	Yes	No			
11	Lessa (2020)	[10]	F	Right	Yes	No			
12	Lessa 2020	[10]	M		Yes	No			
13	Lessa (2020)	[10]	M		Yes	No			
14	Lessa (2020)	[10]	M		No	No			
15	Uchikawa (2011)	[11]	F	Right	No	Yes	6 right-5 left	Microphtalmia and colobomatous cyst Right	
16	Mayou (1981)	[12]	M	Right	No	Np	6a right-6b left		ABS
17	Morovic (2004)	[13]	F	Right	No	Np	6a Right-6b left		ABS
18	Walker (1961)	[14]	M	Right	No	Np	6a Left-4 Right		
19	Walker (1961)	[14]		Left	No	Np	6a Right-4 Left		

(continued)

Table 12.1 (continued)

Case #	Authors	References	Sex	Side	Epibulbar choristoma	Lateral rim bone defect	Associated cleft	Associated craniofacial pathology	Miscellaneous
20	Fijałkowska (2015)	[15]	M	Bilat.	No	Np	6a Right-6b Left-UCLP		
21	Racz (2017)	[16]	M	Right	Yes	Yes	6a Right- 4 Left	Microphtalmia left	
22	Tessier (1977)	[17]	M	Left	Yes	Np		CFM	
23	Baum (1973)	[18]	M	Right	Yes	Np		CFM	
24	Adeosun (2017)	[19]		Left	No	Np	4 left, cheek atypical right		ABS
25	Becerra-Solano (2018)	[20]	F	Left	No	Yes	13-2 Right-13-2 Left	Cranial encephalocoele	ABS
26	Bouguila (2007)	[21]	F	Right	No	Np	Cheek atypical left- cleft palate		ABS
27	Chavane (1890)	[22]		Left	No	Np	6a right-5 Left	Cranial encephalocoele	ABS
28	Hukki (2004)	[23]	F	Right	No	Np	9 Left, oculo nasal, medial upper lip	Bilateral temporal cranial aplasia	ABS
29	Richardson	[24]	M	Right	No	Yes	10 left	Bilateral temporo parietal cutis aplasia	ABS
30	Schramm (2013)	[25]	F	Left	Yes	Np	3 left-UCLP right	Severe ocular staphyloma	ABS
31	Marchand (1897)	[26]		Right	No	Np	6right, BCLP		ABS
32	Ganesh, (1999)	[27]	F	Left	Yes	No			
33	Antonio Fuente del Campo	[28]							
34	Antonio Fuente del Campo	[28]							

35	Antonio Fuente del Campo	[28]							
36	Antonio Fuente del Campo	[28]							
37	Antonio Fuente del Campo	[28]							
38	Antonio Fuente del Campo	[28]							
39	Antonio Fuente del Campo	[28]							
40	Antonio Fuente del Campo	[28]							
41	Sato (2014)	[29]	F	Right	Yes	No			
42	Pitanguy (1967)	[30]	M	Bilat.	No	Yes	8 bilat.		

12.3 Our Cases of Cleft 8 (Table 12.2)

For this research, we reviewed the files of 18 of our patients, which can be seen in Table 12.2.

Table 12.2 Clinical series

Case #	Sex	Side	Epibulbar choristoma	Lateral rim bone defect	Associated cleft	Associated craniofacial pathology	Miscellaneous
1	F	Bilat.	No	Yes	6 bilat.		
2	F	Right	No	Yes	6 right, 5 right, 4 left.	Microphtalmia right, ocular malf. Left	
3	F	Left	No	Yes	8 left.		
4	F	Right	No	Yes	8right, 5 left	Bilateral microphtalmia	
5	M	Left	No				
6	F	Bilat.	No	Yes	6 right, 4 left, BCL		ABS
7	F	Right	No		6 right, 4 left	Microphtalmia left	
8	F	Left	No		6 left, 4 right	Microphtalmia right	
9	F	Left	No		6 left		
10	M	Left	Yes				
11	M	Right	Yes	Yes			
12	M	Right	No	Yes	4 right, 6 right, UCLP right	CFM	
13	F	Left	No	Yes	6c right, 4 left, uclp left		ABS
14	M	Left	No	No	7 bilat.	CFM	
15	F	Left	No			CFM	
16	M	Right	Yes			CFM	
17	F	Left	No	?	4 left		
18	F	Left	Yes	?	3 right	CFM	

Sex: m for male, f for female. Side: bilat. for bilateral. Associated cleft: number for the rare cleft number, UCLP for unilateral cleft lip and palate, BCLP for bilateral cleft lip and palate. Associated craniofacial anomaly: CFM for craniofacial microsomia. Miscellaneous: ABS for amniotic band syndrome

12.4 The Spectrum of Cleft 8

12.4.1 Cleft Affects the Soft Tissues

Compared to other clefts, the spectrum of cleft 8 is quite simple: The cutaneous cleft is a coloboma of the lateral canthus, which means that the two lateral extremities of both the upper and lower palpebrae are not attached together. The lateral fornix is missing.

According to the associated pathology, the area between the lateral ends of lids could be:

- A cleft lined by an epithelium that could be conjunctival mucosa (Fig. 12.2), but it had never been histologically assessed. In our series and the literature, this cleft has been seen only associated with cleft 6a (see the corresponding chapter). Whenever associated with cleft 6, the canthus is dystopic with a downward slanting.
- Usually, the choristoma is located between the palpebral ends in cases associated with a choristoma (Fig. 12.3a).

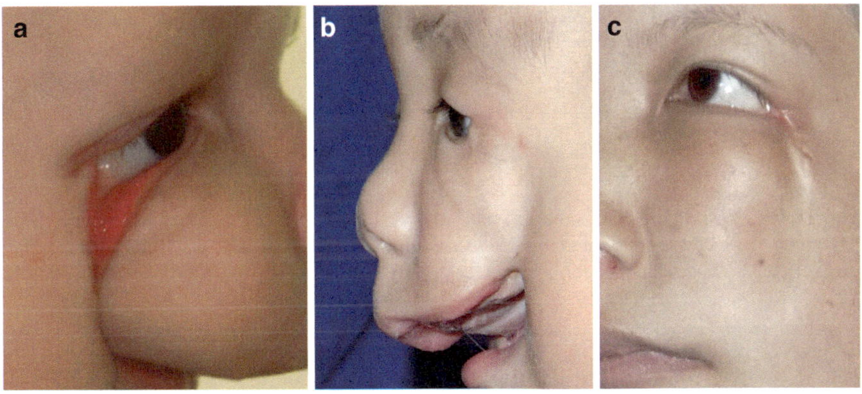

Fig. 12.2 Combination between cleft 8 and 6: (**a**) total; (**b**) mean severity; (**c**) light severity

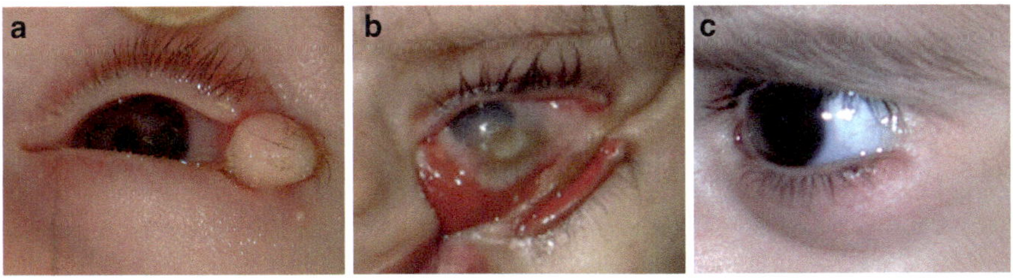

Fig. 12.3 Cleft 8 non associated to cleft 6: (**a**) cleft 8 and choristoma; (**b**) cleft 8 in the setting of an amniotic band syndrome; (**c**) cleft 8 in the setting of Goldenhar syndrome, without conjunctival choristoma

- It is a band of skin in cases isolated or associated with Goldenhar but without choristoma (Fig. 12.3c).
- In cases occurring in the setting of Amniotic Band Syndrome (ABS), the tissue has a cicatricial aspect (Fig. 12.3b).

12.4.2 Cleft Affects the Skeleton

The osseous cleft, when existing, is a defect on the lateral orbital wall. In our series and the literature series, we found a defect of the lateral orbital wall only in cases associated with Cleft 6a (Fig. 12.4) or in complex ABS situations, but we did not have a CT scan for all of the studied patients (Figs. 12.5).

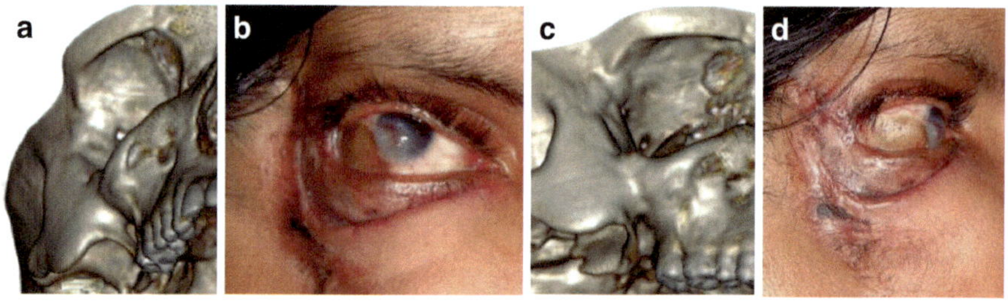

Fig. 12.4 Cleft 8 onto the skeleton: (**a**) and (**c**) reveal the defect of the lateral orbital rim in the patient having a cleft 6 associated to cleft 8 that could be seen in (**b**) and (**d**)**.** (full thickness graft done elsewhere under the palpebra)

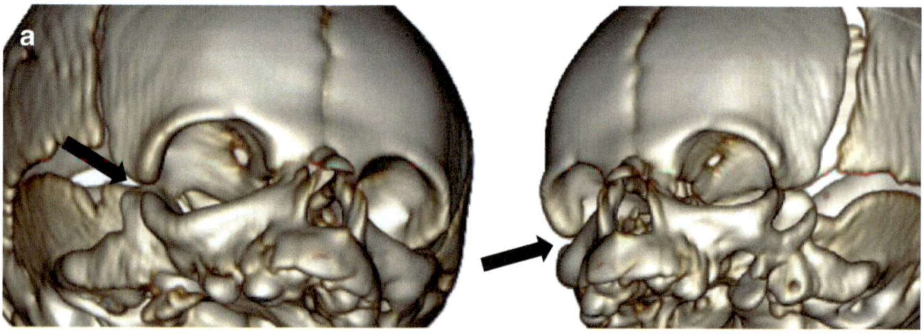

Fig. 12.5 (**a**) Cleft on the skeleton in a bilateral cleft 6 patient. Right side cleft 6a and 8; left side cleft 6b. Arrow to the lateral orbital wall defect. (**b**) Patient with a cleft 8 associated with hamartoma in the setting of CFM. The superposition in vestibular orientation of the patient CT scan (red) with the CT scan of a normal, age matching patient's CT scan (green) demonstrates the defect of the lateral orbital rim

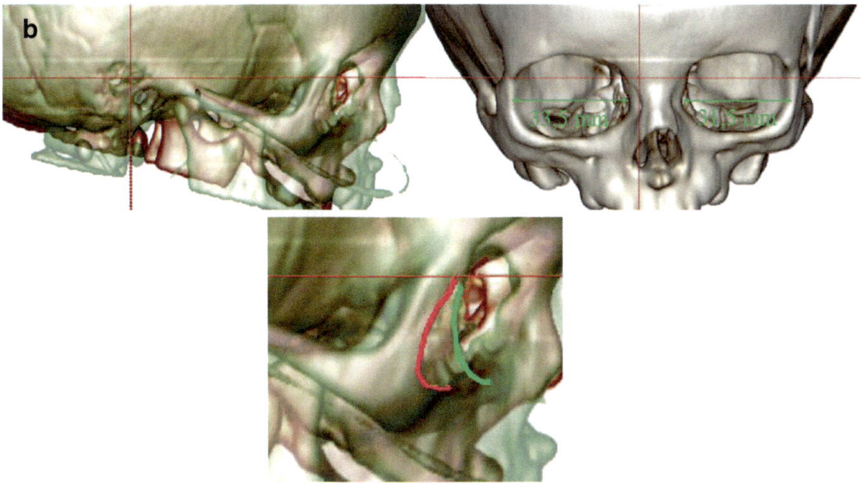

Fig. 12.5 (continued)

12.5 The Phenotypes of Clefts 8

12.5.1 Association Between Clefts 6 and 8 (Fig. 12.2)

It makes sense to give some importance to this association. According to Tessier's rule: the sum of the number of the facial cleft with the corresponding cranial cleft on the same diameter makes 14. Under this condition, 8 is the cranial correspondent to cleft 6.

During the research for cleft 6 (see Chap. 10) [34], we found 55 reported cases of cleft 6 in the literature. Among those 55, 10 were associated with cleft 8. The 10 were 6a under our classification (see Chap. 10).

In our clinical series, 8 out of the 18 patients with cleft 8 were associated with cleft 6.

12.5.2 Association with Other Clefts

The association of cleft 8 with clefts other than Cleft 6 was found 7 times in the literature. All those complex associations were in the setting of the Amniotic Band Sequence. Were associated: clefts 4, 5, 9, 10, and 13.

In our series, 10 out of the 18 were associated with other rare clefts different from cleft 6: clefts 4,5 and 7.

12.5.3 *Association with Ocular Choristomas [35] (Fig. 12.3a)*

The term choristoma designs a congenital tumor of normal histologic components situated in an abnormal location. In the ophthalmologic literature, two types of ocular choristoma are described: epibulbar choristomas and extra conjunctival choristomas.

It happens that epibulbar choristoma: dermoid, lipodermoid could be either isolated or part of a syndrome, as we will see below:

12.5.3.1 In Goldenhar's Syndrome (GS) or (CFM). (Fig. 12.3c)

Several authors report the occurrence of coloboma associated with Goldenhar's syndrome (GS). The most comprehensive papers on this topic were Baum's [18] and Mansour's [36] articles.

Few of the colobomas occurring in GS affect the lateral canthus. Therefore, the association between cleft 8 and current craniofacial microsomia does not come since the association of ocular anomalies with craniofacial microsomia is mandatory for diagnosing GS [37].

In our series, 5 out of 18 cases had a CMF.

12.5.3.2 Cleft 8 and Genodermatosis

Some rare congenital diseases mainly affecting the skin are known to include coloboma in their features. Among them, the encephalocraniocutaneous lipomatosis [7, 8] frequently consists of an association between conjunctival dermo lipoma and cleft of the lateral canthus. Colobomas are also frequent in cases of nevus epidermal syndrome, including lateral canthus splitting.

12.5.3.3 Cleft 8 and Isolated Choristoma

The association of Cleft 8 with choristomas is relatively frequent and has already been quoted above. This association is usually encountered in Goldenhar's syndrome, in which choristoma is one of the cardinal signs, but it can be isolated.

12.5.4 *Cleft 8 and ABS (Fig. 12.3b)*

Out of the 60 cases (42 from the literature and 18 from our clinical series), 14 were in the setting of ABS, noticeably the older observation of Chavane where it was associated with Cleft 6 [22]. Coady, in his paper: *Amniotic Band Syndrome: The Association Between Rare Facial Clefts and Limb Ring Constrictions* [38], did not find a case of cleft 8, but the patients in his series were the same that in Moore's series [31] and in Epley's series [39] which did not include cases with cleft 8.

Assigning a diagnosis to the eyelid alterations in the setting of ABS is an arduous problem. They usually come as a scarring band, oblique across the face from the bottom to the top and from inside to outside, toward the temporoparietal area of the scalp, where they leave a bald line.

This path runs across the orbitopalpebral area, but only a slight difference in its direction will change the number of the rare cleft we will attribute to its diagnosis. Still, this difference is unimportant: the treatment will be almost the same, and the underlying process that induces such malformation is the same, whatever the cleft number.

12.5.5 Isolated Cleft 8

In its paper: "Congenital Craniofacial Anomalies of Ophthalmic Importance" [40] Fries stated, "*Cleft number 8 runs laterally from the lateral canthal angle toward the frontozygomatic suture. Rare in its isolated form, it usually causes a true lateral canthal coloboma, often with a fusion of the edges of the lid defect to the bulbar conjunctiva. An underlying bony defect may also be present with the number 8 cleft.*"

In fact, out of the literature review as well as in our series, we could not find a case of purely isolated cleft 8 with the exception of a Lessa's patient in his series of 6 lateral canthal clefts in which the 5 other cases had an associated choristoma [10]. In our series, we tried to find a single case of this kind.

12.6 Differential Diagnosis

The differential diagnoses for Cleft 8 are with the neighbouring coloboma, cleft 5 and cleft 9.

12.6.1 Cleft 5 (Fig. 12.6)

The association of Cleft 6 with Cleft 8 could be easily confused with Cleft 5, and it has been a standard error in our series to missort cleft 6 as cleft 5 before having a better knowledge of the Cleft 6 anatomy. The position of the cleft on the lip is very close, and it could be difficult to recognize the lateral part of the upper lip in cleft 5, the lateral oral commissure being unfolded in the posterior edge of the cleft. The position of the cleft on the lip is very close, and it could be challenging to recognize the lateral part of the upper lip in cleft 5, and the being of lateral oral commissure unfolded in the posterior edge of the cleft.

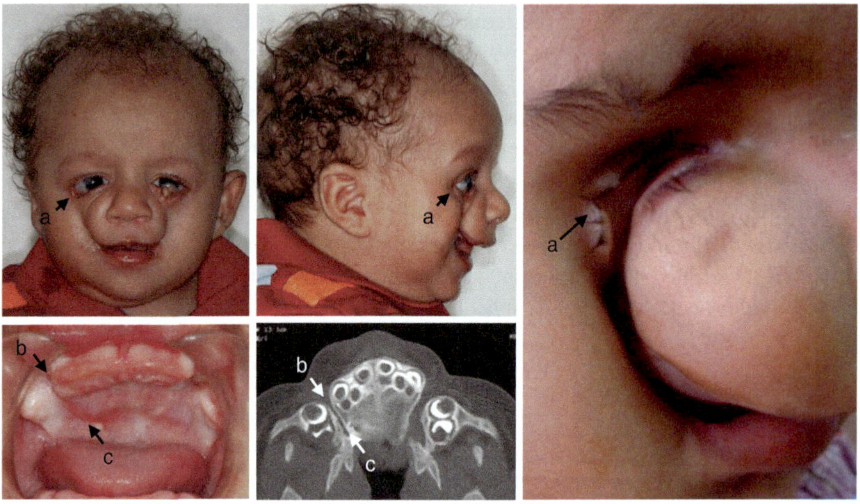

Fig. 12.6 Differences between cleft 5 and 8: (**a**) the coloboma respects the lateral canthus and let a lateral stump of inferior palpebra laterally to the coloboma. (**b**) The alveolar cleft is through the decidual molar area (do not confuse with the sulcus between the tuberosity and an osteo-dental ectopic appendage). (**c**) The cleft plate involve the hard palate from the alveolar cleft

It is easier with the lateral canthus but not evident at any time. The best way to find out is to check the intraoral part of the cleft: Cleft 5 comes across the alveolar ridge at the level of the molar area. In contrast, cleft 6 lets the alveolar ridge alone, crossing the skeleton behind the maxillary tuberosity. When existing, the cleft palate involves a part of the hard palate laterally and the soft palate asymmetrically. The point is that the alveolar ridge is involved since the oblique soft palate cleft looks remarkably like the one of cleft 6. In case of persisting doubt, certainty would come along with the CT scan.

12.6.2 Choristoma Without Canthus Cleft

If a cleft 8 could be observed in Goldenhar syndrome, even in the absence of choristoma (which is a strong argument for denying the responsibility of choristoma for the canthus clefting.), it is most frequent that a choristoma, even large, would be present without consequence for the canthus.

12.6.3 Cleft 9 (Fig. 12.7)

The differential diagnosis with cleft 9 could be discussed in some ABS since, in ABS, the defect is usually irregular with a scarring aspect, and the position of the coloboma onto the upper lid is very close to the lateral canthus; a careful

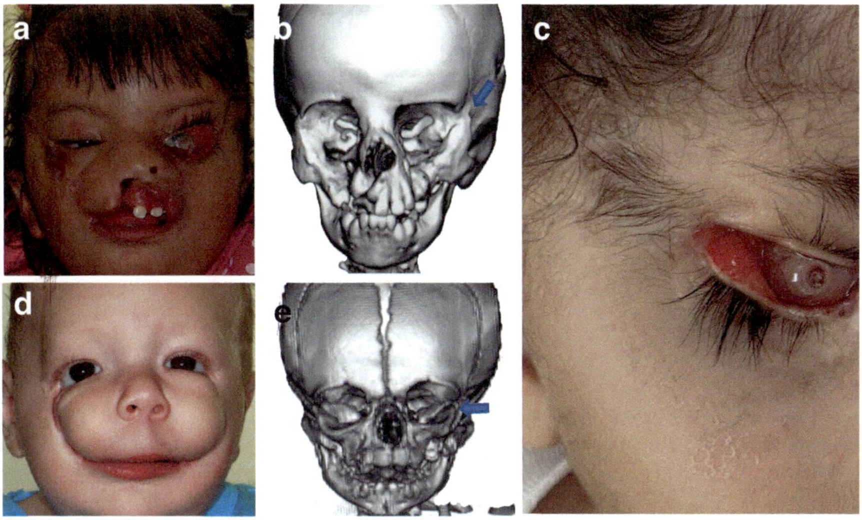

Fig. 12.7 Differences between cleft 8 and 9: (**a–c**) patients with bilateral cleft 9. (**d** and **e**) Patient with bilateral cleft 8. Blue arrows point toward the skeletal defect

examination would recognize an intact lateral canthus laterally to the coloboma. In the end, the distinction is not very important and is of little consequence for the treatment. When existing, the skeletal defect is pathognomonic.

12.7 Treatment of Cleft 8

12.7.1 Cleft 8 Associated with Cleft 6 (Figs. 12.8 and 12.9)

When associated with cleft 6, cleft 8 has to be addressed in the same procedure. There is not only a lateral canthal coloboma but a dystopia due to a double mechanism: shortening of the distance between the oral commissure and the lateral canthus as well as a defect of the lateral orbital rim with a lack of attachment of the lateral canthus. Thus, the correction must address the soft-tissue defect and the osseous defect.

The soft-tissue shortening could be corrected along the whole length of cleft 6–8 by combining a Z-plasty (double opposition cutaneous and mucosal Z-plasty, see macrostomia in Chaps. 10 and 11) to the level of macrostomia with to the canthus level, a hetero-palpebral flap.

The osseous defect is repaired with a bone graft, and we like a large on-lay cranial cortical bone graft over the cleft malar bone. A lateral canthopexy is then performed through the reconstructed lateral orbital rim.

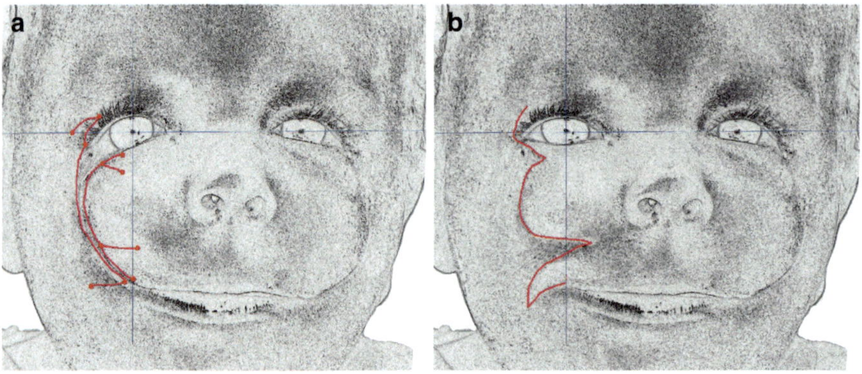

Fig. 12.8 Drawing in case of cleft 8 association to cleft 6a: cutaneous Z-plasty (as part of a double Z-plasty, the second Z-plasty is intra-buccal mucous opposite Z-plasty) to the level of macrostomia and hetero-palpebral flap which, in fact has the shape of a Z-plasty. (**a**) pre-operative drawing; (**b**) position of the flaps to the end. A third Z-plasty could be necessary at cheek level

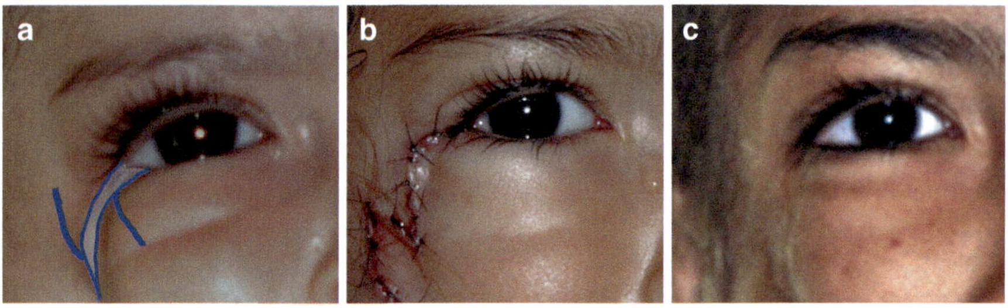

Fig. 12.9 A different flap design for repair of cleft 8 associated to cleft 6, the Z-plasty is drawn in zygomatic area: (**a**) pre-surgical drawing; (**b**) after surgery completion; **c** long term aspect

12.7.2 Cleft 8 and Epibulbar Choristoma (Fig. 12.10)

The choristoma is usually a dermoid or lipodermoid that has to be resected previously to the canthopexy and suture of the two lids to reconstruct the lateral canthus. If requested, the resection of the epibulbar choristoma must be conservative. Most are limbal or subconjunctival. Very few cases are corneal; in this occurrence, most authors prefer excising the dermoid by a superficial keratectomy [18]. The resection of dermo lipoma, which presents itself as a subconjunctival adipose tissue overlaid with some conjunctiva that is sometimes thickened, keratinized and wearing hair follicles, must be conservative. The posterior limit of lipoma is mostly uncertain, seemingly to continuity into the orbital fat without a clear limit.

The resection must take care of several points [41]: respecting the area of lachrymal ducts to avoid xeropthalmia; keeping as much as conjunctiva that could be

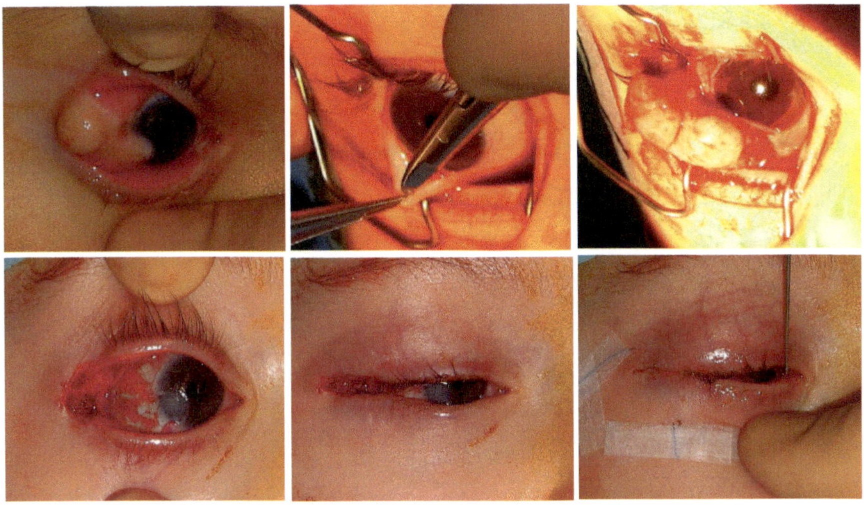

Fig. 12.10 Resection of a choristoma and canthoplasty

dissected off the underlying lipoma; removing only the anterior part of the lipoma without any attempt to dissect the orbital fat.

When hairs and keratinized conjunctiva have had to be respected, the conjunctival suture could require some tension, and authors have advised local flaps or even free conjunctival graft [42]. When the resection is over, the lateral canthus can be repaired.

After excessive resection of dermo lipoma, the complications could be xerophthalmia, palpebral ptosis, or strabismus.

12.7.3 Cleft 8 Isolated with a Large Band of Skin (Fig. 12.11)

Two authors have published specific techniques for reconstructing lateral canthus in cases in which a large band of skin was interposed between the two lateral ends of lids. Tessier [17] and Fuente del Campo [28]. Tessier raises the skin band as a flap, closes the conjunctiva by direct approximation, and performs a canthopexy through a hole in the lateral orbital rim. Fuente del Campo splits the cutaneous band into two flaps that he inserts in two incisions along the palpebral ciliary edge. The underlying fibrous tissue, considered as being what would have been the lateral canthal ligament, is secured to a hole drilled in the lateral orbital rim, and the upper and lower orbicularis muscles are interdigitated. The two flaps fulfil the gaps created by the rotation of the lateral palpebral rims.

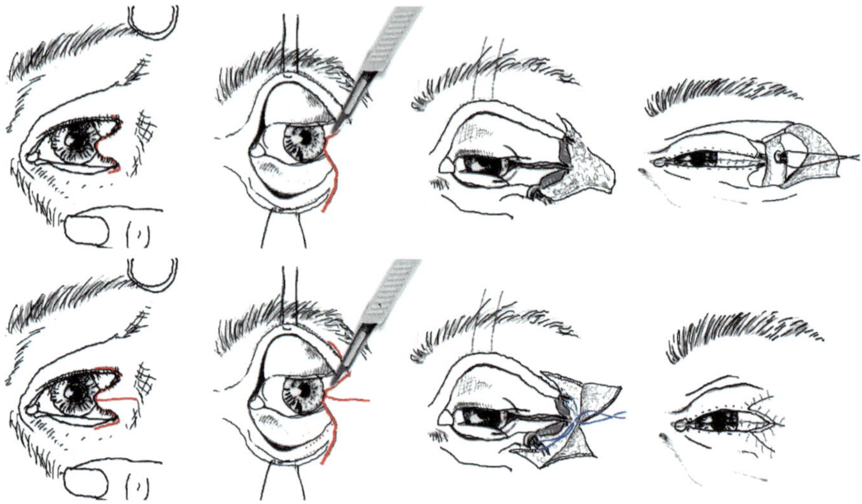

Fig. 12.11 Top: canthoplasty for cleft 8, after Tessier. Bottom: Double Z-plasty after Campos dos Santos

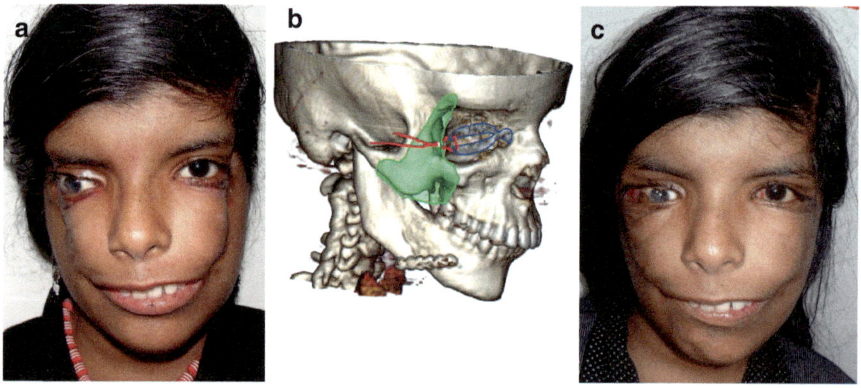

Fig. 12.12 Split cranial cortical graft to reconstruct the malar bone defect and lateral canthopexy through it. (**a**) Before surgery; (**b**) technical sketch; (**c**) after surgery

12.7.4 Reconstruction of Skeletal Defect (Fig. 12.12)

The need for reconstruction of the lateral orbital rim is not usually met in isolated cleft 8. To the contrary, in the association of cleft 8 with cleft 6, there is a considerable defect affecting both the orbital rim and the body of the malar bone. Our preferred technic for repair is, then, to perform a cortical graft, harvested from the parietal area and a canthopexy through the part of the graft that reconstruct the lateral orbital rim.

12.8 Discussion

12.8.1 Cleft 8 and Mandibulo Facial Dysostosis

Tessier's cleft 8 original description [1, 17], which, one has to remember, was published before the availability of CT scans and macromolecular genetics, was a bit confusing. He quoted cleft 8 as part of Treacher Collins syndrome (TCS) together with clefts 6 and 7: "*No. 6, 7 and 8 belong together and comprise the Treacher Collins-Franceschetti syndrome. N°. 7 is more specifically related to hemifacial microsomia, and N°. 8 to Goldenhar syndrome*." He quoted TCS as including a cleft 8 because of the gap between the hypoplastic malar bone and the orbital process of the frontal bone that was misinterpreted in the first artist drawing of his 1977 publication. This drawing of a presumptive Treacher Collins skeleton is erroneous; it displays a cleft between the maxillary and the malar bone when we know that the hypoplastic malar is attached to the hypoplastic maxillary and that the gap is between the malar and the orbital process of the frontal bone. It could indeed be considered a defect of the lateral orbital rim and a cleft 8, but it is not correlated to a cleft of soft tissues.

On the other hand, we now know the TCS setting due to the TCS gene mutation responsible for default in Neural Crest Cells (NCC) migration, and we prefer to remove TCS and other mandibulofacial syndromes from the category of rare clefts.

12.8.2 The Role of Choristoma in Clefting the Lateral Canthus

According to Baum, according to Goldenhar's syndrome (GS), most colobomas were associated with dermolipoma (92% in his series and literature review). It is not surprising since, according to Gorlin [43], an epibulbar dermoid is mandatory to assess GS diagnosis. Mansour [36] describes a lower proportion of coloboma in GS and underlines cases where the dermolipoma could not be held responsible for the occurrence of the coloboma.

So, the hypothesis that the presence of choristoma was a mechanical cause for the default of lids fusion at the level of lateral canthus started to be disputed.

It was a tremendous intuition from Mann in 1937 [44], which was corroborated by Sinha and Mishra in 1950 [45], that the cleft should not be due to the choristoma presence but to a common origin and identic mechanism. From analyzing the literature and cases and research on rare clefts in general, particularly those arising in the setting of ABS, we should tend to this opinion.

References

1. Tessier P. Anatomical classification of facial, cranio-facial and latero-facial clefts. J Maxillofac Surg. 1976;4:69–92. https://linkinghub.elsevier.com/retrieve/pii/S0301050376800136.
2. Mcmullen WH. Congenital malformation in the outer canthus. Proc R Soc Med. 1920;13(Sect_Ophthalmol):85–6. https://doi.org/10.1177/003591572001301738.
3. Craniofacial clefts. Plastic Surgery key; 2023. https://plasticsurgerykey.com/rare-craniofacial-clefts-2/.
4. Boy born with no eyes cleft palate. https://www.thesun.co.uk/news/5755759/boy-born-with-no-eyes-cleft-palate/.
5. Muraskas JK, McDonnell JF, Chudik RJ, Salyer KE, Glynn L. Amniotic band syndrome with significant orofacial clefts and disruptions and distortions of craniofacial structures. J Pediatr Surg. 2003;38(4):635–8. https://linkinghub.elsevier.com/retrieve/pii/S0022346802631501.
6. Cas diagnostic fac. 2023. https://forum.facmedicine.com/attachments/81faec3bf06fbb79ea039b5efcd05c6f-jpg.21965/.
7. Sharifi M, Namdari M. Encephalocraniocutaneous lipomatosis (Fishman syndrome): a rare neurocutaneous syndrome. J Curr Ophthalmol. 2016;28(3):155–8. https://linkinghub.elsevier.com/retrieve/pii/S2452232516300695.
8. Moog U. Encephalocraniocutaneous lipomatosis. J Med Genet. 2009;46(11):721–9. https://doi.org/10.1136/jmg.2009.066068.
9. Chandravanshi S. Encephalocraniocutaneous lipomatosis: a case report and review of the literature. Indian J Ophthalmol. 2014;62(5):622. https://doi.org/10.4103/0301-4738.133521.
10. Lessa S, Sebastiá R, Pontello J. Lateral Canthal clefts of the eyelid. Ophthal Plast Reconstr Surg. 2019;35(5):491–4. https://doi.org/10.1097/IOP.0000000000001353.
11. Uchikawa Y, Ogata H, Hattori N, Miyamoto J, Nakajima T. Palatoplasty for bilateral oblique cleft of the soft palate accompanied by Tessier number 5–7 cleft. Cleft Palate Craniofac J. 2011;48(2):231–5. https://doi.org/10.1597/09-068.
12. Mayou BJ, Fenton OM. Oblique facial clefts caused by amniotic bands. Plast Reconstr Surg. 1981;68(5):675–81. http://journals.lww.com/00006534-198111000-00001.
13. Morovic CG, Berwart F, Varas J. Craniofacial anomalies of the amniotic band syndrome in serial clinical cases. Plast Reconstr Surg. 2004;113(6):1556–62. http://journals.lww.com/00006534-200405000-00003.
14. Walker G. Malformations of the face. Edinburgh and London: E&S Livingstone Ltd.; 1961. p. 202.
15. Fijałkowska M, Antoszewski B. Rare facial clefts. Pol J Surg. 2015;87(8):389–94. https://www.degruyter.com/view/j/pjs.2015.87.issue-8/pjs-2015-0077/pjs-2015-0077.xml.
16. Racz C, Dakpé S, Kadlub N, Testelin S, Devauchelle B, Rachwalski M, et al. Phenotypic spectrum of Tessier facial cleft number 5. J Cranio-Maxillofac Surg. 2018;46(1):22–7. https://linkinghub.elsevier.com/retrieve/pii/S1010518217303517.
17. Tessier P. Nouvelle Classification Anatomique Des Fentes Faciales Cranio-Faciales Et Latéro-Latérales, Leur Rëpartition Autour De L'orbite. In: Rougier J, Société française d'ophtalmologie, editors. Chirurgie plastique orbito-palpébrale. Paris; New York: Masson; 1977.
18. Baum JL, Feingold M. Ocular aspects of Goldenhar's syndrome. Am J Ophthalmol. 1973;75(2):250–7. https://linkinghub.elsevier.com/retrieve/pii/0002939473910209.
19. Adeosun OO, James O, Akinmoladun VI, Owobu T. Amniotic band syndrome associated with orofacial clefts: a report of two cases: amniotic band syndrome. Oral Surg. 2012;5(4):185–9. https://doi.org/10.1111/j.1752-248X.2012.01163.x.
20. Becerra-Solano LE, Castañeda-Cisneros G, Corona-Rivera JR, Díaz-Rodríguez M, Figuera LE, López-Muñoz E, et al. Severe craniofacial involvement due to amniotic band sequence. Fetal Pediatr Pathol. 2018;37(1):27–37. https://doi.org/10.1080/15513815.2017.1392663.
21. Bouguila J, Ben Khoud N, Ghrissi A, Bellalah Z, Belghith A, Landolsi E, et al. Maladie des brides amniotiques et malformations faciales. Rev Stomatol Chir Maxillofac. 2007;108(6):526–9. https://linkinghub.elsevier.com/retrieve/pii/S0035176807002148.

22. Chavane A. Malformation faciale (section par bride amniotique). Bull Société Anat Paris. 1890;5(4):137–41. https://gallica.bnf.fr/ark:/12148/bpt6k6327302h/f159.item#.
23. Hukki J, Balan P, Čeponiene R, Kantola-Sorsa E, Saarinen P, Wikstrom H. A case study of amnion rupture sequence with Acalvaria, blindness, and Clefting: clinical and psychological profiles. J Craniofac Surg. 2004;15(2):185–91. http://journals.lww.com/00001665-200403000-00002.
24. Richardson S, Khandeparker RV, Pellerin P. Amniotic constriction band: a report of two cases with unique clinical presentations. J Korean Assoc Oral Maxillofac Surg. 2017;43(3):171. https://doi.org/10.5125/jkaoms.2017.43.3.171.
25. Schramm C, Rohrbach JM, Reinert S, Mau-Holzmann UA, Aisenbrey S, Bartz-Schmidt KU, et al. Amniotic bands as a cause of congenital anterior staphyloma. Graefes Arch Clin Exp Ophthalmol. 2013;251(3):959–65. https://doi.org/10.1007/s00417-012-2197-z.
26. Marchand F. Missbildungen. In: Eulenburg A, editor. Real-Encyclopädie der gesammten Heilkunde. Wien; Leipig.: Urban and Schwarzenberg; 1897. p. 423–596; (Medicinisch-chirurgisches Handwo}rterbuch fu"r praktische Aerzte).
27. Ganesh A, Rangaswamy M. Pedunculated dermolipoma with overlying upper lid coloboma and absent lateral canthus: cause and effect? Eye. 1999;13(5):687–9. http://www.nature.com/articles/eye1999194.
28. Fuente-del-Campo A. Surgical correction of Tessier number 8 cleft. Plast Reconstr Surg. 1990;86(4):658–61; discussion 662–663.
29. Sato N, Kuroki T, Tosa Y, Shimizu Y, Kusano T, Yoshimoto S. A case of orbital lipoma that occurred in the lateral Canthal region of the Tessier no. 8 craniofacial cleft. Mod Plast Surg. 2014;04(02):32–4. https://doi.org/10.4236/mps.2014.42007.
30. Pitanguy I, Franco T. Nonoperated facial fissures in adults. Plast Reconstr Surg. 1967;39(6):569–77. http://journals.lww.com/00006534-196706000-00005.
31. Moore MH. Rare craniofacial clefts. J Craniofac Surg. 1996;7(6):408–11. http://journals.lww.com/00001665-199611000-00003
32. Monasterio FO, del Campo AF, Dimopulos A. Nasal clefts. Ann Plast Surg. 1987;18(5):377. http://journals.lww.com/00000637-198705000-00004.
33. Lessa S, Pontello J, Duarte D, Costa W, Persichetti P. Lateral canthal choristomas associated with colobomas of lateral canthus. Eur J Plast Surg. 2021;44(2):269–74. https://doi.org/10.1007/s00238-020-01701-4.
34. Pellerin P, Tonello C, da Silva FR, Tang XJ, Alonso N. Tessier's cleft number 6 revisited: a series of 26 new cases and literature review of 44. Cleft Palate Craniofac J. 2022;60:105566562210864. https://doi.org/10.1177/10556656221086459.
35. Mansour AM, Barber JC, Reinecke RD, Wang FM. Ocular choristomas. Surv Ophthalmol. 1989;33(5):339–58. https://linkinghub.elsevier.com/retrieve/pii/0039625789900118.
36. Mansour AM, Wang F, Henkind P, Goldberg R, Shprintzen R. Ocular findings in the Facioauriculovertebral sequence (Goldenhar-Gorlin syndrome). Am J Ophthalmol. 1985;100(4):555–9. https://linkinghub.elsevier.com/retrieve/pii/0002939485906816.
37. Tuin J, Tahiri Y, Paliga JT, Taylor JA, Bartlett SP. Distinguishing Goldenhar syndrome from craniofacial Microsomia. J Craniofac Surg. 2015;26(6):1887–92. https://journals.lww.com/00001665-201509000-00020.
38. Coady MSE, Moore MH, Wallis K. Amniotic band syndrome: the association between rare facial clefts and limb ring constrictions. Plast Reconstr Surg. 1998;101(3):640–9. http://journals.lww.com/00006534-199803000-00010.
39. Eppley BL, David L, Li M, Moore CA, Sadove AM. Amniotic band facies. J Craniofac Surg. 1998;9(4):360–5. http://journals.lww.com/00001665-199807000-00013.
40. Fries PD, Katowitz JA. Congenital craniofacial anomalies of ophthalmic importance. Surv Ophthalmol. 1990;35(2):87–119. https://linkinghub.elsevier.com/retrieve/pii/0039625790900676.
41. Beard C. Dermolipoma Surgery, or, "An ounce of prevention is worth a pound of cure". Ophthal Plast Reconstr Surg. 1990;6(3):153–7. http://journals.lww.com/00002341-199009000-00001.

42. Choi YJ, Kim IH, Choi JH, Lee MJ, Kim N, Choung HK, et al. Early results of surgical management of conjunctival dermolipoma: partial excision and free conjunctival autograft. Br J Ophthalmol. 2015;99(8):1031–6. https://doi.org/10.1136/bjophthalmol-2014-306328.
43. Gorlin RJ, Jue KL, Jacobsen U, Goldschmidt E. Oculoauriculovertebral dysplasia. J Pediatr. 1963;63(5):991–9. https://linkinghub.elsevier.com/retrieve/pii/S0022347663802334.
44. Mann I. Developmental Abnormalities of the Eye. London: Cambridge Univ. Press.: British Journal of Ophtalmology; 1937. p. 379. (out of 444). https://wellcomecollection.org/works/cgvguccx.
45. Sinha PN, Mishra S. Corneal dermoid, report of a case. Am J Ophthalmol. 1950;33(7):1137–41. https://linkinghub.elsevier.com/retrieve/pii/0002939450917326.

Chapter 13
Cleft 9

Philippe Pellerin, Cristiano Tonello, Renato da Silva Freitas, and Nivaldo Alonso

Pearl
Cleft 9 is the last lateral cleft of the cranial series; it is the less frequent. Most of the time, it occurs in the setting of Amniotic Band Syndrome (ABS).

13.1 Original Tessier's Classification (Fig. 13.1)

The Tessier's cleft number 9 has a special place among craniofacial malformations. In the original publication of his classification [1], he stated that he had never met such a condition by himself but that in the logic of his system, it has to exist and be found along the described path. He credited Morian [2] for describing a case in which he made a drawing out of the original Morian's patient picture to illustrate his paper (Fig. 13.2).

P. Pellerin
Plastic Surgery Department, University of Lille, Lambersart, France

C. Tonello (✉)
Craniofacial Surgery Department, Universidade de São Paulo, Bauru, São Paulo, Brazil
e-mail: cristianotonello@usp.br

R. da Silva Freitas
Plastic Surgery Unit, Hospital de Clínicas, Universidade Federal do Paraná, Curitiba, Brazil

Craniofacial Surgery, Assistance Center for Cleft Lip and Palate (CAIF), Hospital do Trabalhador, Curitiba, Brazil

N. Alonso
Department of Plastic Surgery, Universidade de São Paulo, São Paulo, Brazil
e-mail: nivalonso@usp.br

N. Alonso et al. (eds.), *Facial Reconstruction of Unusual Facial Clefts*,
https://doi.org/10.1007/978-3-031-40926-4_13

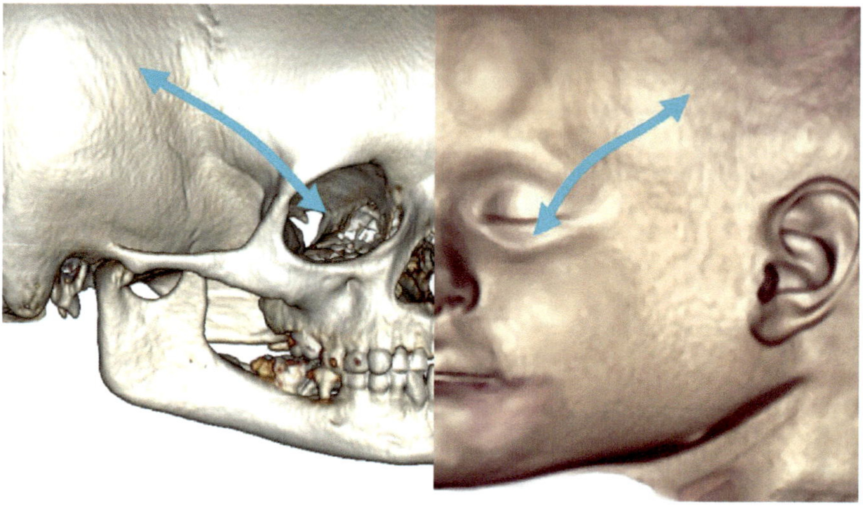

Fig. 13.1 Cleft 9 Situation

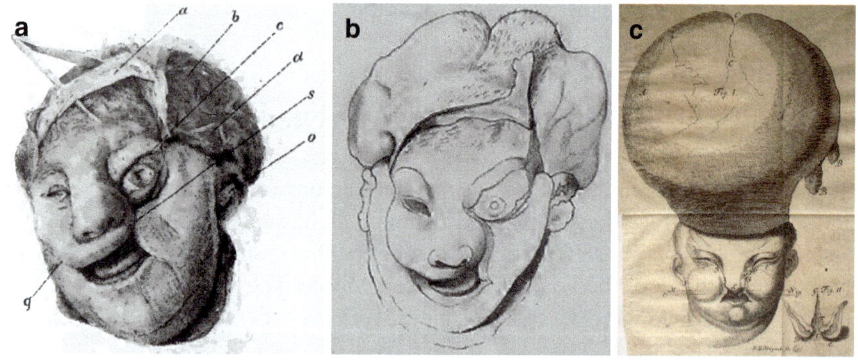

Fig. 13.2 (**a**) Drawing of Morian's patient (1887), in model for the Tessier's drawing of cleft 9. (**b**) Drawing of Nicoti's foetus (1822) in Ahlfeld's atlas. Considering the similarity in both drawings, one can wonder if it is the same subject… (**c**) Walther's case in 1732

It was a clever foreseeing since we now have sufficient cases to bolster his premise.

Tessier gave a few details and quoted Hogeman for personal communication and Sanvenero Rosselli [3], but there needs to be a picture for those two publications.

His statements about cleft 9 were: "*No. 9 is an upper 'lateral' orbital cleft with the cleft in the lateral third of the upper eyelid and the supra-lateral orbital angle [...] in the central part of the ridge and orbital roof*".

13.2 History

The Morian's patient, in 1887, was not the first to be found in the literature.

It looks as if the report by Constant Nicati [4], in his 1822 thesis, of a fetus from the collection of his master, Pr Vrolik, can claim primacy (Fig. 13.2).

In the Ahlfeld atlas [5], a compilation with references of all the cases of human malformations previously published, along with the Vrolik-Nicati observation, two other cases could be seen. One from Bartkov in 1871 [6] and the other from Vrolik in 1849 [7].

13.3 Etiology

Cleft 9 occurs most of the time in the setting of ABS. Thus, we will return the reader to the discussion about ABS etiology in the chapter Aetiology, mechanism and classification of rare clefts. But what is striking in such a limited series of cases is that three patients display appendages evocating the disorganization in mice (Ds.) phenotype, which we will discuss below.

13.4 Cases from Literature (Table 13.1)

The Monasterio publication [8] in 2008 gave a good idea of the cleft 9 frequency. Out of 495 patients with rare clefts, including the cases of Treacher Collins Syndrome, he listed 826 clefts. There were only 5 patients in this series with cleft 9; all were in the setting of multiple clefts in the same patient. This rarity did not come as a surprise since Tessier had yet to meet a case before his 1976 publication. Moore [9] counted 8 patients with cleft 9 out of 438 patients examined at the Australian craniofacial unit.

We kept 23 cases from the literature with valuable data compiled in Table 13.1.

Table 13.1 Literature cases of clefts 9

					Soft tissue				Skeletal						
Observation#	Author	Bib. Ref.	Sex	Side	Palpebra	Eyebrow	Hair line	Temporal	Temporo-parietal defect	Lateral orbital rim	Sphenoidal wing	Hypertelorism	Associated cleft	Associated Cfanomaly	Associated general condition
1	Antoniades	[10]	F	R	Y	Y	Defect	N	Y			II	UCLP homol	Appendage	Ds
2	Al-Ani	[11]	M	R	N	Y	N		Y	Y	y	n		Microphtalmia coronal stenosis	?
3	Balaji	[12]	M	B-as	Y	Y	Defect	Y	?	?		n	Cleft 3 bil		ABS
4	Bubanale	[13]	M	R	Y	Y	Defect	Defect	Y	Y	y	n	Cleft 1-13 right		ABS
5	Cortez-Ortega	[14]	M	R	Y	Y	Peak	N	Y	?	?	II	Cleft 3-BCLP		ABS
6	Adeosun	[15]	F	L	Y	Y	?	?	?	Y	?	n	Cleft 5l, 6 r	Microphtalmia	ABS
7	Darzi	[16]	M	L	Y	Y	Defect	Defect	?	?	?	n	Cleft 4,UCLP	Microphtalmia appendage	Ds
8	David	[17]	F	B-sy	Y	Y	Defect	Defect	Y	Y	y	II	cleft 4r-5l	microphtalmia	?
9	David	[17]	M	R	Y	Y	Peak	N	Y	Y	y	I	cleft 10	Encephalocele	?
10	Hukki	[18]	F	B-sy	Y	Y	Defect	Defect	Y	N	n	n	cleft 4b-O	Blindness Encephalocele	ABS
11	Muraskas	[19]	F	L	y	Y	Defect	Defect	?	?	?	n	Cleft 4l		ABS
12	Obdejin	[20]	M	R	N	Y	N	Defect	Y	?	?	I	BCLP	Encephalocele	ABS
13	Pereira	[21]	?	L	Y	Y	Peak	N	?	?	?	n	Cleft 5l, 6 r		nothing
	Olasoji	[22]												See #6	same case adeosun
14	Perlyn	[23]	F	B-as	Y	Y	Defect	Defect	Y	Y	y	n	Cleft 3b, BCLP	Encephalocele	?

15	Cassio Raposo	[24]	M	R	Y	Y	Defect	?	?	?	?	y	UCLP-Cleft 2-12	Encephalocele	?
16	Cassio Raposo	[25]	M	R	Y	Y	Defect	Defect	?	?	?	y	n	Encephalocele	?
17	Cassio Raposo	[25]	?	r	Y	Y	Defect	Defect	Y	Y	y	III	Cleft 3 bil-BCLP	Encephalocele	ABS
18	Ross	[26]	M	B-sy	Y	Y	Peak	N	?	?	?	I	Cleft 3 bil	Encephalocele	ABS
19	Sakurai	[27]	F	l	Y	Y	Defect	Defect	Y	?	?	III	Cleft 3b-BCLP	Encephalocele	ABS
20	Lies	[28]	F	B-as	Y	Y	Peak	?	?	?	?	I	cleft3-UCLP		ABS
21	Morovic	[29]	M	B-sy	N	Y	Peak	Defect	?	?	?	I	cleft3-BCLP		ABS
22	Morovic	[29]	?	B-sy	Y	Y	Peak	?	?ss	?	?	I	Cleft3 b	Mental retardation	ABS
23	Schramm	[30]	F	l	Y	Y	?	?	?	?	?	I	Cleft 3-BCLP-10r	Ocular staphyloma	ABS

Sex: m or f
Side: l=left; r=right; b-sy=bilateral symmetric; b-as=bilateral asymmetric
Peak=when the airline send a peak toward the eyebrow cleft; defect when there is a line of alopecia
?= when you don't have a data
UCLP= unilateral cleft lip; BCLP=bilateral cleft lip
ABS=amniotic band syndrome; Ds.=disorganization in mice mutation

13.5 Our Clinical Series (Table 13.2)

We have the data of 14 patients with cleft 9, compiled in Table 13.2.

Thus, our statistics will be grounded in 37 cases.

Table 13.2 Our clinical series of clefts 9

Observation#	Sex	Side	Soft tissue				Skeletal			Hypertelorism	Associated cleft	Associated CF anomaly	Associated general condition
			Palpebra	Eyebrcw	Hair line	Temporal	Temporo-parietal defect	Lateral orbital rim	Sphenoidal wing				
1	F	R	Y	y	Peak	N	Y	?	?	II	N	Encephalocele	Nothing
2	M	B-sy	Y	Y	Peak	N	N	Y	N	N	N	N	Nothing
3	M	L	Y	Y			N	Y	?	N	N	Microphtalmia	?
4	M	B-as	Y	Y	Defect	Defect	N	Y	?	N	Cleft 3 bil	N	Nothing
5	F	R	Y	Y	Peak	N	?	?	?	?	Cl 3-UCLP	Microphtalmia	?
6	M	B-sy	Y	Y	Defect	Defect	?	?	?	N	UCLP	Appendages	Ds.
7	F	R	N	N	N	N	N	N	Y	N	N	N	Nothing
8	F	L	Y	?	Defect	Defect	?	?	?	N	UCLP	N	?
9	F	L	Y	Y	Defect	Defect	?	?	?	III	Cleft 1-13	Encephalocele	ABS
10	?	B-as	Y	Y	Defect	Defect	?	?	?	III	cleft3-BCLP	?	?
11	F	B	Y	Y	Peak	?	?	?	?	III	Cleft 3b-BCLP-10l	N	?
12	F	L	Y	Y	Defect	Defect	?	?	?	N	Cleft4 l-cleft 5 r	N	?
13	F	L	Y	Y	Defect	N	?	?	?	N	Cleft 4		ABS
14	F	B	Y	Y	Defect	Defect	N	N	N	N	cleft 3	Epibulbar choristoma	

Sex: m or f
Side: l=left; r=right; b-sy=bilateral symmetric; ɔ-as=bilateral asymmetric
Peak=when the airline send a peak toward the eyebrow cleft; defect when there is a line of alopecia
?= when you don't have a data
UCLP= unilateral cleft lip; BCLP=bilateral cleft lip
ABS=amniotic band syndrome; Ds.=disorganization in mice mutation

13.6 The Spectrum of the Cleft 9

The sex ratio is balanced, with 15 males for 18 females (the sex could not be known for 4 patients).

13.6.1 *Soft Tissue Involvements*

13.6.1.1 The Eyelid (Fig. 13.3)

The coloboma of the upper eyelid is a significant symptom of cleft 9. Its location is on the lateral third of the upper eyelid. It was present in 33 patients. The severity of this coloboma goes from a discreet notch, which would have been missed, if not associated with other symptoms, to the most severe condition, where the upper lid is missing in a setting of ablepharia.

13.6.1.2 The Eyebrow

The eyebrow is affected in most of the patients as well. It could be a cleft in the form of a linear defect in the lateral third of the hairline or a disorganization of the lateral third of the eyebrow. In the most severe situation, the lateral third is missing and can be replaced by a peak of the hairline. The eyebrow was affected 35 times. It is impressive that the eyebrow can be concerned when the eyelid is expected, which happened two times.

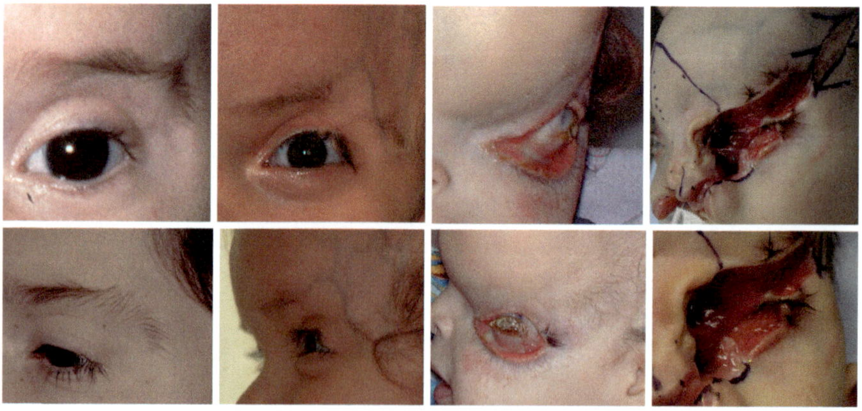

Fig. 13.3 The upper lid coloboma and eyebrow anomalies: From left to right: increasing severity for coloboma

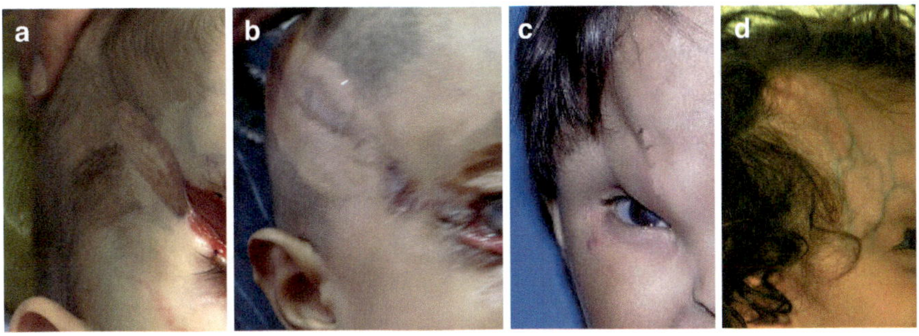

Fig. 13.4 Hair line and scalp anomalies. (**a**) Scaring area; (**b**) Scaring and alopecia. (**c**) Hairline peak. (**d**) Large zone of alopecic and atrophic scalp

13.6.1.3 The Hairline (Fig. 13.4)

A hairline peak is considered a classical marker along the path of rare clefts. For cleft 9, the hairline presents itself in three ways. It was normal in three patients; it was marked 11 times by a peak and 20 times by a defect. This last condition is the most frequent.

13.6.1.4 The Frontotemporal Scalp

A defect of the fronto-parieto-temporal scalp area is typical of the cleft 9. It is most frequently a bald line mimicking a scar. Sometimes, it presents itself as a wider cutaneous defect, which is then interpreted as a cutis aplasia, all the more when it is associated with an underlying skeletal defect and an encephalocele. In 18 patients of the series, the scalp was affected.

13.6.1.5 The Ds. Appendage (Fig. 13.5)

The hypothesis of a gene in man homologous to the gene affected by the disorganization in mice mutation syndrome (Dis) has been discussed below. Thus, we will not redo this research here and let the reader return to the corresponding chapter if interested. Nonetheless, three cases in this research have been associated with cleft 9, some very unusual appendages associated by many authors [31, 32] to the equivalent in Man of the Dis.

They are one of our clinical cases and two from the literature. One from Darzi [16] with the appendage arising from the cheek, the other from Antoniades [10] with an appendage attached to the lateral third of the eyebrow on the side of the cleft 9 and along its path.

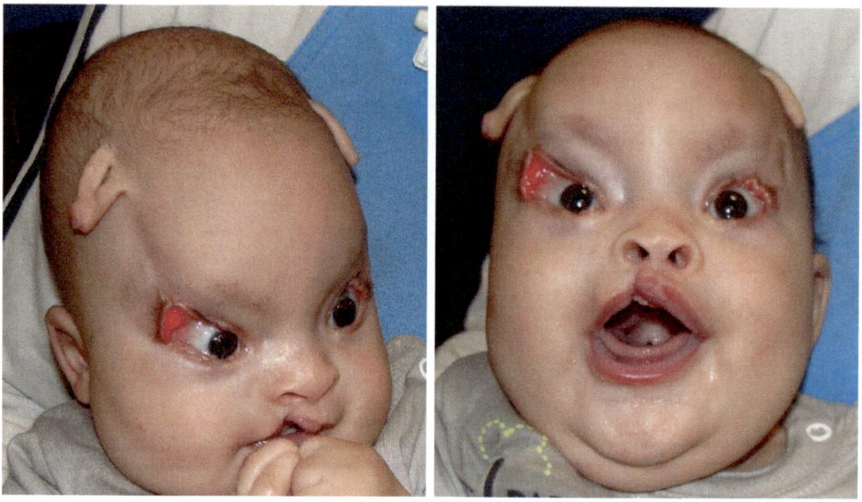

Fig. 13.5 Typical aspect of appendages advocated as belonging to the homologous of Ds. in man

Our case is displayed in Fig. 13.5. The patient has a bilateral cleft nine; on both sides, he presents appendages, two on the right and one on the left.

13.6.2 The Skeletal Symptoms

13.6.2.1 The Orbital Rim (Fig. 13.6)

Cleft 9 affects the superolateral angle of the orbit, mainly at the expanse of the lateral orbital process of the frontal bone.

13.6.2.2 The Skull Base (Fig. 13.7)

The wings of the sphenoid bone are hypoplastic, as shown in Fig. 13.7. Some cases show a full-thickness defect, as in Al-Ani's patient [11], which can be associated with a temporoparietal defect and an encephalocele.

13.6.2.3 The Skull Vault (Fig. 13.8)

Defects of the vault are frequent in Cleft 9, mainly along the cleft path but could be found elsewhere on the skull, giving room for the hypothesis of dysgenesis as the cause for ABS.

An encephalocele was present 11 times associated with vault defects, but we have at least one skull defect without an encephalocele outside of the path of cleft 9.

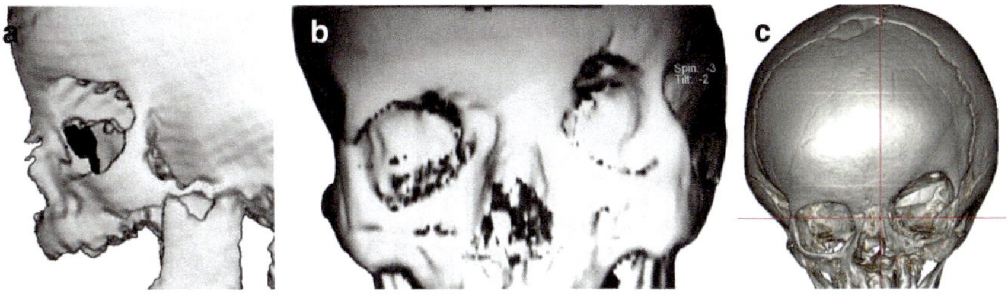

Fig. 13.6 The skeleton in the cleft 9: orbital rim deformities. (**a**) Small notch onto the lateral orbital process of the frontal bone. (**b**) More severe condition associated with microphtalmia. (**c**) Global deformity of the supero-lateral orbital angle, and vertical dystopia assessed thanks to vestibular orientation (red lines are display of horizontal vestibular plane and sagittal plane)

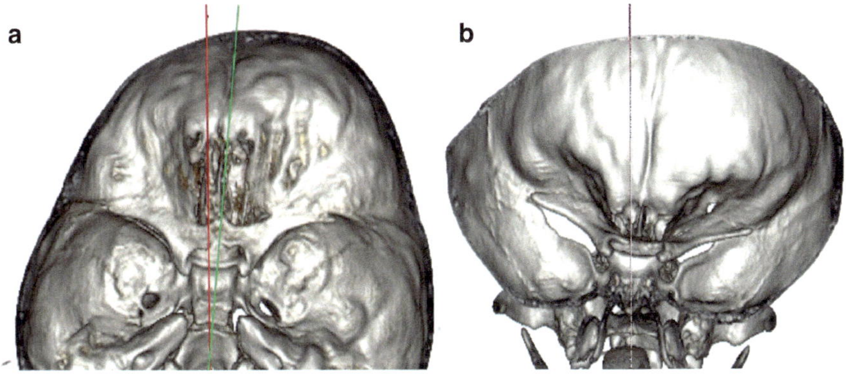

Fig. 13.7 The skull base in cleft 9. (**a**) Axial view. (**b**) Backward view. Both views display the hypoplastic upper sphenoidal wing, with the enlargement of the superior orbital fissure

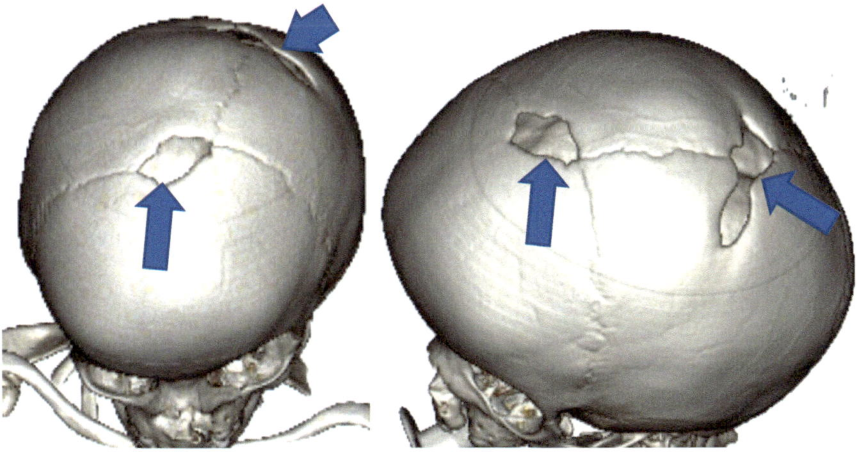

Fig. 13.8 The vault defects. In this case of left Cleft 9, two skull defects appear (blue arrows)

13.6.3 Malformations Associated with the Cleft 9

13.6.3.1 The Setting of Cleft 9

Two constatations are impressive when it comes to the cleft 9 settings.

First, contrary to other rare clefts, it never occurs in the setting of CFM. With the knowledge of the importance of NCCs in the etiology of CFM, we would look at other mechanisms involved in producing cleft 9.

Second, as for other rare clefts, the frequency of the ABS setting in cases of cleft 9 is noticeable. But, for cleft 9, this frequency is overwhelming.

13.6.3.2 Clefts Associated with Cleft 9

Cleft 9 is infrequently isolated; only 6 out of the 37 cases reviewed were not associated with another facial cleft.

Cleft 3 is the most usually encountered, with 15 occurrences; BCLP comes to second place, being met 9 times; then after UCLP 7 times; cleft 4, 5 times; cleft 5, 4 times; cleft 10, three times; cleft 6 and 1–13, 2 times and cleft 0 and 2–12 once.

Cleft 14, 7 and 8 have never been associated.

13.6.3.3 Other Craniofacial Anomalies

As previously noticed, encephalocele is a frequent association, close to 50%. Cerebral anomalies also seem to be frequent, but their frequency is unclear, and we cannot give statistics.

Hypertelorism is not supposed to be a part of the cleft 9 spectrum since it is not an inter-orbital cleft, but albeit there were 5 patients with grade III and 4 patients with grade II. And only 1 could be related to the presence of another inter-orbital cleft.

There were 7 cases of microphtalmia or severe ocular malformation.

Vertical orbital dystopia is present in some cases but difficult to assess. We have been pleased to use the vestibular orientation [33] to demonstrate such displacement, which is difficult to appreciate otherwise.

13.6.4 Differential Diagnosis (Fig. 13.9)

As usually, the neighbouring clefts are the ones to be discussed.

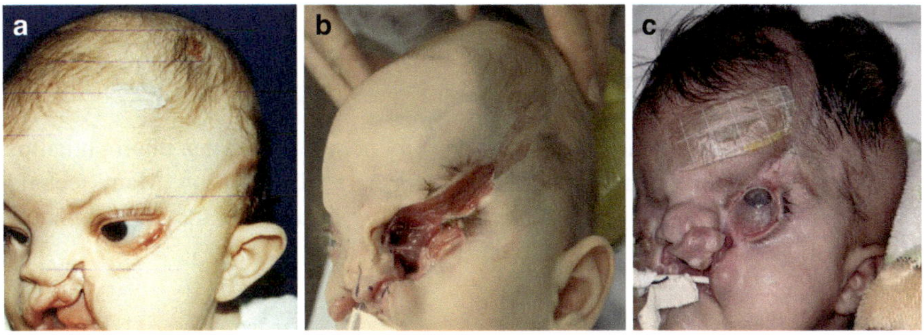

Fig. 13.9 Differential diagnosis. In the ABS setting, a slight change of position yields a different type of rare cleft, but the mechanism is the same. (**a**) Cleft 8. (**b**) Cleft 9. (**c**) Cleft 10

13.6.4.1 Cleft 8

The cleft 8 is very close to the orbital rim, but it never affects the sphenoid bone (even for those who would prefer to keep TCS in the stretch of rare clefts), nor does it sway the skull vault.

About the soft tissues, it could be confusing when there is a huge disorganization of the outer part of the upper eyelids, and we cannot say where the canthus is.

13.6.4.2 Cleft 10

The skeletal defect, in cleft 10, when it is involved, is in the middle of the orbital roof and is frequently associated with a frontal defect yielding an encephalocele.

The coloboma is in the mid-third of the palpebra, but, when the coloboma is very wide, it could be difficult to sort between 9 and 10.

Cleft 10 is very often associated with a hair peak.

For both diagnoses, the careful analysis of medical imaging is very determining. The setting is, too, to be considered since ABS could be a cue.

13.7 Treatment

There are too few cases to build up a codified strategy for cleft 9 treatment, all the most because of the many combinations with other conditions. For most patients, a tailored strategy must be invented, and we would have to apply specific technics to face different situations.

13.7.1 *Technics*

13.7.1.1 The Coloboma

When the eyeball is functional, which is usually not the case when microphthalmia is associated, the eyelid has to be repaired for corneal protection. Many technics have been described. They will be reviewed more in detail in the cleft10 chapter (Chap. 14) since there is little difference between them.

13.7.1.2 The Eyebrow

Depending on the size of the defect, the eyebrow will be repaired either by local flap or by free hair grafts.

13.7.1.3 The Scalp

In some cases of severe cutis aplasia, when the dura-mater is exposed, and at risk, large scalp flaps could be required. Otherwise, the repair of the bald area could be deleted and, when wide, necessitate skin expansion. A narrow linear defect could be fixed by excision and direct suture.

13.7.1.4 The Orbit

Transversal dystopia, another way for naming hypertelorism, can be addressed, as usual, with unilateral or bilateral surgery, box-type osteotomy, or bipartition. Most of the time, the technic is selected according to the surgeon's habit and preference, but it would be better to choose according to the analysis of actual deformity. To our knowledge, vestibular orientation is the only one reliable in the setting of severe craniofacial malformations [34].

13.7.1.5 The Skull

Significant defects of the skull must be mended. In paediatric surgery, autologous bone repair is mandatory, but at the same time, there is few available bone in children. In Perlyn's publication [23] the different solutions are reviewed. Interestingly the technic of interdigitating cranial expansion invented by Argenta, which is exposed in David's publication [35], looks like a fair solution for defects up to 50% of the cranial surface.

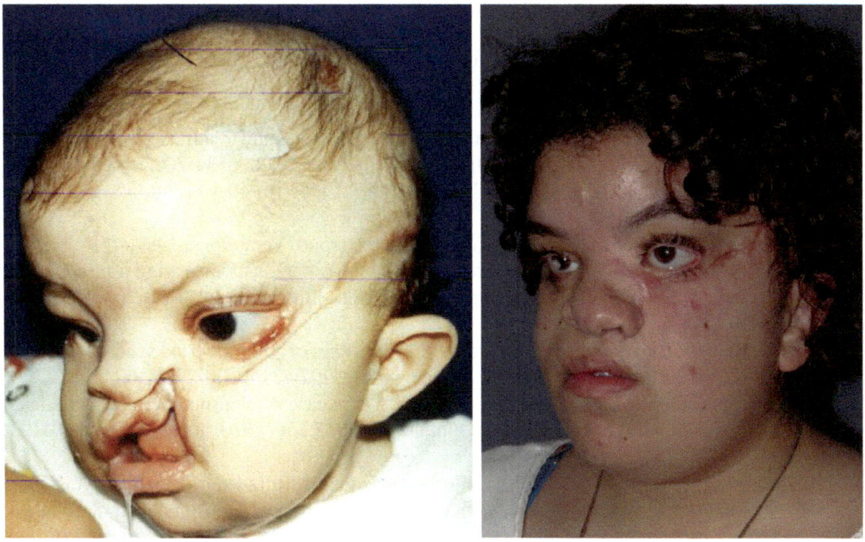

Fig. 13.10 Surgical Treatment long term follow-up after many surgical procedures along life time

13.7.2 Indications

Life-threatening situations, such as cutis aplasia and large encephalocele, came first.

Functional threats, such as corneal exposure of a functional eyeball, must be addressed simultaneously. Aesthetic rehabilitation will then come to permit socialization.

Many surgeries are necessary for different ages to achieve better results, from eye protection to orthognathic surgery to achieve good functional results in these patients. One of the author's patients with long-term follow-up (Fig. 13.10).

References

1. Tessier P. Anatomical classification of facial, cranio-facial and latero-facial clefts. J Maxillofac Surg. 1976;4:69–92. https://linkinghub.elsevier.com/retrieve/pii/S0301050376800136.
2. Morian R. Über die schräge Gesichtsspalte (about oblique facial clefts). Arch Klin Chir. 1887;35:245–88.
3. Sanvenero-Rosselli G. Developmental pathology of the face and the Dysraphic syndrome. Plast Reconstr Surg. 1953;11(1):36–8. http://journals.lww.com/00006534-195301000-00004.
4. Nicati C. Specimen Anatomico pathologicum inaugurale, De Labii Leporini congeniti Natura et Origine. Trajecti ad Rhenum et Amstelodami: Academia Rheno-Trajectina; 1822.
5. Ahlfeld F. Die Missbildungen des Menschen, vol. I. Leipzig: Fr. Wilh. Grunow; 1880. p. 163. http://www.biusante.parisdescartes.fr/histmed/medica/cote?44232x01.

6. Barkow HCL. Beiträge zur pathologischen Entwickelungsgeschichte. Breslau: Nischkowski; 1859.
7. Vrolik W. Embryogenesin Hominis et Mammalium tam Naturalem quam Abnormem. Amsterdam: G. M. P. Londonck; 1849. https://play.google.com/books/reader?id=GlpCAAAAcAAJ&pg=GBS.PP2&hl=fr.
8. Monasterio FO, Taylor JA. Major craniofacial clefts: case series and treatment philosophy. Plast Reconstr Surg. 2008;122(2):534–43. http://journals.lww.com/00006534-200808000-00027.
9. Moore MH. Rare craniofacial clefts. J Craniofac Surg. 1996;7(6):408–11. http://journals.lww.com/00001665-199611000-00003.
10. Antoniades K, Baraister M. Proboscis lateralis: a case report. Teratology. 1989;40(3):193–7.
11. Al-Ani SA, Locke MB, Rees M, de Chalain TM. Our experiences managing a rare Cranio-orbital cleft. J Craniofac Surg. 2008;19(3):819–22. https://journals.lww.com/00001665-200805000-00045.
12. Balaji S, Balaji P. Cicatricial ectropion correction for a case of amniotic band syndrome. Indian J Dent Res. 2020;31(4):644. http://www.ijdr.in/text.asp?2020/31/4/644/298418.
13. Bubanale S, Kurbet S, De Piedade Sequeira LG. A rare case of cleft number nine associated with atypical cleft number two. Indian J Ophthalmol. 2017;65(7):610. https://doi.org/10.4103/ijo.IJO_914_16.
14. Cortez-Ortega C, Garrocho-Rangel JA, Flores-Velázquez J, Ruiz-Rodríguez S, Noyola-Frías MÁ, Santos-Díaz MÁ, et al. Management of the Amniotic Band Syndrome with cleft palate: literature review and report of a case. Case Rep Dent. 2017;2017:7620416.
15. Adeosun OO, James O, Akinmoladun VI, Owobu T. Amniotic band syndrome associated with orofacial clefts: a report of two cases: amniotic band syndrome. Oral Surg. 2012;5(4):185–9. https://doi.org/10.1111/j.1752-248X.2012.01163.x.
16. Darzi MA, Chowdri NA. Oblique facial clefts: a report of Tessier numbers 3, 4, 5, and 9 clefts. Cleft Palate Craniofac J. 1993;30(4):414–5. https://doi.org/10.1597/1545-1569_1993_030_0414_ofcaro_2.3.co_2.
17. David DJ, Moore MH, Cooter RD, Chow SK. The Tessier number 9 cleft. Plast Reconstr Surg. 1989;83(3):520–5. http://journals.lww.com/00006534-198903000-00022.
18. Hukki J, Balan P, Čeponiene R, Kantola-Sorsa E, Saarinen P, Wikstrom H. A case study of amnion rupture sequence with Acalvaria, blindness, and Clefting: clinical and psychological profiles. J Craniofac Surg. 2004;15(2):185–91. http://journals.lww.com/00001665-200403000-00002.
19. Muraskas JK, McDonnell JF, Chudik RJ, Salyer KE, Glynn L. Amniotic band syndrome with significant orofacial clefts and disruptions and distortions of craniofacial structures. J Pediatr Surg. 2003;38(4):635–8. https://linkinghub.elsevier.com/retrieve/pii/S0022346802631501.
20. Obdeijn MC, Offringa PJ, Bos RRM, Verhagen AAE, Niessen FB, Roche NA. Facial clefts and associated limb anomalies: description of three cases and a review of the literature. Cleft Palate Craniofac J. 2010;47(6):661–7. https://doi.org/10.1597/09-033.
21. Pereira FJ, Milbratz GH, Cruz AAV, Vasconcelos JJA. Ophthalmic considerations in the Management of Tessier Cleft 5/9. Ophthal Plast Reconstr Surg. 2010;26(6):450–3. https://journals.lww.com/00002341-201011000-00016.
22. Olasoji HO, Tahir C, Isa A. An unusual bilateral oblique facial cleft in a newborn. Int J Pediatr Otorhinolaryngol. 2005;69(7):999–1001. https://linkinghub.elsevier.com/retrieve/pii/S0165587605000686.
23. Perlyn CA, Schmelzer R, Govier D, Marsh JL. Congenital scalp and calvarial deficiencies: principles for classification and surgical management. Plast Reconstr Surg. 2005;115(4):1129–41. http://journals.lww.com/00006534-200504010-00023.
24. Raposo C, Lim R, Jarrahy R. 6 rare craniofacial clefts. Plast Surg Keys:12. https://plasticsurgerykey.com/craniofacial-disorders-8/.
25. Raposo-Amaral CE, Jarrahy R, Lim R, Alonso N. The rare facial cleft. In: Alonso N, Raposo-Amaral CE, editors. Cleft lip and palate treatment. Cham: Springer International Publishing; 2018. p. 325–62. https://doi.org/10.1007/978-3-319-63290-2_21.

26. Ross W. A curious monster which lived for some time after birth. Trans Obstet Soc Lond. 1867;IX:31–2.
27. Sakurai EH, Mitchell DF, Holmes LA. Bilateral oblique facial clefts and amniotic bands: a report of two cases. Cleft Palate J. 1966;3:181–5.
28. Lies S, Beckwith T, Mills J, Butler L, Ezaki M, Oishi S. Case series: amniotic band sequence with craniofacial abnormalities. Birth Defects Res. 2019;111(19):1494–500. https://doi.org/10.1002/bdr2.1576.
29. Morovic CG, Berwart F, Varas J. Craniofacial anomalies of the amniotic band syndrome in serial clinical cases. Plast Reconstr Surg. 2004;113(6):1556–62. http://journals.lww.com/00006534-200405000-00003.
30. Schramm C, Rohrbach JM, Reinert S, Mau-Holzmann UA, Aisenbrey S, Bartz-Schmidt KU, et al. Amniotic bands as a cause of congenital anterior staphyloma. Graefes Arch Clin Exp Ophthalmol. 2013;251(3):959–65. https://doi.org/10.1007/s00417-012-2197-z.
31. Isidor B, Baujat G, Le Caignec C, Pichon O, Martin-Coignard D, Toutain A, et al. Congenital skin pedicles with or without amniotic band sequence: extending the human phenotype resembling mouse disorganization. Am J Med Genet A. 2009;149A(8):1734–9. https://doi.org/10.1002/ajmg.a.32796.
32. Hunter AGW, Carpenter BF, Opitz JM, Reynolds JF. Implications of malformations not due to amniotic bands in the amniotic band sequence. Am J Med Genet. 1986;24(4):691–700. https://doi.org/10.1002/ajmg.1320240414.
33. Vinchon M, Pellerin P, Pertuzon B, Fénart R, Dhellemmes P. Vestibular orientation for craniofacial surgery: application to the management of unicoronal synostosis. Childs Nerv Syst. 2007;23(12):1403–9. https://doi.org/10.1007/s00381-007-0471-x.
34. Pellerin P, Vinchon M, Guerreschi P, Anastassov Y, Zhang ZY, Tang XJ, et al. Crouzon syndrome anatomy, usefulness of vestibular orientation. J Craniofac Surg. 2022;33(6):1914–23.
35. David LR, Taylor RG, Argenta LC. A technique for cranial bone expansion. J Craniofac Surg. 1996;7(2):151–5. http://journals.lww.com/00001665-199603000-00016.

Chapter 14
Cleft 10

Philippe Pellerin, Cristiano Tonello, Renato da Silva Freitas, and Nivaldo Alonso

14.1 Original Tessier's Classification [1] (Fig. 14.1)

« No. 10 is an upper "central» orbital cleft with the cleft occurring in the middle third of the supraorbital ridge, lateral to the supra-orbital nerve. This cleft extends to the orbital roof and frontal bone (encephalocele). There is a coloboma of the middle third of the upper eyelid, sometimes amounting to total ablepharia. The eyebrow is divided into two portions, the lateral portion angulated vertically joining the hairline of the scalp, the medial portion is virtually absent ».

After Tessier's description of the cleft 10, his warning about the variability in the degree of completeness of rare clefts and his advice to look for other components of rare cleft when being faced with a coloboma of the upper eyelid, it became a rule for most of the craniofacial pathologists, to consider them as a cleft 10, as well as the cleft of eyebrow and corresponding anomalies of the hairline. Thus, we included in our research everything concerning colobomas of the upper lid, clefts of the eyebrow, and anomalies in the lateral third of the frontal hairline.

P. Pellerin
Plastic Surgery Department, University of Lille, Lambersart, France

C. Tonello (✉)
Craniofacial Surgery Department, University of São Paulo, Bauru, São Paulo, Brazil
e-mail: cristianotonello@usp.br

R. da Silva Freitas
Plastic Surgery Unit, Hospital de Clínicas, Universidade Federal do Paraná, Curitiba, Brazil

Craniofacial Surgery, Assistance Center for Cleft Lip and Palate (CAIF), Hospital do Trabalhador, Curitiba, Brazil

N. Alonso
Department of Plastic Surgery, University of São Paulo, São Paulo, Brazil
e-mail: nivalonso@usp.br

N. Alonso et al. (eds.), *Facial Reconstruction of Unusual Facial Clefts*,
https://doi.org/10.1007/978-3-031-40926-4_14

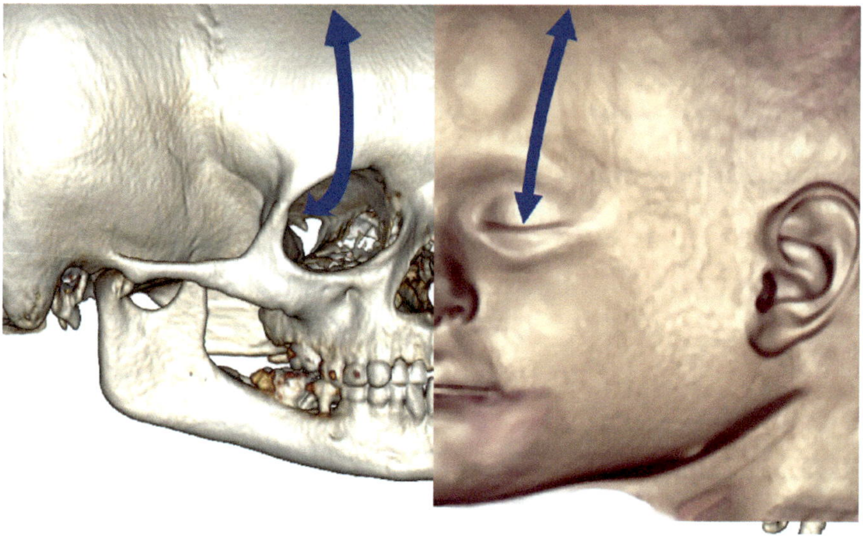

Fig. 14.1 The path of Clefts 10

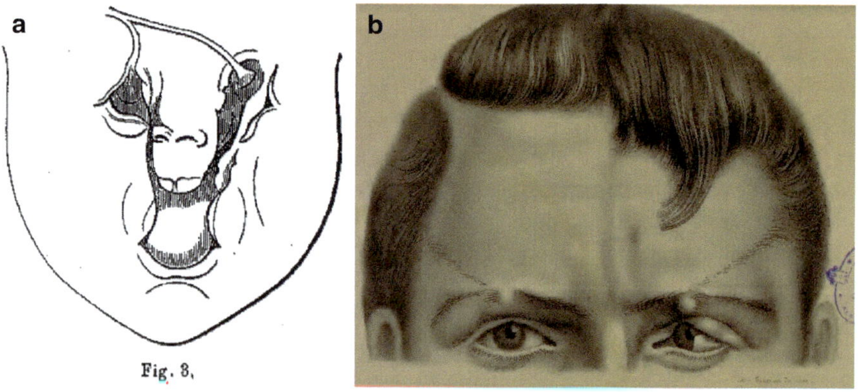

Fig. 14.2 Historical reports. (**a**) Bruns' case in Laroche's thesis 1823. (**b**) Schleich's patient. 1880

14.2 History

Most of colobomas are on the upper eyelid. Observations of coloboma are seldom reported, as in 1823 the Bruns' case in Laroche's thesis [2] (Fig. 14.2a) or Schleich's patient [3] (Fig. 14.2b). Van Duysse in 1882 [4] was the first to make a general review of 23 cases of coloboma. Nicolin, in his 1888 thesis [5], reported the detailed records of 55 cases of coloboma recorded in the literature, plus a personal case. Both authors credit Mayor for the first coloboma report in 1808 in a medical thesis in Montpelier, France. It was the record of a child with an isolated coloboma of the right upper lid with a web attached to the cornea.

The case reported in Nicolin's thesis was successfully operated on, as demonstrated in the pictures of one of the Lumieres brothers, illustrating the idea.

14.3 Etiology

As seen below, the spectrum of cleft 10 is broad, and we can hypothesize that different mechanisms would yield other clinical pictures. In his research [6], Smith made the wise proposition that those colobomas associated with craniofacial malformation are likely to occur early during embryogenesis, when isolated coloboma would arise later, during eyelid separation.

Some syndromes, including palpebral coloboma, are known to be related to specific gene mutations. The Manitoba oculo-tricho-anal syndrome [7] includes, quite frequently (17 out of 37 patients in Chacon-Camacho [8] research), typical features of cleft 10. It is related to a mutation that yields a loss of function of the FREM1 gene, an evolutionarily conserved gene expressed in epithelial/mesenchymal interaction and epidermal remodeling regions. FREM1 protein belongs to the FRAS1/FREM family of extracellular matrix proteins that localizes at the basement membranes and forms a ternary complex that includes FRAS1, FREM1 and FREM2.

On the other hand, FRAS1 and FREM2 mutations result in Fraser syndrome, which is characterised by cryptophthalmos, among other malformations, clinically overlapping with MOTA syndrome. More and more publications of cases of MOTA syndromes or very close-looking patients with pedigree history in different areas around the world [9] drive some authors to associate MOTA with the cleft 10 strongly.

The known macromolecular function of the involved gene gives some ground to the old hypothesis, which stated that coloboma would be consecutive to some deficiency in the ectodermal differentiation.

14.4 Cases from the Literature (Table 14.1)

A bias hampers literature research. On the one hand, isolated colobomas are not infrequent and are usually referred to the ophthalmology departments. Thus, a large series of cases can be found published in the ophthalmology literature, such as the

Table 14.1 Cases from the literature

Patient #	First author	Bib. ref.	Gender	Side	Soft tissues: Eyelid severity	Soft tissues: Eyelid Position	Soft tissues: Eyebrow	Soft tissues: Hair line	Skeleton: Orbital rim	Skeleton: Frontal bone	Skeleton: Orbital roof	Skeleton: Orbital position	Associated ocular anom	Associated cleft	Associated craniofacial anomaly	Other anomaly
1	AD-EL	[10]	M	B	2	Med	N	n	N	N	N	N	N	N	N	N
2	ASSOUAN	[11]	F	L	1	Mid	Y	Defect	?	?	?	Hypertel		Cleft 3 bil-BCLP		ABS
3	GUPTA	[12]	M	R	3	Med	Y	Peak	N	N	N	N	Staphyloma	N	N	N
4	EPPLEY	[13]	M	B	2	Mid	Y	?	1	N	N	Hypertel		Cleft 3 bil-BCLP		ABS
5	EPPLEY	[13]	M	B	2	Mid	Y	?	?	?	?	Hypertel	Microphtalmia	Cleft 3 bil-BCLP		ABS
6	FAN	[14]	?	B	3	Med	Y	?	?	?	?	N	Symblepharon			
7	FAN	[14]	?	L	3	Med	Y	Peak	?	?	?	N	Symblepharon			
8	DAVID	[15]	M	L	2	Mid	Y	Peak	N	N	N	Hypertel		Cleft 1-13-UCLP		CFM
9	GOSLA-REDDY	[16]	F	L	2	Med	Y	N	N	N	N	Vert dyst	Strabismus			
10	GU	[17]	F	L	2	Med	Y	Peak	?	?	?	N				MOTA
11	CHACON-CAMACHO	[8]	F	L	3	Med	Y	Peak	N	N	N	N	Microphtalmia			MOTA
12	PASCASIO	[18]	F	L	2	Mid	Y	Peak	N	N	N	N	Microphtalmia	Cleft 4r-Cleft 6l-UCLP		
13	ORTUBE	[19]	F	B	1	Med	Y	Alopecia	N	N	N	N	Symblepharon			ectodermal dysplasia
14	ORTEGA-MOLINA	[20]	M	B	2	Med	Y	Peak	N	N	N	N	Symblepharon			

15	ORTEGA-MOLINA	[20]	F	R	1	Med	Y	Peak	N	N	N	N	Symblepharon			
16	ORTEGA-MOLINA	[20]	M	L	1	Med	N	N	N	N	N	N				anal imperforation
17	ORTEGA-MOLINA	[20]	M	B	1	Mid	N	N	N	N	N	N	Choristoma			CFM
18	ANKOLA	[21]	M	B	1	Lat	Y	?	N	N	N	N				
19	HOYAMA	[22]	?	L	2	Med	N	N	N	N	N	N	n			
20	KISLAOGLU	[23]	M	R	0	Mid	Y	N	Y	Y	Y	N				
21	LEE	[24]	F	F	1	?	Y	Peak	N	N	N	N				MOTA?
22	McQUILLAN	[25]	?	L	0		N	N	N	N	N	N			Hair lid ectopia	
23	McQUILLAN	[25]	?	R	0		N	N	N	N	N	N			Hair lid ectopia	
24	MARLES	[7]	M	R	1	?	Y	Peak	N	N	N	Hypertel				MOTA
25	MARLES	[7]	M	R	0		Y	Peak	N	N	N	Hypertel	Microphtalmia			MOTA
26	MARLES	[7]	F	L	2	Med	Y	Peak	N	N	N	Hypertel				MOTA
27	MARLES	[7]	F	L	3	Med	Y	Peak	N	N	N	Hypertel				MOTA
28	MARLES	[7]	F	L	2	Lat	Y	Peak	N	N	N	Hypertel				MOTA
29	MARLES	[7]	F	R	2	?	Y	Peak	N	N	N	Hypertel				MOTA
30	MOROVIC	[26]	?	B	1	Mid	Y	Peak	?	?	?	Hypertel		BCLP		ABS
31	MOROVIC	[26]	?	B	1	Mid	Y	Peak	?	?	?	Hypertel		Cleft 3 bil		ABS
32	CASSIO-RAPOSO	[27]	?	B	2	Med	Y	Y	?	?	?					
33	CASSIO-RAPOSO	[27]	?	B	0		Y	Peak	?	?	?	Hypertel		Cleft 3 bil		ABS
34	CASSIO-RAPOSO	[27]	?	L	?	?	Y	Peak	?	?	?	Hypertel		Cleft 2-12		
35	CASSIO-RAPOSO	[27]	M	R	?	?	Y	Peak	?	?	?	Hypertel	Microphtalmia	Cleft 2-12		

(continued)

Table 14.1 (continued)

Patient #	First author	Bib. ref.	Gender	Side	Soft tissues				Skeleton				Associated ocular anom	Associated cleft	Associated craniofacial anomaly	Other anomaly
					Eyelid		Eyebrow	Hair line	Orbital rim	Frontal bone	Orbital roof	Orbital position				
					severity	Position										
36	SEAH	[28]	M	B	3	Med	Y	Peak	?	?	?		Symblepharon	Cleft 0	Frontal lipoma	
37	SEAH	[28]	M	L	2	Mid	N	N	?	?	?		Choristoma	UCLP		CFM
38	SEAH	[28]	F	L	2	Mid	N	N	?	?	?				Spina bifida	CFM
39	SEAH	[28]	M	L	2	Mid	?	?	?	?	?		Choristoma	Cleft 1-13-UCLP		CFM
40	VISTNESS	[29]	F	R	3	Mid	Y	Peak	Y	Y	Y	Vert dyst	Symblepharon			
41	VULOVIC	[30]	M	R	3	Med	Y	?	N	N	N					
42	YEUNG	[31]	?	B	3	Mid	Y	Peak	N	N	N					MOTA
43	YEUNG	[31]	?	L	2	Mid	Y	Peak	N	N	N					MOTA
44	VAN DER MEULEN	[32]	M	R	1	Mid	?	?	N	N	N	Hypertel		Cleft 1-13-BCLP		
45	FONTAINE	[33]	F	R	1	Lat	Y	Peak	?	?	?	Hypertel		Cleft 1-13-UCLP		

46	HUANG	[34]	M	L	3	Mid	Y	Peak	Y	Y	Y	Hypertel	Microphtalmia	Cleft 1-13-UCLP	CFM	CFM
47	LEHALLE	[35]	?	R	1	Med	N	N	?	?	?	Hypertel		Cleft 1-13		CFM
48	LEHALLE	[35]	?	B	3	Med	Y	N	?	?	?	Hypertel		Cleft 1-13		CFM
49	LEHALLE	[35]	?	R	3	Med	Y	N	?	?	?	Hypertel	Symblepharon	Cleft 1-13		CFM

Gender: m for male, f for female
Side: r for right, l for left and b for bilateral
Severity: according to Shao's grading, 0 nothing, 1< to 33%, 33% < 2 < 50% and 3 > 50%
Position: med for medial, mid for middle and lat for lateral
Hypertel for hypertelorism
UCLP for unilateral cleft lip and palate, BCLP for bilateral cleft lip and palate
CFM for craniofacial microsomia, ABS for amniotic band syndrome and MOTA for Manitoba oculo-tricho-anal syndrome

59 case series from Shao in Shanghai [36], the 55 case series from Smith [6], the 51 case series published by Grover [37] or the 21 cases published by Lohdi [38]. On the other hand, patients with complex issues associated with other rare clefts or with skeletal defects and encephaloceles are referred to craniofacial centres and are scarce. Thus, those cases are less frequently found in the literature.

The Monasterio's series [39] included 20 Tessier's rare clefts 10, 10, 3 isolated and 17 associated with other clefts. David's series, reported by Moore [40], 14 of whom 6 were isolated.

Some cases from our series were previously published, they will be counted in our clinical series.

Because of those biases, getting statistics out of the literature will not be hazardous. We could find 376 reported clefts 10 by merging the large series with the small or isolated cases. Out of those cases, we got 49 cases whose pictures and data were available in the publications and which we used for statistics in combination with our clinical series.

14.5 Our Clinical Series (Table 14.2)

We found 76 patients among our cases of rare clefts with one of the symptoms usually related to cleft 10. Those patients are reported in Table 14.2.

Table 14.2 Clinical series

Patient #	Gender	Side	Soft tissues				Skeleton				Associated ocular anom	Associated cleft	Associated craniofacial anomaly	Other anomaly
			Eyelid		Eyebrow	Hair line	Orbital rim	Frontal bone	Orbital roof	Orbital position				
			Severity	Position										
1	F	L	2	Mid	Y	Y	N	N	N	Hypertelorism	Ptosis	Cleft 1-13	N	N
2	M	R	1	Med	N	N	N	N	N	N	Epibulbar choristoma	UCLP	Arachnoid cyst	N
3	F	R	2	Mid	Y	N	N	N	N	Hypertelorism	n	UCLP-cleft 1-13	n	N
4	F	L	0		Y	Y	N	N	N	Hypertelorism	n	Cleft 1-13		CMF
5	M	L	1	Mid	N	N	N	N	N	N	Epibulbar choristoma	Cleft 7		CMF
6	M	L	3	Mid	Y	N	N	N	N	Hypertelorism	Epibulbar choristoma	N	Cranionasal fistula	CMF
7	M	B	2	Med	Y	Y	N	N	N	N	Symblepharon	N		
8	F	R	1	Med	Y	N	N	N	N	N	N	UCLP	Microtia	
9	M	L	3	Med	N	N	N	N	N	N	N	n		CMF
10	M	L	1	Med	N	N	N	N	N	N	N	Cleft 5 bilat	Microstomia	
11	M	R			Y	Y	Y	Y	Y	Dystopic	N	UCLP	Encephalocele	
12	F	L	0		Y	Y	N	N	N	Hypertelorism	N	Cleft 1-13		
13	F	R	3	Med	N	N	N	N	N		N	N		
14	M	R	1	Med	Y	N	N	N	N	Hypertelorism	N	Cleft 1-13		
15	F	R	1	Mid	Y	Y	?	?		Hypertelorism	N	N		
16	F	R	0		Y	Y	Y	Y		Hypertelorism		Cleft12 bilat		Twin(sister unafected
17	M	R	0		Y	Y	N	N	N	N	N	Cleft 3		
18	F	R	1	Med	N	N	N	N	N	N	Epibulbar choristoma	Cleft 3 UCLP		CMF
19	F	R	1	Med	N	N	N	N	N	N	N	Cleft 3 BCLP		

(continued)

Table 14.2 (continued)

Patient #	Gender	Side	Soft tissues: Eyelid: Severity	Soft tissues: Eyelid: Position	Soft tissues: Eyebrow	Soft tissues: Hair line	Skeleton: Orbital rim	Skeleton: Frontal bone	Skeleton: Orbital roof	Skeleton: Orbital position	Associated ocular anom	Associated cleft	Associated craniofacial anomaly	Other anomaly
20	?	B	1	Mid	Y	Y	?	?	?	Hypertelorism	Epibulbar choristoma-microphtalmia		Hydrocephaly	ABS?
21	M	B	0		Y	Y	N	N	N	Hypertelorism	N	Cleft 3 BCLP		Dis?
22	F	L	1	Med	N	N	N	N	N	N		Cleft 3		
23	M	R	1	Med	N	N	N	N	N	N	N	Cleft 3 UCLP		
24	F	B	2	Med	Y	N	N	N	N	hypertelorism				
25	F	L	1	Med	N	N	N	N	N	n	N	Cleft 3 cleft0		
26	F	L	0		Y	Y	N	N	N	Hypertelorism	Right microphtalmia	Cleft 3 UCLP	Right eyebrow - hairline	
27	F	L	2	Mid	Y	Y	Y	Y	Y	Hypertelorism		Cleft 1-13, UCLP	Mental retardation	
28	F	R	0		Y	Y	Y	Y	Y	Hypertelorism		Cleft 3 UCLP		
29	F	R	1	Mid	N	N	N	N	N			cleft 3		
30	M	R	0		Y	N	N	N	N			Cleft 3 BCLP		
31	M	L	2	Lat	Y	?	?	?	?	Hypertelorism	Right microphtalmia	Cleft 9-Cleft3-BCLP	Mental retardation	
32	F	B	0		Y	Y	?	?	.	Hypertelorism		Cleft 3 UCLP	Frontal encephalocele	
33	M	L	0		Y	N								

34	F	B	0		Y	Y	N	N	N			Cleft 3 BCLP		
35	F	L	0		Y	Y	N	N	N			Cleft 3 BCLP		
36	F	L	3	Mid	Y	Y	N	Y	N	Hypertelorism		Cleft 1-13 UCLP		ABS
37	M	L	3	Med	Y	Y	N	N	N			Cleft 3 cleft 1à		
38	M	R	1	Mid	Y	N	N	N	N			Cleft 3 BCLP		
39	M	B	1	Med	N	N	N	N	N			Cleft 3 BCLP		
40	F	L	3	Mid	Y	Y	Y	Y	?	Hypertelorism		Cleft 1-13 UCLP	Frontal encephalocele	ABS
41	F	R	3	Mid	Y	Y	?	?	?		Symblepharon, microphtalmia	Cleft 1-13 BCLP cleft7		CMF
42	M	L	1	Lat	Y	N	N	N	N		microphtalmia	Cleft 3 BCLP		ABS
43	F	R	0		Y	N	N	N	N			Cleft 3 UCLP	Hydrocephaly	cardiac malformation
44	M	R	3	Mid	Y	Y	Y	Y	Y	Hypertelorism	Anophtalmia	Cleft 3 BCLP cleft 1-13	Encephalocele	
45	M	B	3	Med	Y	Y	?	?	?	Hypertelorism	Epibulbar choristoma-microphtalmia	1-13 bilat-BCLP		ABS?
46	F	R	0		Y	N	Y	Y					Encephalocele	
47	M	R	0		N	N	Y	Y	Y	Dystopic	Lateral canthal dystopic			
48	F	B	3	Lat	Y	Y	?	?	?	Hypertelorism	symblepharon	Cleft 1-13	Encephalocele	ABS

(continued)

Table 14.2 (continued)

Patient #	Gender	Side	Soft tissues: Eyelid Severity	Eyelid Position	Eyebrow	Hair line	Skeleton: Orbital rim	Frontal bone	Orbital roof	Orbital position	Associated ocular anom	Associated cleft	Associated craniofacial anomaly	Other anomaly
49	F	R	1	Med	N	N	N	N	N			Cleft 4-cleft6		
50	F	R	1	Mid	N	N	N	N	N		Microphtalmia	Cleft 4-cleft6		
51	F	B	1	Med	N	N	N	N	N		Epibulbar choristoma	Cleft 4 BCLP		
52	F	R	1	Mid	N	N	N	N	N			Cleft4		
53	F	L	1	Med	N	N	N	N	N		Epibulbar choristoma	Cleft4		
54	F	L	1	Med	N	N	N	N	N			Cleft4-cleft 8		
55	M	R	1	Med	N	N	N	N	N			Cleft4		
56	M	R	1	Med	N	N	N	N	N			Cleft 4 UCLP		
57	F	R	1	Med	N	N	N	N	N		Microphtalmia	Cleft4		
58	F	L	1	Med	N	N	N	N	N		Epibulbar choristoma	Cleft 4 bilat		
59	M	L	1	Mid	Y	N	N	N	N			Cleft 4 bilat		
60	M	L	1	Med	N	N	N	N	N			Cleft 4 bilat		
61	M	B	1	Mid	N	N	N	N	N		Microphtalmia	Cleft 4 bilat		
62	M	B	1	Mid	N	N	N	N	N		Microphtalmia	Cleft 4 bilat		
63	M	B	1	Med	N	N	N	N	N			Cleft 4 bilat		
64	F	R	1	Med	N	N	N	N	N			Cleft4		
65	F	R	1	Med	N	N	N	N	N			Cleft 4 bilat		
66	M	R	1	Med	N	N	N	N	N			Cleft 4 bilat		

67	F	R	1	Med	N	N	N	N	N			Cleft 4 bilat		
68	M	L	1	Med	N	N	N	N	N			Cleft4		
69	F	R	1	Mid	N	N	N	N	N		Microphtalmia	Cleft 4 bilat		
70	F	R	1	Med	N	N	N	N	N			Cleft 4 bilat		
71	F	R	1	Med	N	N	N	N	N		Microphtalmia	Cleft 3 cleft8		CMF
72	M	R	1	Med	N	N	N	N	N			Cleft 4 bilat		
73	F	L	1	Med	N	N	N	N	N		Microphtalmia	Cleft4		
74	F	B	3	Med	Y	Y	Y	?	?	Hypertelorism		Cleft 3 BCLP		CMF
75	F	B	3	Mid	Y	Y	Y	?	?	Hypertelorism	Microphtalmia	Cleft 3 bilat		ABS
76	F	L	3	Med	Y	Y	Y	Y	Y	Hypertelorism		BCLP		ABS

Gender: m for male, f for female
Side: r for right, l for left and b for bilateral
Severity: according to Shao's grading, 0 nothing, 1< to 33%, 33% < 2 < 50% and 3 > 50%
Position: med for medial, mid for middle and lat for lateral
Hypertel for hypertelorism
UCLP for unilateral cleft lip and palate, BCLP for bilateral cleft lip and palate
CFM for craniofacial microsomia, ABS for amniotic band syndrome and MOTA for Manitoba oculo-tricho-anal syndrome

14.6 The Features of Cleft 10

14.6.1 Soft Tissue Involvement

14.6.1.1 The Eyelid

Since it is the most apparent, upper eyelid coloboma is the main symptom of cleft 10. It will drive attention to the path where the other components of the cleft are to be looked for.

Two pieces of research have yielded accurate descriptions of the symptoms: Smith [6] in a general study about a series of 55 colobomas whom 93% were onto the upper lid, and Shao [36] in a more specific series of 59 patients (85 eyes) with cleft10 have analyzed the details of ophthalmologic symptoms of cleft 10.

All the cases of Shao's series have an eyelid coloboma, an eyebrow deformity and a hairline peak. Only two in the series have a skeletal cleft.

The Coloboma itself (Fig. 14.3)

Position

The colobomas are supposed to be located in the mid-third of the upper lid, leaving equal stumps of the palpebra on both medial and lateral sides, but it has not been what we found, neither in our series nor in the 59 pictures available from the published cases that we had access to. Some ones are more medial, and others more lateral. This information was absent from Shao's paper and Smith's. Thus, we must rely on our clinical series and pictures from the literature. Out of the 100 colobomas, only 37 were in the mid-third of the upper palpebra, while 77 were in the medial third and 6 in the lateral third.

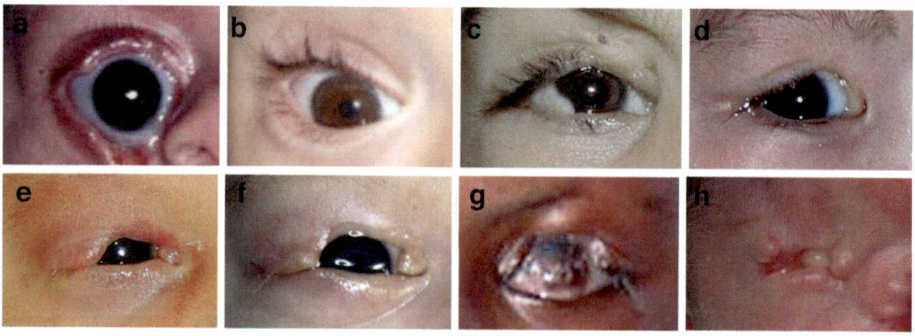

Fig. 14.3 Eyelid colobomas. (**a**) Type of eyelid rim defect frequently associated with cleft 3 or 4. (**b**) Canthal dystopia associated with typical skeletal cleft 10. (**c–f**) Colobomas of increasing severity, (**c** and **d**) are Shao's grade 1; (**e**) Grade 2 and f grade 3. (**g**) Grade 3 coloboma with symblepharon and choristoma. (**h**) Grade 3 coloboma, anophtalmia and choristoma

Width

Smith has a grading into small($S < 33\%$), medium ($33\% < S < 50\%$), and large ($s > 50\%$) but did not give his statistics. Shao's grading includes four grades: grade 0 when no eyelid defect comes with other symptoms of cleft 10. Grades 1, 2 and 3 are the same as Smith's grade 1 for slight, grade 2 for medium, and grade 3 for large. The interest in having a grade 0 is that some patients with a setting of cleft 10, even with severe ocular-palpebral anomalies, are found free of coloboma. Shao gives his statistics of the 85 eyes in 59 patients: none of those patients was in grade 0, 12 were in grade 1, 25 were in grade 2, and 43 (54%) were in grade 3.

Our statistics found 20 grade 0, 54 grade 1, 23 grade 2, and 25 grade 3.

The Symblepharon and Cutaneous Pterygium

Symblepharon, and cutaneous pterygium or local synechiae, symptoms that witness the lack of differentiation of ectoderm into tarsal and bulbar conjunctiva, are usually associated with colobomas. Shao noticed this defect in 76 out of the 85 affected eyes.

In our statistics, we found it 11 times.

The Lower Lid Ectropion

It was an original Shao's observation that the inferior eyelid was frequently abnormal in association with cleft 10. He remarked the presence of a significant lower eyelid ectropion in 34 out of 85 eyes. Due to the high number of lower eyelid clefts associated in our series this point could not be verified.

The Epibulbar Choristomas

In Smith's statistics, but it was not focused on cleft 10 as in Shao's, an association with CMF setting was noticed 13 times out of 55 patients, and most of them had epibulbar choristomas.

Our statistics found choristomas in only 12 out of the 125 patients. CFM was present 17 times, and all the choristomas were in this setting.

Associated Ocular Anomalies

Associated ocular anomalies are of two kinds: primary and secondary.

Primary ocular malformations are colobomas of the primary ocular cleft with or without cyst, iris colobomas, microphthalmia or anophthalmia and staphyloma.

Secondary are strabismus, amblyopia and corneal ulcer.

22 out of the 125 patients had microphthalmia.

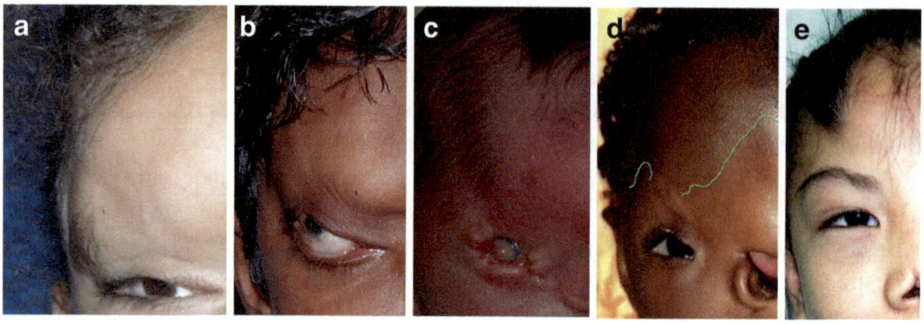

Fig. 14.4 Hairline and eyebrow in cleft 10. (**a**) The medial part of the eyebrow is missing, the lateral part is vertical toward the hairline peak. (**b**) Same as a. (**c**) Wide hairline peak associated with eyebrow cleft, coloboma, microphtalmia and choristoma. (**d**) Very wide hairline wedgeshaped peak (shaved off, green lines show the hairline). (**e**) Association of a cleft 10 peak with a 13 peak, in a patient with several clefts

14.6.1.2 The Eyebrow. (Fig. 14.4)

The eyebrow deformity was constant in Sheo's series since it was a criterion for inclusion.

Tessier's original description was that of an eyebrow severely disorganised: the lateral part verticalised, heading toward the hairline peak and the medial part almost absent.

This point is not detailed in Sheo's research or Smith's.

From the pictures from the published cases and from our clinical series, the eyebrow cleft may come in different shapes: it could be an inverted V-shape, a defect in the midline with different distortions of the edges, or the eyebrow can be completely missing.

77 out of the 125 had an eyebrow anomaly.

14.6.1.3 The Hairline (Fig 14.4)

In cleft 10, some patients have a peak of the hairline, which is a cardinal symptom, but it is a most striking component of the MOTA syndrome in which it becomes a wide band of hairs across the frontal area down to the eyebrow. It becomes a double band in several cases of association between cleft 1 and 13 with cleft 10 that we observed in each of the 13 cases of association of cleft 10 with cleft 1–13.

Of the 125 patients, 27 had a typical hairline peak.

14.6.1.4 The Skeletal Involvement (Fig. 14.5)

Even if a case with a skeletal cleft illustrates Tessier's original cleft 10 descriptions, it is a very infrequent occurrence. In Sheo's series, they have only two patients

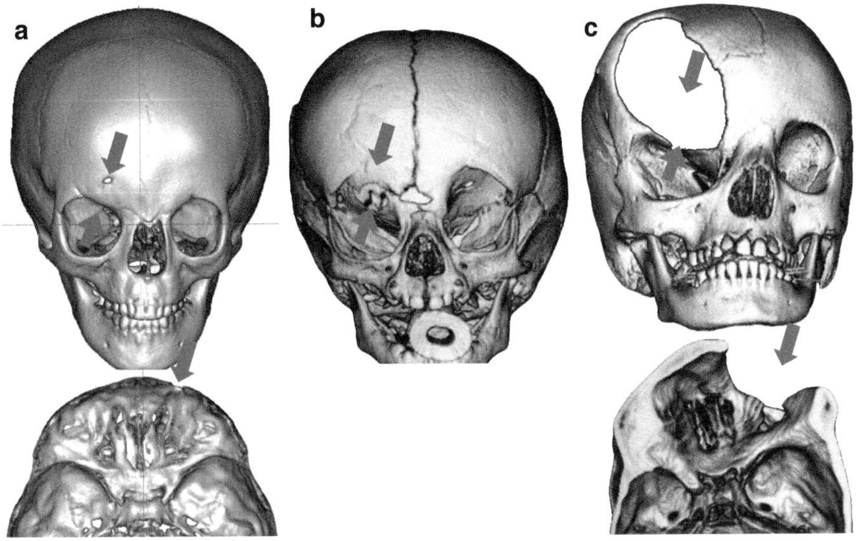

Fig. 14.5 Skeletal defects of cleft 10. (**a**) Minimal defect: hole in the frontal bone, the superior orbital rim is enlarged and smoothed, the orbital roof is swelling downward. (**b**) Mid defect, encephalocele through a frontal defect, the orbital rim is interrupted, defect of the orbital roof at the expand of the frontal bone. (**c**) Severe combined defect and orbital dystopia. (**d**) Less severe form without eyelid coloboma

among 59, a bit over 3%. In the 49 that we get with sufficient information to figure in the statistics, there were 3 patients with a skeletal cleft, a bit over 6%.

The skeletal defect in cleft 10 is very close to what is described in cleft 9, and we wonder if the same condition would not be described similarly under the two appellations and be the consequence of the same pathological process.

Unfortunately, few high-resolution CT scans are available to give ground to a detailed description of the skeletal cleft 10. Among the 125 patients, only 10 of them had proof of a complete skeletal cleft.

14.6.1.5 The Orbital Rim

Typically, the cleft interrupts the superior orbital rim in its middle part, but when an encephalocele goes through the defect, it distorts so much area that it makes it difficult to analyze the anatomy.

The more discrete form of disruption is a change in the orbit's shape, which is elongated in its vertical diameter, as seen on the CT scan displayed in Eppley's report [13].

14.6.1.6 Orbital Roof

The defect of the orbital roof lies in its middle part, mainly through the frontal bone. From the high-resolution CT scan we have, it respects the upper wing of the sphenoidal bone.

The roof is displaced downward, reducing the orbital volume, which yields exophthalmia and vertical orbital dystopia. One patient had an isolated defect of the orbital roof.

14.6.1.7 Frontal Bone

The frontal bone defect leaves room for an encephalocele when it is present. One of the patients had an isolated defect of the frontal bone without an orbital roof or rim alteration.

14.7 Associations with Cleft 10

14.7.1 Association with Craniofacial Clefts

87 out of the 125 cases from our statistics (70%) have cleft associated with the cleft 10.

Cleft 4 is the most frequent, found 27 times (22%). In second place comes the cleft 3 present 23 times, then after cleft 1–13 13 times.

Other rare clefts seldom occur. Two times for clefts 6, 7 and 8. Once for clefts 1, 2–12, 5 and 9.

For the usual cleft lip and palate, they are seen 17 times for bilateral cleft lip and palate (BCLP) and 11 times as unilateral cleft lip and palate (UCLP).

Another way to appreciate those associations is to calculate the relative frequency of the cleft 10 in patients with another rare cleft. Then it is striking to find that in 43 out of 65 clefts 4 (66%) and in 31 cases out of 49 clefts 3 (63%), there is an association with cleft 10.

In our series of 35 clefts 1–13, 14 were associated with cleft 10 (40%).

Such frequencies for those three varieties of rare clefts drive the hypothesis of a common mechanism in the pathogeny of the observed malformations.

14.7.2 Cleft 10 in the Setting of Syndromes

14.7.2.1 The MOTA Syndrome

Manitoba-Oculo-Tricho-Anal syndrome (MOTA) is a rare disease, initially described by Marles [7] in 1992 in about 6 cases in a family of an isolated Indian population in Manitoba. The facial presentation is typical with its association of coloboma with symblepharon (thus: Oculo-) and wedge-shaped hairline peak (thus: Tricho). Those probands are affected at the same time by an anal anomaly (thus: Anal).

In 2007, a new series of 7 patients were reported by Li [41], and in 2009, Yeung published a report of two more cases.

Slavotinek [42] 2011 led a thorough macromolecular collaborative research on the cases previously reported and a new family. This research yields the discovery that mutations in the FREM1 gene were the cause of MOTA, even if the two Yeung's cases did not have the mutation.

In the 49 UCL, we have 10 MOTA, which is a bias since the cases of MOTA are over-represented in this series. The reason is that they fully described in publications and that the publications include a picture of the patients, but, we found cases of cleft 10, which are probably non-diagnosed MOTA as patient number 16 in Table 1 from Ortega-Molina [20] who had anal imperforation and bifid nose.

It was a Yeung [31] hypothesis that much of the cleft 10 would be due to a genetic rather than environmental cause. We will side with it.

14.7.2.2 Cleft 10 and Craniofacial Microsomia

CFM was present in 17 of the 125 recorded cases. Among those 17 patients, 8 were associated with clefts 1–13, and the hairline wedge-shaped peak looked very much as in MOTA but heading toward the cleft 1–13 rather than the coloboma.

14.7.2.3 Cleft 10 and ABS

12 patients out of the 125 were in the setting of ABS. It is striking that all of them were associated with cleft 3 and/or BCLP.

14.8 The Cleft 10 Phenotypes

A few phenotypes can be described among the combinations that can be ascertained.

- Isolated coloboma of the upper eyelid, either uni or bilateral, occurs in about half of the time.
- The rest of the cleft 10 comes in association with a syndrome.
- The association of upper eyelid coloboma with eyebrow anomaly, hairline anomaly and digestive tract malformation are MOTA syndromes, but discrete digestive anomaly could be missed, and seemingly isolated cleft 10 are probably MOTA and should be tested for a FREM1 mutation. It is believable that other mutations will be found to explain the Yeung [31] cases.
- Craniofacial microsomia is known as frequent association with rare clefts, but, interestingly, a cleft that is frequently associated with this condition is the cleft

1–13, which has an anomaly of the frontal hairline very similar to the hairline anomaly met in the MOTA syndrome. We could infer a close mechanism.

- Amniotic band syndrome as well, even considered by some ones as a typical cause of rare clefts, is often associated with cleft 10, but, again, it is not any of the clefts associated there, but bilateral cleft 3 and BCLP. Here again, we could imagine a common mechanism.
- The skeletal cleft 10, the prototype of Tessier's description, is the rarest of all. The original description of the skeletal defect matches our cases, but the upper eyelid is usually free of defect, and the eyebrow deformity is quite different from the other clefts 10. We even have a patient in which a typical skeletal cleft 10 was associated with a soft tissue cleft similar to cleft 9. To the contrary, in another patient, a typical skeletal cleft 9 was associated with a typical cleft 10 in soft tissues.

There is more in common between this phenotype and the cleft 9 than between this phenotype and the cleft 10.

14.9 The Differential Diagnosis

14.9.1 The Cleft 11

We tried to find a very distinctive path for the cleft 11. In theory, it could be the coloboma of the medial third of the upper lid, but it looks like it is more convenient to sort them with the cleft 10 since the consequences and treatments are the same.

14.9.2 The Cleft 9 (See the Corresponding Chapter)

Colobomas of the outer part of the eyelid are difficult to differentiate. We better rely upon the general orientation of the defects along the path toward the temporal area for cleft 9 and toward the frontal area for cleft 10, but it is a subtle distinction for most patients.

About the skeletal cleft, as said above, whether it affects or not the superolateral orbital corner does not make a big difference. We are unable to differentiate the skeletal defects involving the superior orbital rim together with its roof and the frontal bone when it extends a bit toward the lateral orbital process of the temporal bone, process which makes the border between the two paths.

14.10 Treatments

We will discuss the elementary procedures available for each specific anatomical defect before considering the indications for considered phenotypes.

14.10.1 Eyelid Repair (Fig. 14.6)

The need for surgical repair of upper lid coloboma yielded many technics described in treatises and journal publications. They can be classified into direct sutures, local flaps and free grafts.

14.10.1.1 Direct Sutures

According to Shao's classification [36], colobomas of grade 1, with a width inferior to one-third of the upper eyelid, can be repaired directly. The tarso-conjunctival layer is better approximated by a continuous suture with a non-absorbable monofilament (5/0) left for 10 days, the orbicularis muscles by absorbable sutures. We used to put a suture to the free eyelid margin onto the grey line and a subcuticular continuous suture with non-absorbable monofilament to the skin that will be removed by the tenth day, as well as the tarsoconjunctival suture and free margin stitch. We used to make a Z-plasty on the cutaneous layer (Fig. 14.6), which releases more efficiently the mechanical constraints and shifts the plane of sutures.

Thanks to the Z-plasty, we can also fix the grade 2 colobomas.

Others prefer to adjunct a release of the lateral canthal ligament (cantholysis) and an incision along the palpebral crease to ease the advancement of the cutaneous-muscular flap. The Tenzel procedure (Fig. 14.7) [43] combines such a cantholysis with a rotation advancement of a musculocutaneous flap, including the orbicularis muscle, harvested from the lateral area.

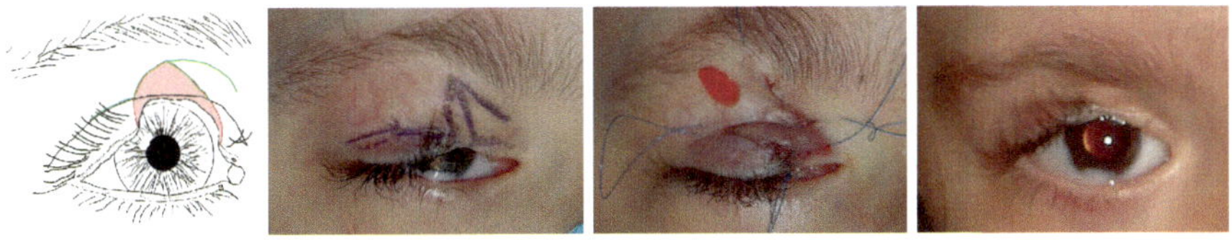

Fig. 14.6 Coloboma repair with Z-plasty. The area tinted pink shows the excision to refresh the coloboma edges. The green lines show the incisions, notice their position in relation with the palpebral crease

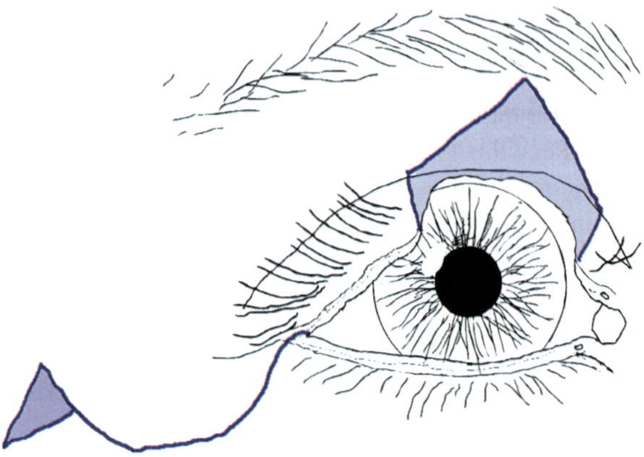

Fig. 14.7 Tenzel procedure: cantholysis, lateral rotation-advancement flap

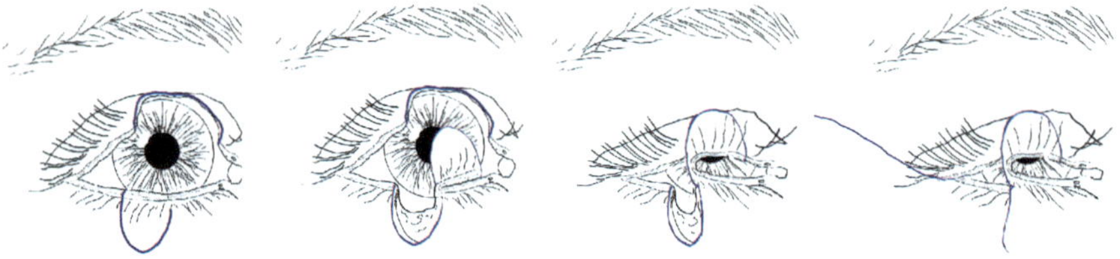

Fig. 14.8 Mustarde's procedure. Hetero-palpebral full-thickness flap. Advancement flap to close the donor site

14.10.1.2 Local Flaps

The more popular flap for the repair of significant palpebral defects, which can be used for Grade 3 coloboma or after the failure of a more conservative technic, is the Mustarde heteropalpebral rotation flap nicknamed the "switch flap" published in 1971 [44] (Fig. 14.8). It was initially designed for upper lid defects after tumor resection, but some advocate it as a coloboma repair technique.

For the same indication, the Cutler-Beard flap has been used [45] as it was initially by the authors for colobomas. Contrary to Mustarde's flap, it does not replace the missing eyelashes.

14.10.1.3 Free Grafts

To avoid the temporary bridging by those heteropalpebral flaps, someones prefer using free composite tarsoconjunctival grafts. Those grafts can be harvested from the lower lid on the same side or the upper lid on the opposite side. Different regional flaps then cover the free graft.

Fibromucous grafts can be harvested from the hard palate to reconstruct the posterior lamina of the palpebra, instead of the tarsoconjunctival tissue, in conjunction with local flaps.

Those technics derived from the oncological repair or trauma repair for very large defects are practical in ablepharia or in cases of severe symblepharon associated with the coloboma that are more frequent in Fraser's syndrome, which is a disease close to MOTA but that we did not include in our study of the cleft 10.

14.10.2 Eyebrow Repair

The repair of eyebrow defects depends upon its nature. Distortion with narrow gaps can be fixed by Z-plasty-type procedures aiming at relocation and straightening of the eyebrow line (Fig. 14.9).

Broader defects will necessitate a reconstruction. The wise idea is to use the abnormal frontal band of hairs, as recommended by Fan [14], when it reaches the eyebrow area as a local flap.

When there is no available local hairs-bearing flap, it could be brought on a long facial pedicle from the temporal area. The inconvenience with scalp flap is the fast growth of hairs, which necessitates almost daily trimming.

After the disappointing results of scalp flaps, free grafts have gained in popularity, and the skill gained with follicular unit transplantation for baldness has been applied, with nice results for eyebrow reconstruction as advocated by Ergün [46]. It could be used alone or in combination with plasty of relocation.

14.10.3 Hairline Repair

A major ectopic streak of hairs heading down to the distorted eyebrow is afflicting, and most of the patients cannot stand it; most are used to shaving it. The technic,

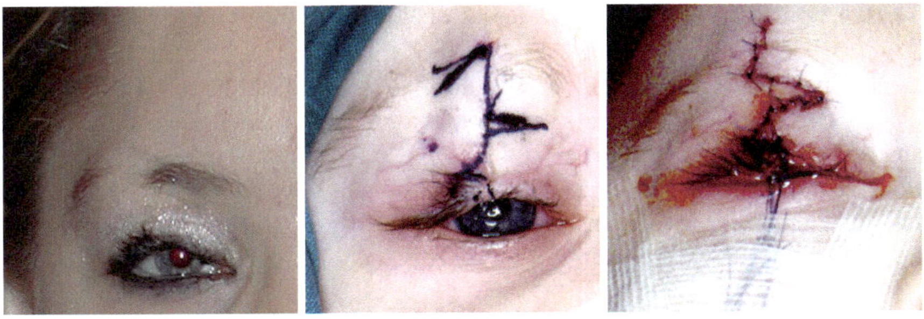

Fig. 14.9 Z-plasty to set in line the two parts of the eyebrow

advocated above by Fan, to use this abnormal hair-bearing area as a flap to reconstruct the eyebrow defect, hits two birds with the same stone.

Tessier's historical patient with the first transcranial approach to hypertelorism treatment has had such a condition treated by resection and full-thickness graft before being referred to Tessier.

Unfortunately, the graft could be as conspicuous as the treated condition. Thus, resection, which nowadays can be facilitated by a previous skin expansion, is usually the best choice.

Our advice would be to keep this part for the end of the treatment and use it, if necessary, to repair a missing eyebrow.

An epilation by electrolysis can be attempted but is unsuitable for large areas.

14.10.4 Skeletal Repair

The repair of skeletal malformations has two aspects: orbital dystopia and bone defects.

14.10.4.1 Surgery for Orbital Dystopia

There are two kinds of dystopia: hypertelorism and vertical dystopia.

Hypertelorism is not directly related to the cleft 10, but out of the 125 cases statistics, 24 had hypertelorism, usually dues to an associated inter-orbital rare cleft, most of the time a cleft 1–13. As for any hypertelorism, the technic can be a box osteotomy, a facial or craniofacial bipartition, or a unilateral mobilization according to combined anomalies.

A vertical dystopia of the orbit is frequently associated with the skeletal cleft 10 and secondary to the encephalocele through the orbital roof, pushing down the orbital content and could require an osteotomy, especially when it is associated with hypertelorism.

14.10.4.2 Repair of the Bone Defect

Bone defects are responsible for encephaloceles and need reconstruction. Since it is usually performed as a pediatric surgery, autografts are better. Depending on the surgical team's habits and the age of the patient at the time of surgery, it could be an iliac bone graft or cranial graft, split when feasible of full thickness associated with interdigitated calvarial expansion as advocated by Argenta in David's publication [47].

14.10.5 *Surgical Planning and Indication*

In complex conditions, when several malformations must be addressed in the same patient, it is only sometimes possible to fix everything in the time of the same procedure.

The functional risk for an eye that is exposed because of a large coloboma must be addressed first.

When there is an association with skeletal deformities and no functional emergency, we tend to prioritize the skeletal repair to have a reliable frame before performing the soft tissue surgery.

14.11 Discussion

Our observations during the research for Cleft 10 brought some reflections about two topics: the nosological place of upper lid coloboma, on the one hand, and skeletal defect involving the upper orbital rim, the orbital roof and the supraorbital part of the frontal bone in another.

Firstly, the coloboma. According to the original Tessier classification, upper lid coloboma could be part of cleft 10 as well as of clefts 9 or 11. Our research did not find a specific setting for cleft 11. Colobomas of the upper lid come indifferently as colobomas in the medial, mid or lateral part of the eyelid. Broad colobomas, Shao's grade three, are frequently met as isolated, while the colobomas associated with clefts 3, clefts 4 and clefts 1–13, which are very common, occurring in almost 50% of cases, are narrow colobomas, more as a simple notch or just some irregularity of the eyelid edge. Here again, the location is indifferent to the lateral third, mid-third of the medial third of the eyelid.

As a principle, we have considered that colobomas of the upper lid would be a sign of cleft 10. The coloboma location on the lid is usually indifferent, with the exception of the cleft 9.

For cleft 9, we need to refer to the skeleton and to the cutaneous symptoms and hairline anomalies seen further, but the boundary lakes, sometimes, of clearness. As already said above, we have seen cases where the path of soft tissue defects was typically the one of cleft 9 when the path of the skeletal defect was the one of cleft 10 and the contrary. This leads to the topic of the skeletal defect.

Secondly, the skeletal defect. Patients with skeletal defects along clefts 9 and 10 paths are extremely rare. Thus, there is no literature on this matter, and the question comes from the beginning since Tessier did not speak about cleft 9.

We are lucky to have a sufficient number of observations to support our opinion that patients with combined skeletal defects of the roof, orbital rim and lateral part of the frontal bone, which usually gives room for an encephalocele, whether they cross or not through the superolateral orbital corner are of the same meaning, belonging to a common pathological phenomenon. That the path would head a bit upper or lower does not matter.

References

1. Tessier P. Anatomical classification of facial, cranio-facial and latero-facial clefts. J Maxillofac Surg. 1976;4:69–92. https://linkinghub.elsevier.com/retrieve/pii/S0301050376800136
2. Laroche V. Essai d'anatomie pathologique sur les monstruosités ou vices de conformation primitifs de la face. Paris: Thése de medecine,Faculté de Médecine de Paris; 1823.
3. Schleich G. Ängebornes Colobom der Augelider. 1880. https://archive.org/details/b21645103/page/16/mode/2up.
4. Duyse V. Bride dermoide oculo-palpébrale et colobome partiel de la paupière avec remarques sur la génese de ces anomalies. Ann Ocul. 1882;LXXXXVIII(3 & 4):101–32.
5. Jules NICOLIN. Du Colobome des Paupiéres. Medical Thesis. Lyon: Faculté de Médecine; 1888.
6. Smith HB, Verity DH, Collin JRO. The incidence, embryology, and oculofacial abnormalities associated with eyelid colobomas. Eye (Lond). 2015;29(4):492–8. http://www.nature.com/articles/eye2014335.
7. Marles SL, Greenberg CR, Persaud TVN, Shuckett EP, Chudley AE. New familial syndrome of unilateral upper eyelid coloboma, aberrant anterior hairline pattern, and anal anomalies in Manitoba Indians. Am J Med Genet. 1992;42(6):793–9. https://doi.org/10.1002/ajmg.1320420609.
8. Chacon-Camacho OF, Zenker M, Schanze D, Ledesma-Gil J, Zenteno JC. Novel FREM1 mutations in a patient with MOTA syndrome: clinical findings, mutation update and review of FREM1 -related disorders literature. Eur J Med Genet. 2017;60(3):190–4. https://linkinghub.elsevier.com/retrieve/pii/S1769721216304438.
9. Karanam SR. Manitoba oculotrichoanal syndrome: first case report from India. DJO. 2016;27(2):111–3. https://doi.org/10.7869/djo.220.
10. Ad-El DD, Moor EV, Newman A, Weinberg A, Meir PB, Wexler MR. Bilateral isolated upper eyelid coloboma ? An infrequent entity with rare clinical presentation. Eur J Plast Surg. 1994;17(5) https://doi.org/10.1007/BF00208844.
11. Assouan C, Ambroise B, de Boutray M, Labbé D, Bénateau H, Veyssiere A. Tessier number 4 bilateral craniofacial cleft associated with amniotic band syndrome: 22 years of follow-up. J Stomatol Oral Maxillofac Surg. 2018;119(3):208–11. https://doi.org/10.1016/j.jormas.2017.12.005.
12. Gupta PC, Peralta D, Parker M, Crowe C, Clark B, Traboulsi EI. Bilateral microphthalmia with cyst, facial clefts, and limb anomalies: a new syndrome with features of Waardenburg syndrome, cerebro-oculo-nasal syndrome, and craniotelencephalic dysplasia. Am J Med Genet. 2003;117A(1):72–5. https://doi.org/10.1002/ajmg.a.10154.
13. Eppley BL, David L, Li M, Moore CA, Sadove AM. Amniotic band facies. J Craniofac Surg. 1998;9(4):360–5. http://journals.lww.com/00001665-199807000-00013.
14. Fan X, Shao C, Fu Y, Zhou H, Lin M, Zhu H. Surgical management and outcome of Tessier number 10 clefts. Ophthalmology. 2008;115(12):2290–2294.e3. https://linkinghub.elsevier.com/retrieve/pii/S0161642008004466.
15. David DJ, Hemmy DC, Cooter RD. Craniofacial clefts. In: Craniofacial deformities. New York: Springer; 1990. p. 63–92. https://doi.org/10.1007/978-1-4612-3232-2_5.
16. Gosla Reddy S, Acharya AP. Rare facial clefts. In: Bonanthaya K, Panneerselvam E, Manuel S, Kumar VV, Rai A, editors. Oral and maxillofacial surgery for the clinician. Singapore: Springer; 2021. https://doi.org/10.1007/978-981-15-1346-6_77.

17. Gu S, Khoong Y, Huang X, Zan T. Facial cleft? The first case of manitoba-oculo-tricho-anal syndrome with novel mutations in China: a case report. BMC Pediatr. 2021;21(1):46. https://doi.org/10.1186/s12887-021-02506-5.
18. Pascasio DCG, Denadai R, Tansipek BU. Tessier number 3, 4, 7, and 10 clefts, microphthalmia, and duplicated zygomatic arch: a rare association. Eur J Plast Surg. 2020;43(1):79–82. https://doi.org/10.1007/s00238-019-01557-3.
19. Ortube MC, Dipple K, Setoguchi Y, Kawamoto HK, Demer JL. Ocular manifestations of oblique facial clefts. J Craniofac Surg. 2010;21(5):1630–1. https://doi.org/10.1097/SCS.0b013e3181ecc4cd.
20. Ortega Molina JM, Mora Horna ER, Salgado Miranda AD, Rubio R, Pérez S, de Larraya A, Salcedo CG. Congenital upper eyelid Coloboma: clinical and surgical management. Case Rep Ophthalmol Med. 2015;2015:1–4. http://www.hindawi.com/journals/criopm/2015/286782/.
21. Ankola PA, Abdel-Azim H. Congenital bilateral upper eyelid coloboma. J Perinatol. 2003;23(2):166–7. https://doi.org/10.1038/sj.jp.7210872.
22. Hoyama E, Limawararut V, Malhotra R, Muecke J, Selva D. Tarsomarginal graft in upper eyelid coloboma repair. J AAPOS. 2007;11(5):499–501. https://doi.org/10.1016/j.jaapos.2007.04.011.
23. Kislaoglu E, Yüksel F, Uçar C. Tessier number 10 cleft. Eur J Plastic Surg. 1998;21(2):108–9. https://doi.org/10.1007/s002380050040.
24. Lee HM, Noh TK, Yoo HW, et al. A wedge-shaped anterior hairline extension associated with a tessier number 10 cleft. Ann Dermatol. 2012;24(4):464. https://doi.org/10.5021/ad.2012.24.4.464.
25. MacQuillan A, Hamilton S, Grobbelaar A. Angiosomes, clefts, and eyelashes. Plastic Reconstr Surg. 2004;113(5):1400–3. https://doi.org/10.1097/01.PRS.0000112793.45806.7A.
26. Morovic CG, Berwart F, Varas J. Craniofacial anomalies of the amniotic band syndrome in serial clinical cases. Plastic Reconstr Surg. 2004;113(6):1556–62. https://doi.org/10.1097/01.PRS.0000117185.25173.38.
27. Raposo-Amaral CE, Jarrahy R, Lim R, Alonso N. The rare facial cleft. In: Alonso N, Raposo-Amaral CE, editors. Cleft lip and palate treatment. Springer International Publishing; 2018. p. 325–62. https://doi.org/10.1007/978-3-319-63290-2_21.
28. Seah LL, Choo CT, Fong KS. Congenital upper lid colobomas: management and visual outcome. Ophthalmic Plast Reconstr Surg. 2002;18(3):190–5. https://doi.org/10.1097/00002341-200205000-00007.
29. Vistnes LM, Sergott TJ. Surgical reconstruction of a difficult orbital cleft. Ophthalmic Plast Reconstr Surg. 1986;2(4):179-182. doi:https://doi.org/10.1097/00002341-198601070-00001
30. Vulovic D, Novakovic M, Sarenac T, et al. Congenital upper eyelid coloboma with ipsilateral eyebrow hypoplasia. VSP. 2012;69(9):809–11. https://doi.org/10.2298/VSP1209809V.
31. Yeung A, Amor D, Savarirayan R. Familial upper eyelid coloboma with ipsilateral anterior hairline abnormality: two new reports of MOTA syndrome. Am J Med Genet. 2009;149A(4):767–9. https://doi.org/10.1002/ajmg.a.32743.
32. van der Meulen JCH, Vaandrager JM. Facial clefts. World J Surg. 1989;13(4):373–83. https://doi.org/10.1007/BF01660750.
33. Fontaine G, Walbaum R, Poupard B, et al. Fronto-nasal dysplasia (apropos of 4 cases). J Genet Hum. 1983;31(Suppl 5):351–65.
34. Huang X, Zhu B, Jiang H, et al. A de novo 1.38Mb duplication of 1q31.1 in a boy with hemifacial microsomia, anophthalmia, anotia, macrostomia, and cleft lip and palate. Int J Pediatr Otorhinolaryngol. 2013;77(4):560–4. https://doi.org/10.1016/j.ijporl.2012.12.006.
35. Lehalle D, Altunoglu U, Bruel A, et al. The oculoauriculofrontonasal syndrome: Further clinical characterization and additional evidence suggesting a nontraditional mode of inheritance. Am J Med Genet. 2018; https://doi.org/10.1002/ajmg.a.40662.
36. Shao C, Lu W, Li J, Chen J, Yao Q, Fan X, et al. Manifestation and grading of ocular involvement in patients with Tessier number 10 clefts. Eye (Lond). 2017;31(8):1140–5. http://www.nature.com/articles/eye201739.

37. Grover AK, Chaudhuri Z, Malik S, Bageja S, Menon V. Congenital eyelid colobomas in 51 patients. J Pediatr Ophthalmol Strabismus. 2009;46(3):151–9.
38. Ali Lodhi A, Afzal Junejo S, Alam Khanzada M, Akram Sahaf I, Kamal SZ. Surgical outcome of 21 patients with congenital upper eyelid coloboma. Int J Ophtalmol. 2010;3(1):69–72.
39. Monasterio FO, Taylor JA. Major craniofacial clefts: case series and treatment philosophy. Plast Reconstr Surg. 2008;122(2):534–43. http://journals.lww.com/00006534-200808000-00027.
40. Moore MH. Rare craniofacial clefts. J Craniofac Surg. 1996;7(6):408–11. http://journals.lww.com/00001665-199611000-00003.
41. Li C, Marles SL, Greenberg CR, et al. Manitoba oculotrichoanal (MOTA) syndrome: report of eight new cases. Am J Med Genet. 2007;143A(8):853–7. https://doi.org/10.1002/ajmg.a.31446.
42. Slavotinek AM, Baranzini SE, Schanze D, et al. Manitoba-oculo-tricho-anal (MOTA) syndrome is caused by mutations in FREM1. J Med Genet. 2011;48(6):375–82. https://doi.org/10.1136/jmg.2011.089631.
43. Tenzel RR, Stewart WB. Eyelid reconstruction by the semicircle flap technique. Ophthalmology. 1978;85(11):1164–9. https://linkinghub.elsevier.com/retrieve/pii/S0161642078355780.
44. Mustardé JC. Surgical treatment of malignant tumours of the upper lid. Chir Plast. 1971;1(1):25–33.
45. Cutler NL, Beard C. A method for partial and Total upper lid reconstruction. Am J Ophthalmol. 1955;39(1):1–7. https://linkinghub.elsevier.com/retrieve/pii/0002939455926465.
46. Ergün SS, Sahinoglu K. Eyebrow Transplantation. Ann Plast Surg. 2003;51(6):584–6. http://journals.lww.com/00000637-200312000-00012.
47. David LR, Taylor RG, Argenta LC. A technique for cranial bone expansion. J Craniofac Surg. 1996;7(2):151–5. http://journals.lww.com/00001665-199603000-00016.

Chapter 15
Cleft 30

Cristiano Tonello, Renato da Silva Freitas, Nivaldo Alonso, and Philippe Pellerin

Pearls
- Median cleft deformities of the lower lip and mandible are rare congenital anomalies.
- In our sample, other associated malformations include congenital laryngeal deformities, cleft palate, and hand and foot anomalies like it could be observed in Richieri-Costa-Pereira Syndrome and Oromandibular Limb Hypogenesis Syndrome.
- The operative approach consists of freeing the tongue and closing the lower lip. Osteosynthesis of the lower border of the mandible must be performed, and mandibular osteogenesis distraction is sometimes required.

C. Tonello (✉)
Craniofacial Surgery Department, University of São Paulo, Bauru, São Paulo, Brazil
e-mail: cristianotonello@usp.br

R. da Silva Freitas
Plastic Surgery Unit, Hospital de Clínicas, Universidade Federal do Paraná, Curitiba, Brazil

Craniofacial Surgery, Assistance Center for Cleft Lip and Palate (CAIF), Hospital do Trabalhador, Curitiba, Brazil

N. Alonso
Department of Plastic Surgery, University of São Paulo, São Paulo, Brazil
e-mail: nivalonso@usp.br

P. Pellerin
Plastic Surgery Department, University of Lille, Lambersart, France

N. Alonso et al. (eds.), *Facial Reconstruction of Unusual Facial Clefts*,
https://doi.org/10.1007/978-3-031-40926-4_15

15.1 History

Paul Tessier's traditional publication in 1976 showed a famous drawing among craniofacial surgeons. Although the picture has the median mandibular classified Tessier 30, no mention is described of this cleft. According to Tessier, "*Fifteen locations for clefts (0 to 14) have been determined, using the orbit as the point of reference. They are distributed according to eight time zones, cleft no. 7 being the lateral-most. I have personally observed 14 of the 15 clefts; I have not seen an example of no. 9*" [1].

Maybe Paul Tessier was figuring out that clefts will be found in the mandible location, which may be the reason for this gap between cleft numbers 14 and 30. However, in a historical publication from Morian in 1887 [2], cited in Tessier's classification, no mention of mandibular cleft could be found too.

Karl Grunberg, in his book "*Die Morphologie der Missbildungen des menschen und der Tiere,*" described a spectrum of median lower lip cleft from minor defect to cleft involving the mandible and neck. Curiously, Grunberg describes a special kind of cleft called "healed intrauterine cleft" similar to a case described for us, like a variant of Tessier number 30 (Figs. 15.1 and 15.2) [3, 4].

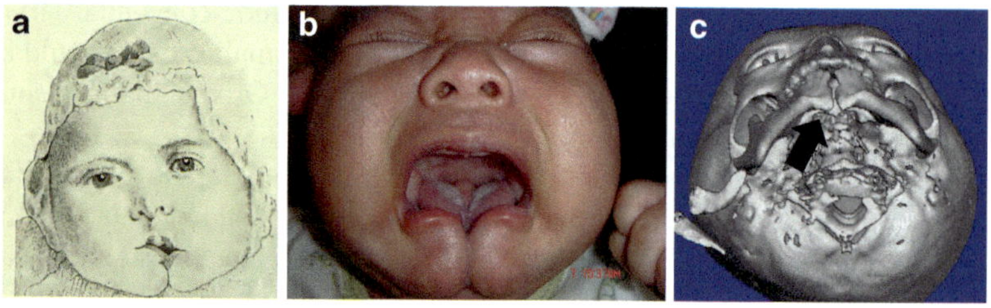

Fig. 15.1 (**a**) Median mandibular cleft in drawing in 1909 from Karl Grunberg in: "Die Morphologie der Missbildungen des menschen und der tiere"; (**b**) Classical median cleft of the lower lip, mandible associated to the bifid tongue (Courtesy Dr. Wang Tao, Chongquing); (**c**) Three-dimensional Computed Tomography reconstruction of the median mandibular cleft

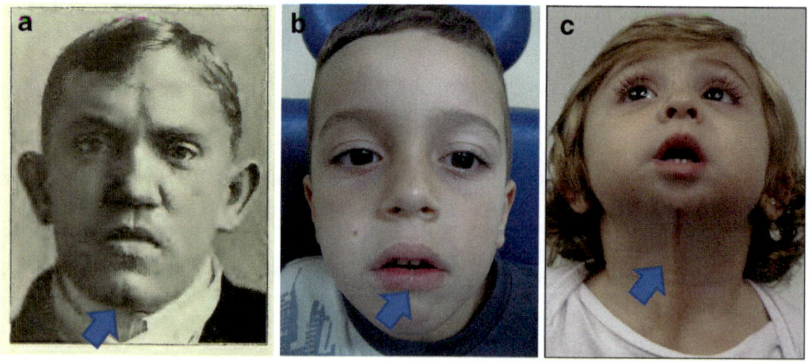

Fig. 15.2 (**a**)"Healed intrauterine cleft" described by Karl Grunberg in: "Die Morphologie der Missbildungen des menschen und der tiere"; (**b**) A small notch in the vermillion very similar to a small defect described by Grunberg like a "healed intrauterine cleft"; (**c**) A notch in the mandibular symphysis and a region of cutaneous retraction with subcutaneous soft tissue thickening in the mandibular midline extending to the neck. A Variant of Tessier Number 30 Cleft described by the authors

15.2 Anatomical Findings

Midline clefts of the lower lip are rare malformations usually associated with clefts of the mandible. No hereditary factors or gender predilection have been identified.

Couronné (1819) [5] was the first author to report this abnormality. Tessier classified the midline cleft of the lower lip as a number 30 facial cleft. Clinical presentation can vary widely in their extent and severity: they can be associated with a midline lower lip cleft, a cleft of the mandibular symphysis, a bifid tongue, ankyloglossia, and in some cases can continue to the manubrium sternum and involve the hyoid bone, thyroid cartilage, and strap muscles of the neck [6].

These clefts are often associated with dental anomalies and soft tissue skin tags and can be markedly asymmetrical [7]. However, they are reported to be as rare as 4 to 5 per million live births [8]. In 1989, a review reported 48 cases, with 37 involving the mandible [9]. By 1996, a further study from Oostrom reported 65 cases [10]. Recently, Valk et al. described a literature review of 72 cases between 1996 and 2020 [11].

Most authors believe cleft results from a failure of fusion of the first pair of branchial arches or a failure of mesodermal penetration into the midline structures. However, Monroe believed that the loss of fusion of the first branchial arch might be followed by the failure of fusion of all the lower arches [12].

However, Oostrom et al. [10] hypothesized that only one first branchial arch develops during the early embryonic period, and two mandibular processes develop within this structure. These mandibular processes do not fuse but merge during the late embryological period (after 7 weeks of development). In the same period, there is the formation of the lower lip and the alveolar process with enlargement and outgrowth of the osteogenic membrane in each mandibular process, resulting in the construction of the mandible and its symphysis.

Proposed descriptions of the pathogenesis of median clefts of the lower lip and mandible include A) hypoplasia of the mandibular processes during the early embryonic period leading to the severe cleft of the mandible extending into the neck; or B) during the late embryonic period, resulting in less severe median clefts. The lower cleft lip, ranging from a notch of the mucosa to a complete cleft, can be explained by insufficient outgrowth of the lip, most probably due to incomplete merging of the mandibular processes.

The bifid tongue can be explained as a persistent intermandibular groove, similar to a merging defect of the tongue. The mandibular cleft is defined as an impairment of the outgrowth of the definitive mandible's osteogenic centers, resulting in the absence of its symphysis [13].

15.3 Associated Malformations

Other associated malformations include congenital laryngeal deformities, cleft palate, and hand and foot anomalies like could be observed in Richieri-Costa-Pereira syndrome and Oromandibular Limb Hypogenesis Syndrome.

15.3.1 Richieri-Costa-Pereira Syndrome (RCPS)

Robin sequence with cleft mandible and limb anomalies (OMIM# 268305), formerly known as Richieri-Costa-Pereira syndrome, is an autosomal recessive acrofacial dysostosis [14] mainly characterized by the cleft mandible, Robin sequence, short stature, and limb defects. It is caused by mutations in the EIF4A3 gene, related to RNA metabolism in mandibular, laryngeal, and limb morphogenesis [15]. In addition, the first and second branchial arches are affected in RCPS, resulting in numerous craniofacial anomalies [14, 16, 17]. Demographic studies indicated that RCPS is a rare condition affecting a few individuals related to parental consanguinity [18]. This new clinical condition was first described by our geneticist Dr. Antônio Richieri-Costa (in memoriam) from the Hospital for Rehabilitation of Craniofacial Anomalies of the University of São Paulo (Fig. 15.3).

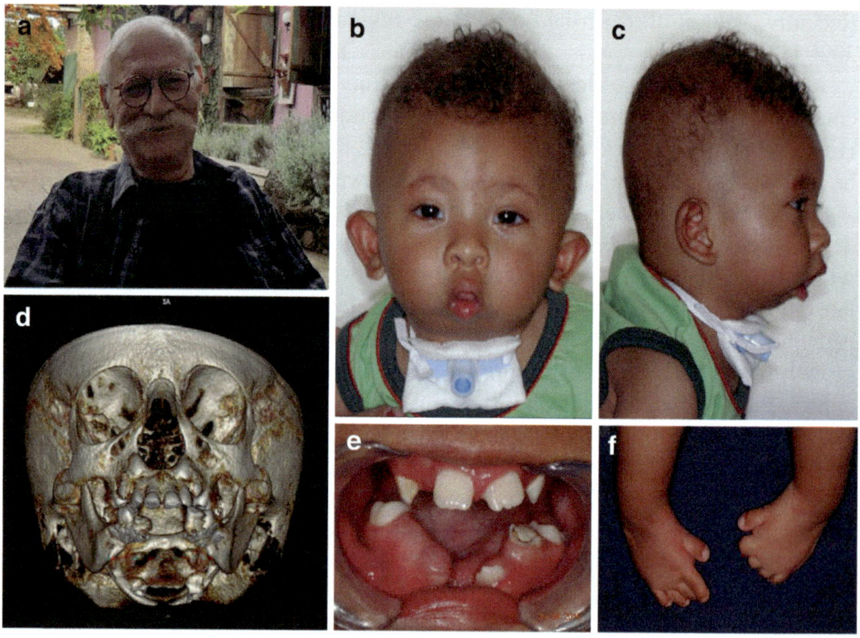

Fig. 15.3 (**a**) Dr. Antônio Richieri-Costa (in memoriam) in: "Obituary: Antônio Richieri-Costa (1946-2019)"- Am J Med Genet. 2019;1; (**b** and **c**) Microgathia in a boy with RCPS. Tracheostomy due to respiratory distress; (**d**) Three-dimensional Computed Tomography reconstruction of the median mandibular cleft; (**e**) Central and lateral incisors absent associated with alveolar cleft; (**f**) Limb defects frequently observed in RCPS

15.3.2 Oromandibular Limb Hypogenesis Syndrome (OLHS)

OLHS is a rare condition, with very few cases reported. This syndrome compromises the mandible, tongue, and jaw. It may also have abnormalities of the limbs or fingers. The clinical presentations with embryological development make it possible to classify OLHS into four significant subgroups according to Chicarilli and Polayes, including in some syndromes [19]. However, the boundaries between these subtypes could be more precise due to overlapping presentations, mainly in those without limb anomalies (Fig. 15.4).

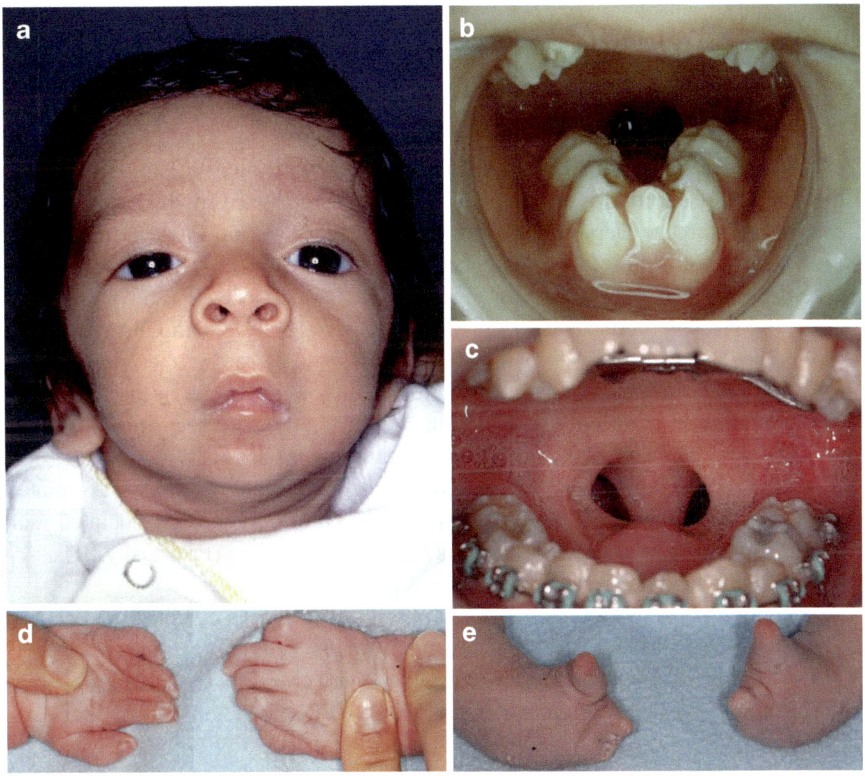

Fig. 15.4 (**a**) Micrognathia and microstomia observed in patients with OLHS; (**b**) Severe transversal deficiency of mandible and teeth absent; (**c**) Severe tongue hypoplasia; (**d** and **e**) Limb defects are frequently observed in OLHS

Table 15.1 Clinical findings in Tessier number 30 cleft

Gender	21 Female	30 Male	
Lip	13 Lower lip clefts	1 Small notch in the vermillion	37 With no lower lip cleft
Mandible	15 Complete clefts	13 Incomplete cleft	14 Transversal deficiency
Tongue	14 Tongue hypoplasia	5 Bifid tongue	
Teeth	42 With teeth absence	9 With no absence	
Neck	3 Clefts	38 With on clefts	
Chest wall	1 Cleft	50 With no clefts	
Associated malformations	16 RCPS	15 OLHS	23 With limb malformation

15.4 Our Cases

This series of patients with Tessier number 30 clefts were analyzed retrospectively. Fifty-one patients with Tessier number 30 clefts were treated by three centers: the Craniofacial Surgery Department from the University of São Paulo (Hospital for Rehabilitation of Craniofacial Surgery and Hospital of Clinics); the Assistance Center for Cleft Lip and Palate (CAIF) in Curitiba, Brazil; as well as the Division of Plastic and Reconstructive Surgery of Centre Hospitalier Régional Universitaire in Lille, France.

Twelve lower lip clefts and one patient with only a tiny notch in the vermillion were identified. In addition, complete mandibular clefts were seen in 15 patients, and 13 incomplete mandibular clefts were seen in other patients.

In 14 patients could be identified mandibular transversal deficiency associated with tongue hypoplasia. All these patients had an OLHS diagnosis associated with micrognathia in most cases. Two patients had ramus agenesis (Pruzansky III) associated with the median mandibular cleft.

Five patients had a bifid tongue. The majority of the cases demonstrated central and lateral incisors absents. Neck involvement was present in 3 patients.

Limb malformations were present in twenty-three cases; these were classified as either Richieri-Costa Syndrome (16 cases) or OLHS (15 patients) (Table 15.1).

15.5 Surgical Treatment

First of all, there are some important considerations regarding mandibular clefts. For example, the relationship between cleft location, developing dentition, the role of bone grafting, growth restriction, and surgical treatment for growth restriction is different between clefts in the midline of the mandible and the maxilla of a patient with unilateral cleft lip and palate [11].

Historically, treatment of this anomaly has remained relatively similar. However, most authors have released the tongue and closed the lower lip in the early stages of life in most patients [20, 21]. This approach is logical since the lip and tongue must suck, swallow, and phonate.

15.5.1 Lip Repair

Most studies report a simple "V" excision of the cleft with direct closure of the lip and the use of a Z-plasty if the cleft extends into the neck. Millard et al. [22] proposed a Z-plasty of the released lingual frenulum and a midline incision vertically to the buccal sulcus. The fibrotic union of the muscle is excised except in the normal chin dimple position, and the muscle is sutured together across the cleft. The excess mucosa and vermilion are trimmed.

Several methods of surgical correction of the mento-sternal band have been described, including linear closure and single or multiple Z-plasties or W-plasties. The success is highly variable depending on the location, size, and length of time before surgical correction and the complete excision of the lesion. Linear closure has been suggested as a possible option for small lesions, and the surrounding skin is lax. However, when used in extended defects, it can result in hypertrophic scarring, contractures, and secondary anterior open bite. Therefore, using single or multiple Z- or W-plasties is recommended for more extended defects to improve the cosmetic and functional results and have less risk of cicatricial contracture formation. Z-plasty is the most commonly used way of incision closure in the literature. It allows the surgeon to [1] lengthen a contracted scar, [2] reorient the direction of a scar or defect, [3] break up a straight line, and [4] shift soft tissue contour. Despite that, Z-plasty can lead to hypertrophic scarring in the oblique limbs along with triangle tip depression and necrosis if the angles are too acute (<30). For that reason, the result of the operation is only sometimes regarded as cosmetically successful by the parents. In general, however, the result is functionally pleasing, and the patient can extend his neck without impediment (Fig. 15.5) [4].

15.5.2 Mandibular Reconstruction and Mandibular Osteogenesis Distraction (MOD)

The ideal timing for treatment of the mandibular cleft remains undetermined. Millard et al. [22] reported a mandible repair using a rib graft, wiring, and Vitallium splint at 8 years of age. In patients without respiratory disturbance, the mandibular defect closure is frequently delayed until 10–12 years of age to prevent tooth bud damage during mandibular surgery [20, 21]. However, careful uni-cortical osteosynthesis of the lower border of the mandible may avoid harm to the tooth buds if

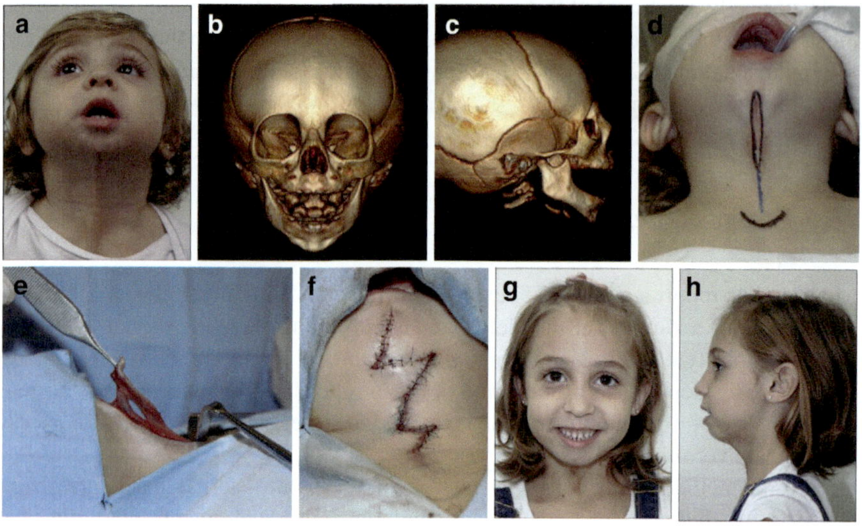

Fig. 15.5 (**a**) Clinical photograph of an 18-month-old girl illustrating mild micrognathia presenting a cutaneous retraction limiting the full extension of the neck. (**b** and **c**) Three-dimensional computed tomographic (CT) images before surgery. (**d**) 4.4cm linear subcutaneous lesion of midline cervical area, extending between the chin and the thyroid's isthmus on magnetic resonance image. (**e**) Intraoperative resection of fibrotic subcutaneous cord followed by a Z-plasty reconstruction (**f**). (**g** and **h**) 3-year follow-up of surgical correction, revealing minimal hypertrophic scar and appropriate functional result

surgery is performed in the early period [10, 23]. Sherman and Goulian [24] successfully treated median mandibular bone defects at 20 months. Moreover, osteosynthesis may benefit mandible development, resulting in critical functional improvements in speech, eating, and occlusion.

The technique consists of subperiosteal dissection through an incision in the lower buccal sulcus, preserving the continuity of the mucosa. The exposed bone ends are freshened with a burr, and a bone graft is used to reconstruct the defect. The donor material may be rib, calvarium, or iliac crest. Screws, mini plates, or wire may be used to fix the graft into position.

Extrusion of a fixation plate and screws after surgery could be observed due to tiny mandible segments or lack of oral soft tissue for coverage.

Ishii et al. [20] performed cleft bone reconstruction in 2 stages: a mandibular fixation at 6 years of age and an iliac graft 1 year after. We prefer single-stage reconstruction at an early age, avoiding multiple procedures and reaping the benefits of improved speech eating and occlusion early on. Our surgical protocol is as follows: in patients without respiratory distress or feeding problems, the continuity of the mandible is assessed. Mandibular osteogenesis distraction may be used for contour improvement if the mandible is contiguous. If the mandible is not contiguous, we

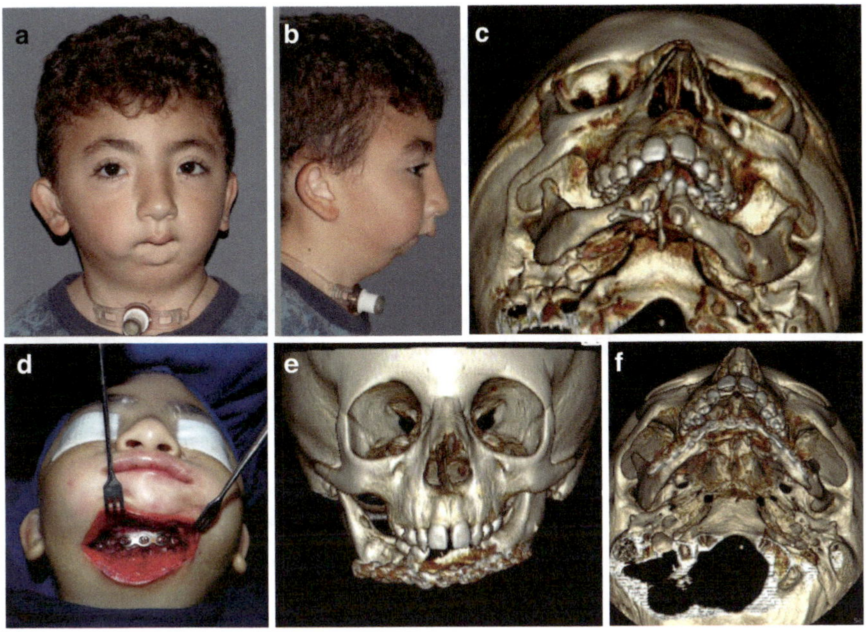

Fig. 15.6 (**a** and **b**) Microgathia in a boy with RCPS. Tracheostomy due to respiratory distress; (**c**) Three-dimensional Computed Tomography reconstruction of the median mandibular cleft; (**d**) Immediate post-operative bone graft (iliac crest). (**e** and **f**) Follow up of bone graft and contiguous mandible in three-dimensional computed tomography reconstruction image

recommend bone grafting with a costal graft or iliac crest at an early. Soft tissue deformities of the lower lip, tongue, and neck should also be corrected at an early age (3–6 months), as indicated (Figs. 15.6 and 15.7) [13].

15.5.3 Mandibular Midline Distraction

Guerrero pioneered rapid surgical mandibular expansion for correcting mandibular transverse discrepancies [25]. Later work by Guerrero and coworkers [26] showed that mandibular symphyseal DO, using both tooth-borne and bone-borne expansion devices, is an effective surgical alternative to orthognathic surgery in treating transverse mandibular deficiency.

Rapid mandibular widening surgery is usually performed under general and local anesthesia. The horizontal incision is made with an electrocuting knife or scalpel 4–6 mm labial to the depth of the mandibular vestibule through the orbicularis oris muscle in the posterior aspect of the lower lip extending from canine to canine.

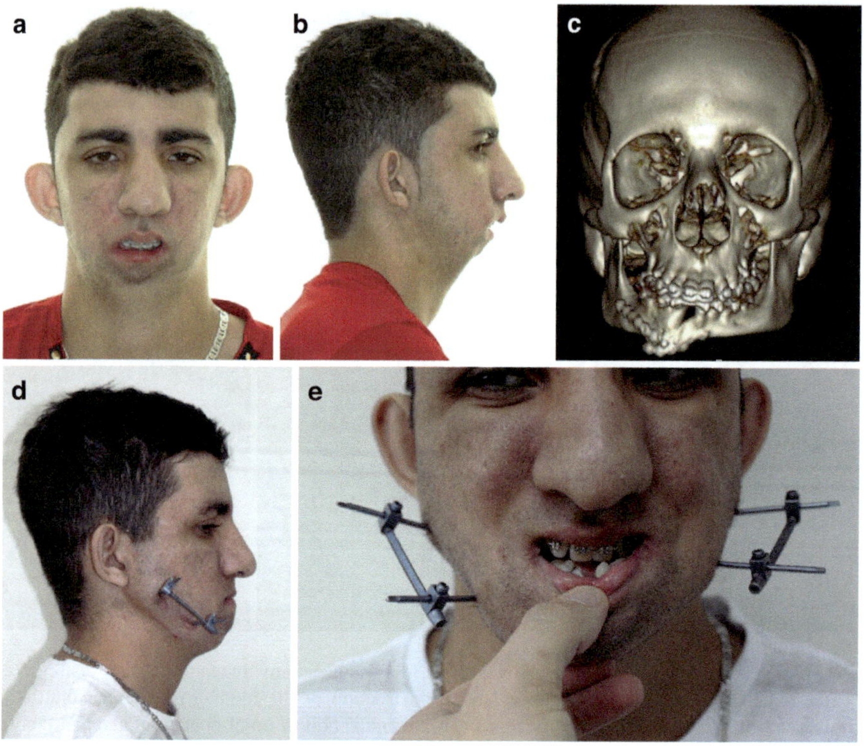

Fig. 15.7 (**a** and **b**) Microgathia in a male, 16 years old with RCPS. (**c**) Three-dimensional computed tomography reconstruction of the median mandibular cleft corrected with bone graft; (**d** and **e**) Mandibular osteogenesis distraction after bone graft in mandibular symphysis

After the muscle is transected, the dissection is directed obliquely, posteriorly, and inferiorly through the mentalis muscle until contact is made with the mandibular symphysis. The tissues are reflected inferiorly in a subperiosteal plane to the lower border of the mandible, where a channel retractor is placed. The superior tissue flap is minimally detached subperiosteally from the planned osteotomy site at the alveolar ridge's crest, and care is taken to avoid tearing the gingival tissue.

The interdental osteotomy must be meticulously performed without vertical pressure on the mandible to obviate displacement of the Hyrax appliance. Once the osteotomy is completed, the expansion appliance is activated. Mandibular widening by intraoral distraction osteogenesis ensures that the interdental bone cut is complete and the margins of the osteotomy site are separated.

The mentalis muscle is reattached to its origins with resorbable sutures placed through the muscle margins to coapt the cut edges. The mucosa is closed with interrupted plain sutures. The patient returns to the surgeon 4–7 days after surgery to begin the distraction at 1 mm per day until the desired widening is achieved. The patient is seen daily until the expansion is completed (Figs. 15.8 and 15.9) [25–27].

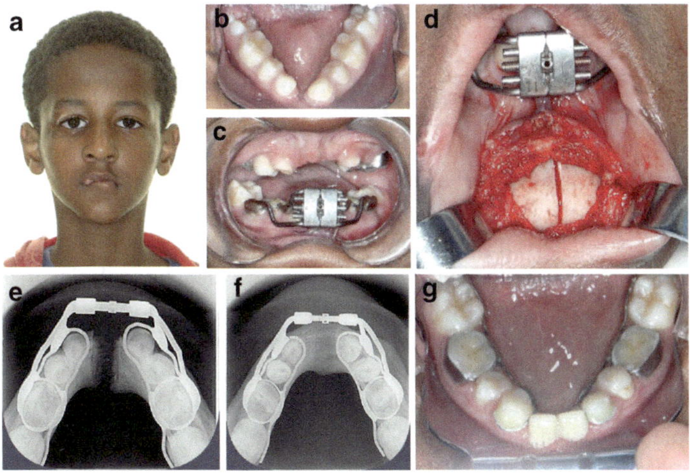

Fig. 15.8 (**a**) Micrognathia and microstomia observed in patients with OLHS; (**b**) Severe transversal deficiency of mandible and teeth absence associated with tongue hypoplasia; (**c**) Hyrax appliance tooth-borne; (**d**) Intraoperative interdental osteotomy with teeth preservation for mandibular midline distraction. (**e**) Initial radiological view of the osteotomy during the expansion process; (**f**) Consolidation of osteogenesis in the osteotomy site. (**g**) Aesthetical refinements after mandibular distraction

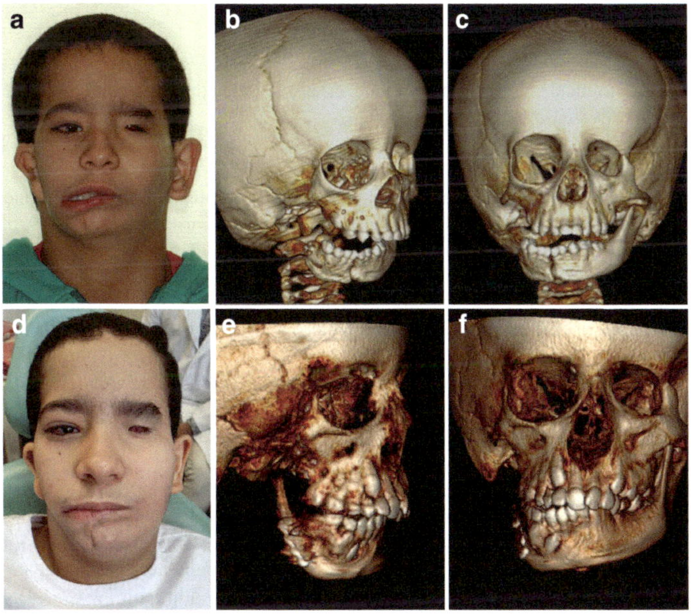

Fig. 15.9 (**a**) Male, craniofacial asymmetry, bilateral preauricular tags, and microphthalmia. In addition, he had an epibulbar dermoid, a Tessier 7 cleft, and microtia. He had a midline cleft of the lower lip with involvement of the mandible. (**b** and (**c**) Three-dimensional computed tomography demonstrated hypoplasia of the mandibular ramus and mandibular cleft. (**d–f**) Long-term follow-up of cleft lip repair, mandibular symphysis fixation, and mandibular reconstruction with bone graft (costal graft)

15.6 Case Description

Male, craniofacial asymmetry, bilateral preauricular tags, and malocclusion. In addition, he had an epibulbar dermoid, a Tessier 7 cleft, hypoplasia of the mandibular ramus, and type II microtia with external auditory canal atresia on the right side and microphthalmia and facial tags on the left side. Furthermore, the patient had a midline cleft of the lower lip with involvement of the mandible (Tessier 30 cleft). Appropriate speech and language, and psychomotor development were observed. A three-dimensional computed tomography scan revealed hypoplasia of the zygomatic bone on the right side, hypoplasia of the zygomatic process of the temporal bone, external auditory canal atresia, agenesis of the glenoid fossa, agenesis of the mandibular condyle and ramus, and hypoplasia of the mandibular body. Decreased orbital volume was observed on the left side. In addition to these findings, images also revealed a median mandibular cleft [28].

Lip repair had been done using a simple "V" excision of the cleft with direct lip closure at 6 months old. After that, wiring fixation of the median mandibular cleft was done.

Single-stage right mandible reconstruction was performed at 5 years old to improve respiratory distress and feeding problems with a costal graft.

References

1. Tessier P. Anatomical classification of facial, cranio-facial and latero-facial clefts. J Maxillofac Surg. 1976;4:69–92.
2. Morian R. Über die schräge Gesichtsspalte (about oblique facial clefts). Arch Klin Chir. 1887;35:245–88.
3. Grünberg K. Chapter IV: Die Mißbildungen des Kopfes. In: Die Morphologie der Missbildungen des menschen und der tiere. Jena: verlag von Gustav Fischer; 1909. p. 113–204. (Die Morphologie der Missbildungen des menschen und der tiere). Disponível em: https://archive.org/details/b21506899_0002.
4. Tonello C, de Matos ICP, Feitosa LB, Peixoto AP, Alonso N. Congenital midline cervical cleft: a variant of tessier number 30 cleft causing Micrognathia. Cleft Palate Craniofac. 2021;58(11):1446–51.
5. Couronné A. Observation d'un bec-de-lièvre, compliqué de fentes à la voûte palatine. Ann Clin Soc Med Prat Montepellier. 1819;6(2s):107.
6. Walker G. Malformations of the face. Edinburgh and London: E&S Livingstone Ltd.; 1961. p. 202.
7. El-Ashmawi NA, ElKordy SA, Salah Fayed MM, El-Beialy A, Attia KH. Effectiveness of gingivoperiosteoplasty on alveolar bone reconstruction and facial growth in patients with cleft lip and palate: a systematic review and meta-analysis. Cleft Palate Craniofac J. 2019;56(4):438–53.
8. Becker MJ. Mandibular symphysis (medial suture) closure in modern Homo sapiens: preliminary evidence from archaeological populations. Am J Phys Anthropol. 1986;69(4):499–501.
9. Erdogan B, Karaca C, Gorgu M, Bozkurt MA. Incomplete midline cleft of lower lip. Eur J Plast Surg. 1989;12(6):279–80.

10. Oostrom CAM, Vermeij-Keers C, Gilbert PM, van der Meulen JC. Median cleft of the lower lip and mandible: case reports, a new embryologic hypothesis, and subdivision. Plast Reconstr Surg. 1996;97(2):313–20.
11. van der Valk R, Magill S, Pellatt A, Ahmadi-Lari N, Hall SP, Cobb ARM, et al. Tessier 30 facial clefts—A literature review of 72 cases (1996-2020), suggested treatment protocol, outcome measures, minimum dataset for future case reports, and registries. Cleft Palate-Craniofac J. 2022;59(5):644–51.
12. Monroe CW. Midline cleft of the lower lip, mandible and tongue with flexion contracture of the neck: case report and review of the literature. Plast Reconstr Surg. 1966;38(4):312–9.
13. da Silva Freitas R, de Oliveira E Cruz GA, Alonso N, Forte AJ, Busato L, Persing J. Tessier number 30 clefts: surgical correction of a rare malformation. Rev Bras Cir Craniomaxilofac. 2010;13(1):12–7.
14. Richieri-Costa A, Guion-Almeida ML, Pagnan NAB. Acro-fronto-facio-nasal dysostosis: Report of a new brazilian family. Am J Med Genet. 1992;44(6):800–s.
15. Favaro FP, Alvizi L, Zechi-Ceide RM, Bertola D, Felix TM, de Souza J, et al. A noncoding expansion in EIF4A3 causes Richieri-Costa-Pereira syndrome, a craniofacial disorder associated with limb defects. Am J Hum Genet. 2014;94(1):120–8.
16. Guion-Almeida ML, Richieri-Costa A. Acrofrontofacionasal dysostosis: report of the third Brazilian family. Am J Med Genet A. 2003;119A(2):238–41.
17. Pinto RO, Peixoto AP, Pinto ADS, Richieri-Costa A, Raveli DB, Tonello C, et al. Hyoid bone position and head posture in patients with Richieri-Costa Pereira syndrome (EIF4A3 mutations). J Craniofac Surg. 2020;31(4):e356–9.
18. Favaro FP, Zechi-Ceide RM, Alvarez CW, Maximino LP, Antunes LFBB, Richieri-Costa A, et al. Richieri-Costa-Pereira syndrome: a unique acrofacial dysostosis type. An overview of the Brazilian cases. Am J Med Genet. 2011;155(2):322–31.
19. Chicarilli Z, Polayes I. Oromandibular_limb_hypogenesis_syndrome. Plast Reconstr Surg. 1985;76(1):13–24.
20. Ishii M, Ishii Y, Moriyama T, Enomoto S, Ono T, Ohyama K, et al. Seventeen-year follow-up of a patient with median cleft of the lower lip, mandible, and tongue with flexion contracture: a case report. Cleft Palate Craniofac J. 2002;39(5):555–9.
21. Millard DR Jr, Lehman JA Jr, Deane M, Garst WP. Median cleft of the lower lip and mandible: a case report. Br J Plast Surg. 1971;24(4):391–5.
22. Millard R Jr, Wolfe SA, Berkowitz S. Median cleft of the lower lip and mandible: correction of the mandibular defect. Br J Plast Surg. 1979;32(4):345–7.
23. Yildirim I, Aydin Y, Cinar C, Ogur S. Management of total lower face cleft. Plast Reconstr Surg. 2002;109(2):683–7.
24. Sherman JE, Goulian D. The successful one-stage surgical management of a midline cleft of the lower lip, mandible, and tongue. Plast Reconstr Surg. 1980;66(5):756–9.
25. Guerrero CA. Rapid mandibular expansion. Rev Venez Orthod. 1990;48:1–4.
26. Guerrero CA, Bell WH, Contasti GI, A.M. Rodriguez mandibular widening by intraoral distraction osteogenesis. Br J Oral Maxillofac Surg. 1997;35:383–92.
27. Guerrero C, Contasti G. Transverse (horizontal) mandibular deficiency. In: Bell WH, editor. Modern practice in orthognathic and reconstructive surgery. Philadelphia: Saunders; 1992. p. 2383–97.
28. Vendramini-Pittoli S, Guion-Almeida ML, Santos JM, Garcia Júnior SM, Yoshida MM, Richieri-Costa A, et al. An unusual presentation of oculoauriculovertebral spectrum with a Tessier 30 cleft: report on two cases. Clinical Dysmorphol. 2015;24(4):144–50.

Index

N. Alonso et al. (eds.), *Facial Reconstruction of Unusual Facial Clefts*, https://doi.org/10.1007/978-3-031-40926-4

GPSR Compliance

The European Union's (EU) General Product Safety Regulation (GPSR) is a set of rules that requires consumer products to be safe and our obligations to ensure this.

If you have any concerns about our products, you can contact us on ProductSafety@springernature.com

In case Publisher is established outside the EU, the EU authorized representative is:

Springer Nature Customer Service Center GmbH
Europaplatz 3
69115 Heidelberg, Germany

Batch number: 10732076

Printed by Printforce, the Netherlands